DE to

alth

Credits

The Rough Guide to Men's Health

Editors: Lois Wilson, Pat Gilbert, Jo Kendall
Layout: Fit4Life Media
Picture research: Sarah Bentley,
Christopher Lewis/RunCity Images
Proofreading: Jason Freeman
Production: Rebecca Short

Rough Guides Reference

Editors: Peter Buckley, Tracy Hopkins, Sean Mahoney,
Matthew Milton, Joe Staines, Ruth Tidball
Director: Andrew Lockett

Publishing Information

This first edition published January 2009 by
Rough Guides Ltd, 80 Strand, London WC2R 0RL
345 Hudson St, 4th Floor, New York 10014, USA

Penguin
Penguin
Penguin Group

Typeset in C

The publis
information in
compiling th
professional
any action, cl
contained in
otherwise making use of the medical information contained in this book.

© Lloyd Bradley, 2009
384 pages; includes index

A catalogue record for this book is available from the British Library

ISBN 13: 978-1-84836-004-4

1 3 5 7 9 8 6 4 2

THE ROUGH GUIDE to
Men's Health

by
Lloyd Bradley

www.roughguides.com

Acknowledgements

The author would like to thank the following, without whom this book would not have been possible: all at Fit4Life Media and RunCity; Derek Yates, Lois Wilson, Pat Gilbert, Jo Kendall, Sarah Bentley, Christopher Lewis and Jason Freeman; Gideon, Sarah, Sarah, Lili and Sandra aka *The Rough Guide to Men's Health*'s panel of experts; Effua Baker, Russell Fairbrother, Pete Muir and Steve Perrine; Ruth Tidball, Andrew Lockett and Peter Buckley; Joel Chernin and Nina Sharman; Simon Kanter, Paul Simpson and Mark Ellingham; Diana, George & Elissa Bradley.

About the author

Lloyd Bradley has been classically trained as a chef, is a regular marathon runner and was formerly Health & Fitness editor at *GQ* magazine and Consultant Editor at *Men's Health* and *Runner's World* magazines. He is also the author of *The Rough Guide to Running*.

Picture credits

All illustrations and graphics supplied by DK Images; except pp. 39, 47, 59, 79, 127 and 326 drawn and supplied by Derek Yates

All still life photography supplied by RunCity Images; except pp. 41 and 221 supplied by DK Images

All other photography supplied by RunCity Images; except pp. 29, 40, 45, 51 and 157 supplied by DK Images

Cover credits: front cover image courtesy of Images.com/Corbis; back cover image courtesy of Hein van den Heuvel/zefa/Corbis; inside cover image courtesy of The Gallery Collection/Corbis.

Contents

Contents

Contents

Why worry?

Why indeed? You've done alright so far. But wouldn't you like to do better? In truth, it's not really a matter of worry, more a case of having concerns. While it would be daft to assume this twenty-first century lifestyle is going to kill us all, it would be equally misguided to think we can live to our fullest potential without putting a bit of effort into how we do it. And if you've got as far as picking this book up and opening it you are probably almost as aware of this as we are.

Welcome to *The Rough Guide to Men's Health*

You are holding in your hands a book that aims to get you fitter and healthier and improve your performance in just about every area of your life. A book that doesn't assume there's necessarily anything wrong with you in the first place, just that, unless you're a professional athlete with a team of psychiatrists and a relationship counsellor with a 24-hour call-out service, everything about you could function considerably better if it all had a bit of a tune-up. Most people could eat better; most people could improve the efficiency of their exercise regime; most people would like to make their relationship run smoother; would like to do better at work; would like better sex; firm up the old midriff; enjoy their holidays to the absolute max; and so on. Which is where we come in: to help you get that bit more out of whatever situations you are probably quite happy with at the moment.

Also, to start from the standpoint that there could be nothing criminally unhealthy in your lifestyle at the moment allows us to add to your life rather than take away. Too many health books – notably men's health books – devote so much energy to telling you what you shouldn't be doing, they immediately alienate potential readers. Here at the *Rough Guide to Men's Health*, we're fairly

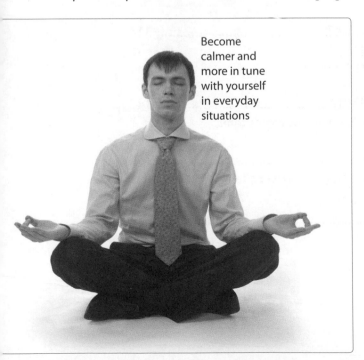

Become calmer and more in tune with yourself in everyday situations

certain we know what it is you get up to and, provided it's in moderation, there's not a great deal of point in us telling you to stop it – cigarette smoking, cocaine, heroin and unprotected sex are about all we draw an unequivocal line through. The idea here is to carry on enjoying yourself, but do so from a standpoint of being able to handle it as you do, and recover quickly afterwards. We want you to live forever, rather than die in the attempt.

How it all works

The *Rough Guide to Men's Health* won't be coming at you like a medical dictionary or targeting specific areas of your body and trying to scare you with all that could go wrong with them. Our approach is we look at the various areas of your life, then look at how they could be maximized, made easier or just kept safe. The first section, **Whatever, Whenever, Wherever**, deals exactly with those situations in a series of chapters with titles like, "At work", "On holiday", "In the bedroom", "In the kitchen", "In later life", then discusses how your maximum health and fitness would improve each aspect of them and help you avoid problems up ahead. The chapter will then explain how to achieve this optimum state. But it does so in a combination of running text, quick tips and bite-sized information panels, allowing you to take something away from each page regardless of how much time you may be able to give it at that moment. And because we know that you'll retain this knowledge better if you understand the theories behind it, we don't neglect the background science and medical-type diagrams, but we do our best to keep them separate from the rest of the book.

Section two is **Fit For Life**, which takes a longer term and less lifestyle-specific view of your health and fitness. One chapter, "A man for all seasons", takes you through life decade by decade, letting you know what you may have to look forward to – pros as well as cons – and how you can continue to live the best life you can whatever it might

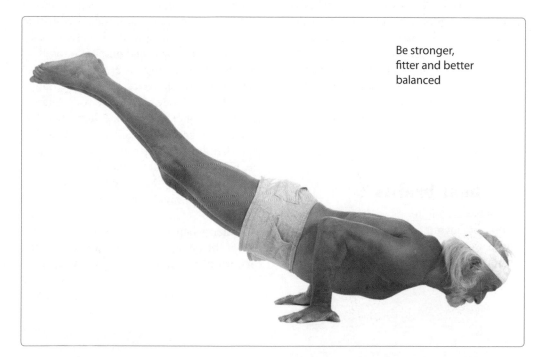

Be stronger, fitter and better balanced

throw at you. In another chapter, "Looking after Number One", the simple question posed is, Why do so many men leave it so late before going to the doctor? We detail how to get round all those excuses and then how to make sure you get the best out of it when you get there. While the final chapter in that section, "Improve your performance", is devoted to getting the best out of the advice the book has already given you, as that is the only way you are going to get the best out of your life.

The final section, **Reference**, pretty much does what it says on the tin. The main part of it is a straightforward guide to common complaints, how to spot them, what to do and how to prevent them coming back. It also carries a symptoms grid chart that allows you to find out what you might have, based on what symptoms you are showing. This takes so much of the guesswork out of diagnosing yourself, and isn't a service you'll find in too many other men's health books. Then lastly, there is a comprehensive directory of further reading, useful websites and interesting organizations, which also contains a list of the most commonly used alternative therapies, a brief explanation of what they are, and how to find out more about them.

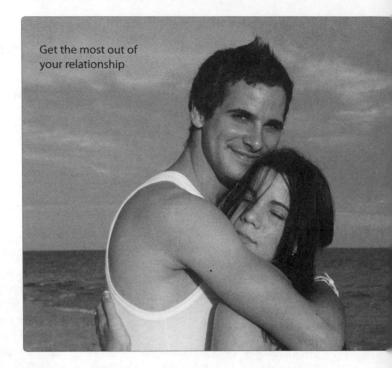

Get the most out of your relationship

The best brains

Of course I couldn't have done too much of this by myself, and I had the support, advice, words of wisdom and perpetual good humour of the most eminently qualified **Panel of Experts**. One of London's top personal trainers; the editor of *Scarlet*, the world's most readable sex magazine; a GP with a busy urban practice; a member of the British Dietetic Association and the Nutrition Society; and a practising psychiatrist who, for seven years, has provided on-site counselling for the *I'm a Celebrity... Get Me Out of Here!* contestants, so she is certainly no stranger to hard work. They are, respectively, Gideon Remfry, Sarah Hedley, Dr Liliana Risi, Dr Sarah Schenker and Dr Sandra Scott, so let's give them a nice big round of applause as we meet them individually (see opposite) and find out why the *Rough Guide to Men's Health* has so much oestrogen on its Panel of Experts.

Then when you've done that, enjoy the rest of the book, drink more water and look forward to a fitter, healthier and livelier life.

Lloyd Bradley (London, 2008)

Meet the panel

The *Rough Guide to Men's Health* panel of experts advised on much of the book and contribute directly with their words of wisdom in the Expert advice boxes and the larger grey quote boxes throughout the text. You'd be advised to pay close attention to what they are saying. And if you're wondering why there are so many women advising on men's health, it's because they always seem to know what's really best for us. Except when it comes to lifting heavy weights, obviously.

Sarah Hedley

Sarah (right) is the editor of *Scarlet* magazine, a national women's glossy specializing in sex and relationships, co-author of *Time Out's 1000 Books to Change Your Life*, and author of *Sex By Numbers*, which has been translated into six languages, and her new book, *Feel Sexy Now* will be out in October 2009. Previous posts include Women's Editor of *Maxim* magazine, Sex Editor of *Cosmopolitan* magazine, agony aunt for *Men's Fitness* magazine, and columnist for *The Sun*. She has appeared as a social commentator on shows including *The Oprah Winfrey Show*, *How to Look Good Naked*, *Richard & Judy* and the *BBC News*. She has enjoyed the role of TV agony aunt on teen shows T4's *Dirty Laundry* and Trouble's *Fancy Me Island*. She lives in London with her husband, and dreams of one day owning a dog.

scarletmagazine.co.uk

Sarah Hedley, our sex and relationships expert

Dr Sarah Schenker

Our second Sarah (pictured overleaf) is a qualified State Registered Dietitian, Accredited Sports Dietitian and Registered Public Health Nutritionist. Sarah works part-time as a nutrition scientist for the British Nutrition Foundation and as a consultant sports dietitian for Delia Smith and Norwich City Football Club. Sarah is a member of the British Dietetic Association and the Nutrition Society and has served on both professional and government committees. Sarah has extensive media experience and regularly writes for magazines, newspapers

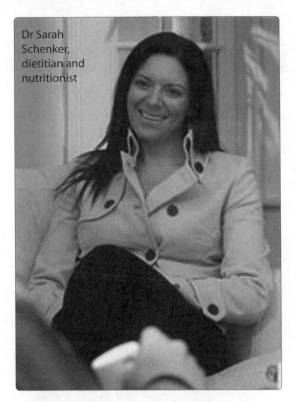

Dr Sarah Schenker, dietitian and nutritionist

Poliquin (a renowned strength training method), spinning (aerobic fitness on a stationary bike), kettle bell (training with traditional Russian cast-iron weights), and pre- and post-natal fitness for women. Gideon is currently guest trainer for *Men's Fitness* magazine, has been a fitness writer for magazines such as *GQ*, *Vogue* and *Red* and was the celebrity trainer on the TV show, *Britain's Top Model*. He has competed in a variety of events including kickboxing, martial arts, marathons, adventure races, and Olympic lifting. His fitness philosophy is simple: apply a holistic approach and through knowledge, fun, empowerment, hard work and commitment, the goal will be achieved and the life change will happen.

kxgym.co.uk

and journals as well as appearing regularly on TV and radio, from news programmes to reality shows. Recently Sarah has worked with Ewan McGregor for his documentary, *Long Way Round* and with Jamie Oliver for *Jamie's School Dinners*.

sarahschenker.com

Dr Sandra Scott

Sandra (pictured opposite) trained as a psychiatrist at the Maudsley Hospital in South London. Her work has included

Gideon Remfry

Gideon (right) is a personal trainer and fitness manager at the KX members club in Chelsea, London. He has been working within the industry for over fifteen years and specializes in strength and conditioning and "functional exercise". His influences are drawn from judo and kickboxing, of which he is a black belt. His fitness qualifications include

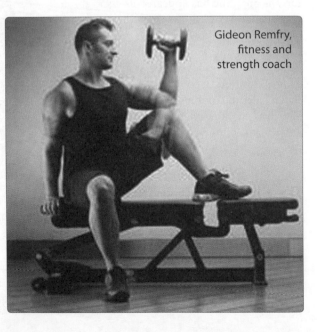

Gideon Remfry, fitness and strength coach

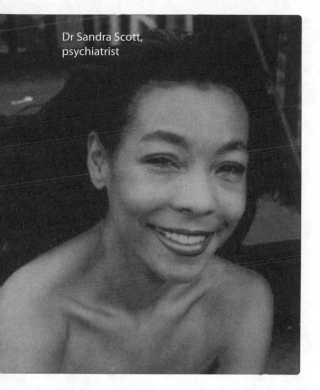

Dr Sandra Scott,
psychiatrist

Boys *Alone*, which followed ten eleven- and twelve-year-old boys living unsupervised for five days and nights and dealt with issues of friendships and group dynamics between them. She is currently preparing a book for publication with the working title, *How Not to Be Perfect*.

Dr Liliana Risi

Lili (below) was born in South Africa and is a sociologist and doctor with an MSc in Sexual Health. She then completed her training in General Practice in the UK. She set up the research programme for Marie Stopes International – the UK's leading provider of sexual and reproductive healthcare – and has published research into what changes people's behaviour. She now works as a GP in London where she recently set up a gardening scheme for patients with chronic health problems, and is a great believer in mindfulness – ancient teachings promoting the idea of being fully aware of one's thoughts or actions in the present, rather than in the past or future – and its potential to improve physical well-being.

bangor.ac.uk/mindfulness

family therapy, cognitive behavioural therapy, parent/child work and acute adult psychiatry. She has worked in the UK on both *Celebrity Big Brother* and *Big Brothers 2, 3, 4* and *5*, and provided psychological support for contestants on two series of *Hell's Kitchen*. Sandra also worked on BBC1's *Tomorrow's World* special, *Lab Rats*, where she took six volunteers and put them through scientific experiments designed to explore the human condition. For seven years, she has been in the Australian jungle, to counsel the celebrities for *I'm a Celebrity... Get Me Out of Here!* and she oversaw the filming and was on hand for any crisis that arose on the ground-breaking C4 documentary

Dr Liliana Risi,
London GP

Part 1
Whatever, whenever, wherever

In the kitchen & on the run

Although healthy eating has never been higher up on the social agenda, the reality is that many of us are gaining less nutrition through our food than in days gone by. This is due to a combination of the demands of our twenty-first century lifestyle; the supply of, and demand for, cheap food across the developed world; and a decline in the amount of education given about food in the schools system. However, it's still not that difficult to eat your way to better health, and the difference it makes will be instantly noticeable.

Cheap food, low value

Why we eat is very straightforward: we need to provide calorific fuel to power our muscles; and to provide our bodies with the necessary nutrients, in the form of vitamins and minerals, to function, self-repair and ward off infections. We expend calories through physical effort and nutrient reserves get used up as our bodies go about their regular business. Then, when we need either more calories or nutrients, we feel hungry and eat to replenish the levels. Thus everything stays evenly balanced and in perfect working order. Or at least that's the theory.

In practice, over the last couple of decades, the time that should be spent on everyday healthy eating and good food habits has gone the way of a good night's sleep – it's seen as time that could be spent doing something much more exciting. Thus the attendant demand for quick, easy, grab-and-go food has led to an industry boom in the production of processed food, ready meals, takeaways and snacks. These products often sacrifice nutritional content for greater volume, bulking themselves up with sugar, salt and trans fats (see p.26).

As a result, the present love affair with quick and inexpensive food means it's surprisingly easy to be very well fed

F *Fact: In the twenty-first century, single men between the ages of 20 and 35 have been statistically shown to have worse diets, in terms of lack of nutrition and number of damaging ingredients, than any other demographic… on both sides of the Atlantic. While this might not appear to be doing them too much harm, as at that age the metabolism tends to be super efficient, the concern is that their habits are storing up trouble for later life.*

How it all works: nourishment

By the time food leaves the stomach, it has been reduced to a thick oozing liquid called chyme. This allows it to pass easily into the small intestine, which is where the absorption into the system of ninety percent of its nutrient content takes place. Nutrients are separated from the waste product and taken up by the millions of microscopic tendril-like projections – villi – that line the small intestine's internal walls allowing them to pass through into the bloodstream. Once in the bloodstream they are delivered to the liver which stores, processes and controls their release into the system, once again via the bloodstream, to whatever organ requires them. The liver also regulates the flow of sugar into the bloodstream and filters out any toxins – this is why the liver is so affected by excess alcohol consumption, as the body sees that as a poison to be removed.

The first stage of the small intestine is the duodenum, where the chyme is mixed with bile and pancreatic juice fed in by the liver and pancreas, respectively. These liquids will neutralize stomach acid to allow the digestive enzymes to function more efficiently. The iron, calcium and folic acid content of the food is transferred into the bloodstream through the duodenum walls, but the majority of nutrient absorption takes place further down the intestinal tract at the very end of the duodenum and in the second section of the small intestine, the jejunum.

Once in the jejunum, the process is known as "active absorption" because it uses energy to select what is needed from the chyme, hence feelings of drowsiness after a big meal. In this central section, protein, fat and the fat-soluble vitamins A, D, E and K are absorbed through the walls, and carbohydrate is broken down into glucose and glycogen to be stored in the liver or the muscles or burned immediately for energy (see p.20).

In the third section of the small intestine, the ileum, the digestion process started in the previous sections will be completed, and any vitamin B12 will be absorbed. Also, any excess bile will be taken back into the system and taken to the liver for reprocessing.

What is left then passes into the large intestine, where it is dried out and, as the water is removed, the water-soluble B (all except B12) and C vitamins are absorbed into the system. They are not taken to the liver, but directly to the tissues or organs in which they will be utilized. This means the body has no storage capability for these vitamins and they need to be taken every day.

1. Food taken in through mouth

3. Further broken down by bile and pancreatic juice

2. Broken down in stomach

4. Nutrients are extracted and moved to the liver via the bloodstream

6. From the liver nutrients are distributed around the body

5. Waste matter is passed on to the colon

Portions or servings?

In the UK, according to the Food Standards Agency, the five portions of fruit and veg a day guideline refers to 80g helpings. In spite of this, most food labels give nutrition advice per 100g.

In the US, a "serving" is one medium-sized fruit; half a cup of raw, cooked, frozen or canned fruits or vegetables; 6 fl oz (170ml) of one hundred percent fruit or vegetable juice; half a cup of cooked, frozen or canned beans or peas; one cup of raw leafy vegetables.

but remain undernourished, often without realizing it. In reality you'll be functioning well below your best or struggling to reach previous levels of performance and your immune systems will be severely compromised. It's low nutrition that is at the root of so many of today's inexplicable and almost unquantifiable ailments – those times when we feel "just sort of stressed out" or "a bit under the weather" or are susceptible to any illness going around. The phrase "I just can't seem to shake this cold…" is always a

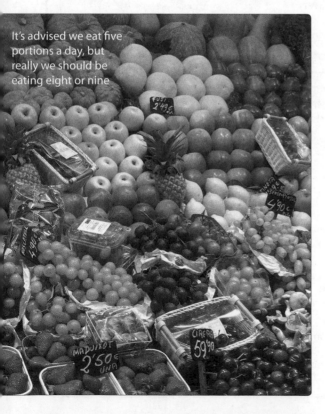

It's advised we eat five portions a day, but really we should be eating eight or nine

telltale symptom. And this is without considering the current obesity crisis and soaring levels of both heart disease and type 2 diabetes, which are both hugely diet related.

So much of today's food is padded out with "empty calories" – calories that provide a fill-up of fuel when we start to flag but very few nutrients, hence the name. These empty calories make us feel hungry again almost immediately, and keen to eat more of the same. You will more than likely need little of this extra fuel. The excess ends up on our bodies as fat, affecting the heart and the blood-sugar levels.

Also, as worrying as the physical damage being done is the long-term psychological effect these changed eating habits are having on us. We are today paying less and less attention to the whole notion of eating as a pleasurable family or social activity – we regularly skip breakfast, snatch lunch on the run, or eat dinner off our knees. As a result, everything to do with food becomes devalued and we are even less likely to take it seriously. Furthermore, the salty or sugary taste of so much processed food will further undermine the important emotional relationship we have with eating.

It's one of the huge ironies of modern life that cooking has never, apparently, been so trendy – witness the number of cookery shows on TV and the level of fame achieved by some actually quite ordinary chefs. Yet we're eating worse

Six significantly damaging dietary habits you may not realize you have got

Habit	How it can affect you
Eating too much	Restaurant portions and pre-packaged servings have increased considerably in size during the last decade or so, so it is very easy to be overeating without thinking you are consuming any more than you have always done.
Eating at strange times	Random eating habits or constant grazing are usually accompanied by a poor nutritional value of the food being consumed, simply because it is convenience rather than routine defining what you are eating. And too often that means processed snacks, junk food and cheese.
Confusing the issues of nutritional health and weight loss	Too many men who aren't noticeably porky assume they are eating well simply because they are not putting on weight. This isn't necessarily the case and an increase in nutrition levels will considerably boost their feeling of general well-being and raise the immunity capabilities of their bodies.
Substituting nutrition through food with supplements	Satisfying your nutritional needs through a balanced diet will always be much more beneficial than eating rubbish and popping vitamin pills. Good whole food affects you in all sorts of ways other than simply supplying, say, vitamin A or fibre, and it's this holistic rather than targeted approach to nutrition the body needs to stay truly healthy.
Believing what it says on the tin	Too much food sloganeering is relative rather than subjective. Simply announcing something as "a healthier option" is meaningless – healthier than what? A tub of lard? "30% fat free!" can also be interpreted as "70% fat". Always read the whole of the label.
Misunderstanding nutritional guidelines	There are so many conflicting eating plans and apparently scientific pieces of dietary advice out there, beyond basic guidelines such as can be found in this book, it will be impossible to find out what is precisely right for you without getting yourself checked out by a professional.

food than we ever have done. In spite of all the sway of the celebrity apron-wearers and the "food porn" cookery shows, we actually seem to care less about what we eat and how we eat it.

However, with a little attention to forward planning and an investment of not very much money and even less time, it's incredibly easy to turn your eating habits around. Or, if you are already off the junk food, get more out of how you eat, whether you think you can cook or not.

What's a well-balanced diet?

There has been a great deal talked and written about how a good diet needs to incorporate the five major food groups (cereal, dairy, meat, fruit, vegetables), and when this theory was first put forward around fifty years ago, it was right for practically everybody. These days, though, a significant proportion of the Western population don't eat meat, and

Water works

Even with the bottled water industry booming to a degree that your parents' generation would find hard to comprehend, it's still not unusual for men not to drink enough water during the course of the day – in the Western world, in the twenty-first century, we should be drinking at least two litres per day. Keeping your water levels replenished is absolutely vital, as around seventy percent of your body is water and making sure it stays that way means everything else has the correct environment within which to function. We lose water through sweat, vapour escaping out of our mouths, urination and through our eyeballs. Yet it has to keep flowing to make sure everything moves around our system as it should and that waste is removed. So water needs to be constantly topped up. In fact, when you think you feel hungry it is more likely you are actually thirsty and in the initial stages of dehydration, so taking regular drinks will go a long way to stopping you snacking between meals.

Don't try and quench your thirst with fizzy or sugary drinks, or even fruit juice, and definitely not beer, as these will not provide the water that your thirst is telling you your body needs and could result in your drinking more of them in an attempt to stave it off. Drink more water if the weather is warm or you have been exerting yourself physically, or if you have a cold, as coughing, sneezing and blowing your nose will use up fluid reserves. Also, a good habit to get into is to take a large drink of water as soon as you wake up in the morning, as your body will have been drying out while you slept.

there are growing numbers that feel better off without dairy. Thus the idea of defining a good diet by actual foods is looking distinctly outdated and these days it makes much more sense to talk about what should be included, in terms of what you need to provide for your body.

The basic building blocks of a healthy diet are carbohydrate, fibre, protein and fat (see below), which need to be supplemented with the micronutrients of vitamins and minerals (see opposite and p.22). As long as this is all in place, what food you obtain these from should be a matter of personal choice.

A

Expert advice: "It's important to vary the fruit and veg you eat. Too many people just eat the stuff they like day in day out and think that will do. It's better than nothing, but it won't give you the range of nutrients you need."
Dr Sarah Schenker

The purpose of a good diet is to supply you with enough energy to go about your daily business, the substances needed for cell growth, repair and healing, and the defences to fight off infection or guard against harmful bacteria. Obtaining the nutrients we need through diet can also go a long way to prevent serious conditions such as arthritis, osteoporosis or heart disease occurring later in life, and eating correctly can even prevent or counteract depression. At the same time, a healthy diet won't offer too much of anything that could have a detrimental effect, like fat, sugar or salt. Eating correctly is what your body is evolved to expect, therefore as soon as you do, your all-round feelings of well-being will increase.

Carbohydrates

Carbohydrates are metabolized into blood glucose to become the body's primary source of energy, and exist in our diet in two forms: simple and complex. The former is also known as simple sugars, and includes fructose (the natural sugar found in fruit) and sucrose

Micronutrients: the vitamins and minerals

Nutrient	Found in	What it does	How deficiencies can affect you
Vitamin A	Liver, fish oil, tomatoes, leafy green veg, oranges	Promotes strong bones and teeth, good eyesight and healthy skin	Spots, acne and itching; poor night vision
Vitamin B1 (thiamine)	Whole grains, nuts, beans, liver, eggs	Supports the metabolization of carbohydrate	Muscle fatigue as the carbs aren't able to fuel them efficiently
Vitamin B3 (niacin)	Liver, poultry, nuts, beans	Metabolizes carbohydrate and fat; produces sex hormones; maintains the nervous system	Fatigue and a low sex drive
Vitamin B12	Liver, red meat, poultry, dairy, eggs	Aids the nervous system; produces red blood cells in bone marrow	Fatigue and anaemia due to low red blood cell count
Folic acid	Leafy green veg, egg yolk, whole grains, nuts	Produces red blood cells	Anaemia
Vitamin B2 (riboflavin)	Eggs, liver, brown rice, leafy green veg, brewer's yeast	Aids digestive process; repairs tissues; helps adrenalin production	Mouth sores; fatigue as energy is not released from food properly
Vitamin C	Citrus fruit, kiwi fruits, blackcurrants, strawberries, green veg	Boosts the immune system; promotes healthy teeth, gums and bones	Fatigue; bad teeth and swollen, sore or bleeding gums
Vitamin D	Fish oils, eggs, liver	Regulates calcium being used for bone growth	Liver and kidney problems and possible osteoporosis
Vitamin E	Vegetable oil, leafy green veg, nuts, meat	Protects red blood cells	Fatigue and anaemia
Calcium	Dairy, sardines and whitebait (because you eat the bones), eggs, leafy green veg	Builds bones and teeth; promotes muscle movement and cell function	Brittle bones and muscle and nerve problems
Magnesium	Nuts, whole grains, soya beans, dairy	Builds bones and teeth; aids the nervous system	An increased likelihood of kidney stones
Iron	Leafy green veg, nuts, whole grains, liver, meat	Transports oxygen to the red blood cells and, with them, to the muscles	Anaemia and chronic fatigue
Zinc	Meat, whole grains, seafood	Aids the prostate gland and sperm production; lowers blood pressure	Hair loss, reduced appetite and fatigue
Chromium	Red meat, dairy, leafy green veg	Acts as a catalyst to many different enzymes	High blood pressure, fatigue, reduced fertility

Recommended daily allowances

	Man 20–29 years old	30–39	40–49	50+
Energy	2800kcal	2500kcal	2500kcal	2300kcal
Protein	58g	55g	55g	58g
Fibre	24g	24g	26g	28g
Carbohydrate	350g	330g	330g	280g
Fat of which is saturates	95g 30g	95g 30g	95g 30g	85g 27g
Salt of which is sodium	6g 2.4g	6g 2.4g	6g 2.4g	6g 2.4g
Vitamin A	1000mcg	1000mcg	1000mcg	1000mcg
Vitamin B1 (thiamine)	1.5mg	1.4mg	1.4mg	1.2mg
Vitamin B2 (riboflavin)	1.7mg	1.6mg	1.5mg	1.4mg
Vitamin B3 (niacin)	19mg	18mg	17mg	16mg
Vitamin B12	3.0mcg	3.0mcg	3.0mcg	3.0mcg
Vitamin C	60mg	60mg	60mg	60mg
Vitamin D	10mcg	7.5mcg	5.0mcg	5.0mcg
Vitamin E	10mcg	10mcg	10mcg	10mcg
Folic acid	400mcg	400mcg	400mcg	400mcg
Calcium	750mg	750mg	750mg	800mg
Magnesium	300mg	300mg	300mg	300mg
Iron	10mg	10mg	10mg	10mg
Zinc	10mg	10mg	10mg	10mg
Chromium	500mcg	500mcg	500mcg	500mcg

A calorie is the energy needed to raise the temperature of one gram of water by ten degrees Celsius.

A kilo calorie (kcal or C) is 1000 calories. It's what's used on food packaging to denote the amount of energy provided.

A milligram (mg) is a thousandth of a gram.

A microgram (mcg) is a millionth of a gram.

Good chol, bad chol

Not all cholesterol is the devil on a dish – in fact it is vital to keep the body functioning. Manufactured by the liver, cholesterol falls into two categories: Low Density Lipoprotein (LDL) and High Density Lipoprotein (HDL), and for natural balance the body requires a 75/25 percent split. Both do the job of transporting nutrients around the system via the bloodstream, but the latter, HDL, known as "good cholesterol", is returned to the liver for reprocessing once it has delivered its load, while LDL, "bad cholesterol", is of a low enough density to penetrate the surface of the artery walls, establish a hold and start building up deposits. The less-flexible HDL particles actually play a big part in keeping the arteries from clogging up by knocking LDL off the inner surfaces.

Although it is only an excess of LDL that is the potential killer – clogged arteries mean high blood pressure and increased risk of heart disease – because we cannot regulate which type our bodies produce, it's safest to cut down on any cholesterol-producing fat.

(refined table sugar) and lactose (milk sugar), maple syrup, corn syrup and honey are also included in these groups. If it is refined, sugar is straightforward calorific energy, offering nothing else in the way of nutrition – empty calories – and because sugar is converted quickly into glucose to power the body, sugar rushes are swift and palpable. The downside is they get used up just as suddenly, resulting in an equally dramatic crash. Simple carbs should be taken on by eating fruit, rather than through the refined sugar found in so much processed food. At least that way they will be accompanied by the nutrients in the fruit.

Complex carbohydrates are found in whole grains, vegetables, pulses and fruit, and exist as sugars that include starches and fibre as part of their molecular make-up. Fibre is an absolutely crucial part of our diet, as it is the part of the plant that is not broken down during the digestion process. This permits it to move through our system, helping to keep intestinal internal walls clear – a kind of scouring pad effect. It will also retain water to deliver to the colon to keep faeces soft, and attract some of the chemicals that create cholesterol and remove them from the system. In doing this fibre prevents constipation, regulates cholesterol and is believed to reduce the risks of bowel and stomach cancer by clearing out accumulative

Ⓜ Mythbuster: tea and coffee have no place in a healthy eating plan

You shouldn't have to give up tea and coffee, but if you're drinking half a dozen cups a day you ought to cut down. Too much coffee, especially after a meal or when taking a vitamin supplement, can impede the absorption of minerals into the system – particularly iron. This means that behind the instant caffeine buzz you will actually be contributing to longer-term fatigue. Also,

to use tea or coffee, particularly with sugar or with a sugary or carb-loaded snack, as a quick pick-me-up may well be allowing you to ignore any underlying nutrition-related causes of your lack of energy during the day. You will find that once you start eating properly you'll have so much more vigour that you'll no longer need all that caffeine. If you are considering giving up tea and coffee, phase it out gradually over two or three weeks, as going cold turkey will lead to bad headaches; also make sure you are eating right to offset the inevitable tiredness.

F

Fact: The only eating plan that will work is the eating plan you stick to. There is no point in devising yourself such a spartan regime it becomes impractical when integrated into your life, therefore you either can't go along with it or you resent it so much it won't last long. Go for something that will disrupt your life as little as possible.

hazardous waste. Potatoes, whole wheat pasta and bread, cereals and beans are great sources of fibre-rich complex carbohydrate.

Protein

Protein is vital to build new tissue and is therefore essential for growth and to repair damage to the body. It is made up of amino acids that are either synthesized within the body (nonessential amino acids) or have to be introduced through the diet (essential). Of the dietary protein, all animal protein – found in meat, fish, poultry, eggs and dairy – contains the essential amino acids, as do all soy bean products. But every other example of vegetable protein – whole grains,

leafy green veg, nuts and pulses – will only contain some. Therefore vegans can only meet their complete protein needs from eating combinations of foods. It's known as mutual supplementation, and dictates that beans, nuts and wholegrain cereals need to be combined with brown rice to tick all the protein requirement boxes, just as brown rice, whole wheat and nuts need to be supplemented with beans.

Protein deficiency is almost unheard of in developed countries, although convalescents will often need to increase their protein intake beyond the "Recommended Daily Allowance" as it will be in greater demand from the body's healing process.

Fats

Fat is the other good source of calorific energy, but is so concentrated a form it is very easy to unwittingly overbalance your personal "calories consumed/calories expended" equation with too much fat. It's because there is far too much fat in the American and, increasingly, the British diet that obesity is such a problem. Ideally, no more than 25 percent of your daily calorific intake should come from fat, and even less if you have a tendency towards weight gain.

Some fat is crucial to an efficiently functioning system as, in the liver, it is

Sell by? Use by? Best by?

These date stamps are not legally required or regulated as part of food labelling, and are there as recommendations rather than tablets of stone:

Sell by is from the manufacturer for the shop's guidance, advising it on the latest it should be on sale. As far as consumers are concerned there will be a few more days – maybe even a week – left in the product.

Best by indicates at which point the product will start to deteriorate and no longer be at its finest in terms of flavour or texture. It will probably still be edible for a couple of days afterwards, but check it by smell first.

Use by is the product's expiration date and it should not even be kept, let alone eaten, beyond this point. Throw it out.

B

Best investments in your larder:

Garlic

Whether it actually wards off vampires is moot, but garlic will help you in so many other ways it's no wonder it was once believed to have super powers. Garlic boosts the immune system, is a powerful anti-fungal agent, reduces blood cholesterol, assists with blood sugar management and lowers blood pressure. Peel each clove, chop finely and add to cooking food.

Salmon

Very high in omega-3, the essential fatty acid that raises HDL cholesterol and protects against heart attacks by reducing blood clotting. Cut into steaks, lightly brush with oil, squeeze a lemon over them and grill.

Black pepper

Use it freshly ground – you should be able to smell the oil being released – and it is a powerful blood purifier, and also acts as a digestive aid, meaning it will help you get more out of the food that it is added to. Mill over food either at the cooking stage or at the table. Or both.

Spinach & kale

The most nutritiously efficient vegetables, they are practically bursting with vitamins A, C and K, plus they have a very high iron, potassium, magnesium and folate content. Steam very quickly or eat raw in a salad.

Sweet potatoes

Nutrition-wise, these are higher performing potatoes as they are a fantastic source of vitamin C, carotenoids, potassium and fibre.

Wash, but don't peel, and bake or steam exactly as you would a regular potato.

Olive oil

By far the best oil to use. As it is so loaded with

monounsaturated fats, it works to lower LDL cholesterol. It has a lower burning point than vegetable oil, so don't use it for frying – not that you were going to fry anything anyway.

Broccoli

Masses of vitamins C and A, folic acid and the carotenoids that boost your immune system and protect your cells against free radicals. Lightly steam or cut into small florets and eat raw.

Bilberries

A super-performing food that will help reduce the strain on your heart as it eases blood circulation by reducing clotting and clearing deposits from your blood vessel walls. Eat raw or use when baking in pies and muffins.

Tomatoes

An excellent source of vitamins A and C, and rich in lycopene – the chemical that is believed to lower the risk of prostate, lung and stomach cancer. Eat raw in salads, use as a base for stews or soups or brush with oil, season with salt and pepper and grill.

Walnuts

The superstar of the nut world, walnuts are rich in monounsaturated fats and omega-3 fatty acid. Walnuts also contain chemicals that keep the artery walls clear, lower the risk of gallstones and help the brain function. Eat them as a snack or chop and add to salads.

Don't eat that, eat this!

Avoid in your diet	Include in your diet
Boiled vegetables	Roast vegetables
Dried herbs	Fresh herbs
Potatoes	Sweet potatoes
Coffee	Green tea
Butter	Olive oil spread
Fried fish	Steamed fish
White flour products	Wholemeal flour products
Carton juice	Fresh squeezed juice
Fried eggs	Poached eggs
Chips	Jacket potatoes
Sweets	Dried fruit
Fried meat	Grilled meat
Crisps	Nuts
Lager	Red wine

turned into cholesterol which promotes cell growth and hormone manufacture and transports the fat-soluble vitamins A, D, E and K around the bloodstream. Dietary fat takes on four different forms, each of which affects the system in a slightly different way. Saturated fats are the mainstay of cholesterol production – notably "bad" LDL cholesterol (see box on p.23) – and are found mainly in meat, dairy and poultry. It is recommended that saturated fats make up less than half of your fat intake. Polyunsaturated fats, found in corn, soy bean and sunflower oils, will actually lower your overall blood cholesterol level, but this is not such a good idea because it also causes your "good" HDL cholesterol levels to drop. Polyunsaturated fat should also be less than half of your fat consumption. Monounsaturated fat is the good guy, as it reduces harmful LDL cholesterol without affecting HDL levels. Olives and olive oil are a rich source of monounsaturated fat, as are nut and vegetable oils. This type of food should make up the majority of your fat consumption.

Trans fat, also known as hydrogenated fat or hydrogenized oil, has risen to great prominence in processed foods recently – especially in the US – and is an acknowledged killer. It is the product of polyunsaturated fats that have been treated with hydrogen to harden the oils in order to make them go further in food manufacture as margarine or shortening. Its potentially deadly side effect is that it will send the LDL concentration in your bloodstream through the roof, while reducing HDL levels. Food containing trans fats should be avoided at all costs.

Reclaim your kitchen

The basis of any healthy eating plan you will be able to follow is having as much control as possible over what is on your plate. The best way to achieve this is to prepare it yourself. The secret of doing it yourself is to keep things simple.

Too many people get put off the idea of cooking because they've watched too many TV chefs in action and thought, "I could never do that". Or, worse still, they bought a tied-in cookery book, attempted a couple of the recipes, which have either gone wrong during the preparation or turned out looking nothing like the picture, meaning both the book and the culinary aspirations have stayed on the shelf ever since. It's why Delia Smith's *How to Cook* and Jeff Smith's *Frugal Gourmet* books have been so massively popular – they don't assume an existing expertise.

Both authors explain the "why" as well as the "what" of food and cookery, and impart a fair amount of theory of how it all works. This is far more important than page after page of beautifully photographed recipes, as the key to all cookery is knowing what will happen to a piece of food when you do something to it. It's this basic understanding that engages your interest in cookery and leaves you far more likely to get into it. Plus it will allow you to keep things interesting as you'll have the knowledge to make up your own dishes.

Once you get into the kitchen and start

T *Tip: Wash, under running water, any fruit or vegetable you are going to eat raw but don't peel first. You have no idea where it's been, who's handled it and how much pesticide residue and wax (to make it look nicer) remains on its surface.*

cooking there are keys to keeping it simple. Start off by using ingredients that you already have, because you know you're going to like them and you'll be familiar with what preparation they need. Or only buy new stuff you know you will use again once you've opened the jar – nothing leads to culinary

Food hygiene

Avoid cross contamination of cooked and raw food Don't allow them to come into contact with each other on the work surface or in the fridge; use different cutting boards to prepare each and wash knives and utensils immediately after contact with raw meat, fish or poultry.

Wash your hands after handling raw meat, fish or poultry Do this immediately, as you can transfer bacteria to fridge door handles, work surfaces or your clothes.

Clean up as you go along Keep a sink full of water (so hot you should barely be able to keep your hands in it) for washing up in and so you can wipe down work surfaces frequently.

Keep your fridge cold enough Below 5°C (41°F).

Make sure reheated food is thoroughly reheated Even if you are in a hurry, as it's too easy to heat it to a point at which the centre is warm enough for bacteria to multiply but not hot enough to kill them.

Make sure frozen food is fully thawed before you start cooking If it isn't this could interfere with the time it takes to cook and it may not get done all the way through.

Don't put hot food in the fridge It will cause the fridge to work too hard to maintain the correct internal temperature, thus overload it and affecting the temperature controls. Also the hot food will warm up whatever else is in there.

Cover everything not in use Either in the fridge or on the work surface, as you never know what might be in the air in your kitchen.

Store raw meat, fish and poultry at the bottom of the fridge It will be cooler down there and will also remove the possibility of blood dripping on to any other foods.

Wash your hands before you start touching food You'd be amazed at how many people don't.

B

Best investments in the kitchen:

Steamer

Steaming vegetables rather than boiling them makes sure you keep as much of the water-soluble vitamin B and C content as possible. It also reduces the likelihood of the food overcooking and going limp and tasteless. Steamers are available as self-contained electrical units or traditional models that need to be put on the stove. Expect to pay from £25 to £50 ($40–$90).

Blender

Smoothies, fruit shakes and puréed vegetable soups should be part of your plan, therefore a blender with a capacity of at least a litre is a must. Look for a model with pulse as well as continuous speeds. Expect to pay £75 ($145).

Wok

Used carefully, this large, round-sided pan will allow you to stir-fry platefuls of vegetables without oil or any water, which will retain the maximum vitamin content and cook to a lovely crispness. Expect to pay £15 ($30).

Juicer

As, from a nutritional point of view, the only juice worth drinking is juice you've squeezed yourself, this is a must. Although a citrus press is a good start, a juice extractor will allow you to blend some very tasty and highly beneficial drinks. Expect to pay about £100 ($180).

Kitchen roll

We all like fried food and nobody expects you to give it up totally; however, before you put it on your plate, put it on a paper towel to blot up the excess oil. Expect to pay 75p ($1).

Sharp knives

Having decent kitchen knives will make cooking much easier and therefore much more pleasurable, each of which means you're likely to do more of it. Knives that fit your hands and perform specific functions are a must, and keeping them sharp reduces the risk of you cutting yourself as you will have to use less pressure. Expect to pay £100 ($190) for a set of four.

Good-quality roasting tray

A tray that distributes heat evenly and doesn't stick will make roasting vegetables a joy. Buy one that can double as a grill pan and with ridges on the bottom to drain fat away from the food. Expect to pay £40 ($70).

Coarse-grinding pepper mill

As soon as peppercorns are cracked they start to lose their flavour and nutrients, therefore grind them directly into/over your food to maximize flavour and benefit. Expect to pay £12 ($20).

Airtight containers

If you are going to cook in advance or prepare snacks to keep in the fridge you will need to store it. Buy containers that can be used in both the freezer and the microwave for maximum efficiency. £10 ($18) for a set of assorted sizes.

Pastry brush

When grilling – or even frying – food, brush it with oil rather than pour it on or, worse still, pour it into the pan. Using a brush can cut around eighty percent from your oil usage. Expect to pay £3 ($5).

What's in a name?

If a food product clearly mentions an ingredient as part of its name – **strawberry yoghurt** – it must have actual strawberries in it. If it calls itself **strawberry-flavoured yoghurt** it doesn't need to have any strawberries in it, but the flavouring must have come from the fruit itself. **Strawberry-flavour yoghurt**, however, can derive its taste from anything, provided it ends up approximating the taste of strawberries. Should the yoghurt have a **picture of strawberries** on the label, it doesn't have to actually contain the fruit, but the flavour must be derived from it rather than from chemicals. Remarkably, fish or meat that announces itself as "smoked" doesn't have to have been near a fire; it only needs to have been treated in some way to make it taste smoky.

A food's country of origin could be different from the country of processing, yet it may be labelled in reference to the latter: a British pork pie doesn't have to have been made with British pork. It's usually good practice to disregard such terms as "Traditional", "Selected" or "Country"; they are essentially meaningless.

resentment quicker than having to buy a kilo jar of capers because you're going to use a teaspoon of them, once. In the beginning, until you become sure of yourself, adorn food as little as possible as this will bring out its natural flavour as much as it will save you time and trouble.

It's always better to cook with a dry heat – on the grill or in the oven – rather than boiling or frying, as they will either dissolve a fair amount of the nutrient content or see it absorb unacceptable levels of fat. Then make sure you cook food for as short a time as possible, as this will preserve flavour, nutrients and texture – if you can eat it raw,

do so. Shop as often as you are able, to make sure what you start off with is as fresh as possible. Don't keep food for too long, even if it's in the fridge, always pay careful attention too the date stamps and use common sense as to when to throw out fresh produce.

But I don't have time to cook healthy food

Of course you do. If you've got time to put a frozen pizza in the oven you've got time to roast a tray of vegetables. If you've got time to open a carton of juice you've got time to squeeze a grapefruit. If you've got time to fry

Have healthy food prepared *before* you get hungry

up a Full English you've got time to knock up a bowl of broccoli soup. If you've got time to meander around the supermarket picking out ready meals, you've got time to stroll through a street market choosing fresh fruit and veg. And you'll get better banter from the stall holders than you will from the checkout operators. True, cooking from scratch will take more time than convenience food – that's why it's called convenience food – but look upon it as a bit of time spent now to allow you much more time later, as you will surely live longer.

The thing to do is prepare food when you have got time and put it in a covered container in the fridge – then cooking will be relatively quick when you do want to eat. Clean and chop some vegetables for your evening meal while your morning cup of tea is brewing; or make enough soup for a

Is organic produce really better for you?

The real answer is "sort of… perhaps". While it won't actually do you a great deal more good than conventionally-farmed food, it certainly won't do you any harm either.

There has been a huge growth in organic produce on both sides of the Atlantic in recent years – in the UK and US in 2006, the market was worth £1.2 billion and $17 billion, with each figure expected to almost double by 2010. Yet, according to research carried out by the Food Standards Agency in the UK and similar organizations in France and Sweden, there is no solid scientific evidence to say that organic food is more nutritious than conventionally farmed food. What actually makes a difference is how fresh the food is – the closer it is to being picked or killed the higher its nutrient content. Because organic food will not contain artificial preservatives and will only have been minimally processed (if at all), it has to be eaten much fresher. Conventionally farmed fruit and vegetables, eaten as soon as they are picked, will offer the name "goodness" measure as organic.

Importantly, however, organic fruit or vegetables or meat is as nature intended, therefore – and admittedly this is purely subjective – many believe it offers a completely authentic and more intense taste experience. Which, by itself, justifies the huge extra cost.

The other big plus point of organic fruit and vegetables has a less personal quality – it is kinder to the environment, because soil won't be over-farmed with the aid of chemical fertilizers, and it won't involve spraying pesticides into the air. Also, and this is a rapidly increasing influence on people's choices, while meat and poultry will not have been pumped full of growth hormones and pesticides, it will have been raised humanely.

It should be mentioned that, in spite of Soil Association regulation, there is good and bad practice on organic farms as well as factory farms.

Agricultural activity	Conventional farming	Organic farming
Promoting plant growth	Chemical fertilizers	Natural fertilizers such as manure or compost
Keeping pests and disease down	Sprayed chemical insecticide	Birds, insects and traps
Killing weeds	Chemical herbicides to target specific plants	Remove by hand, and keep them down with mulch
Refreshing soil	Chemical fertilization	Rotation of fields
Feeding animals	Antibiotics, growth hormones, processed feed	Organic feed, grazing

couple of days and ladle it out of a pot in the fridge when you fancy some. Or, as it takes the same time to cook a big casserole as it does a smaller one, cook for more than one meal and freeze the rest – just make sure, if there are several meals' worth, you freeze it as individual meals because thawing and re-freezing is likely to invite bacteria. Carrying out this batch cooking at times when you have little else to do will repay during busy periods of the week. Also, it's worth noting that regulating your eating patterns will make it much easier to plan meals in advance.

Three quick, delicious and nutritious dishes

Roast vegetables

Wash and peel (where necessary) a selection of vegetables – what you choose is up to you, but aubergines, courgettes, parsnips, garlic cloves and peppers are a good start – chop into five-centimetre pieces; sprinkle with salt and pepper; toss in olive oil and lemon juice; roast in a hot oven for about thirty minutes, tossing three or four times. Sprinkle with chopped flat leaf parsley and serve.

Ratatouille

Chop about 250g of tomatoes; slice a large onion; cut three courgettes into centimetre-thick slices; finely chop three cloves of garlic; combine the ingredients in a saucepan that has a lid; season with salt and pepper and add a splash of olive oil; put the lid on the pan and cook very slowly on a low heat for about twenty minutes, stirring frequently, until it looks like a stew. Serve.

(Either of the above is perfect by themselves or will make a very good-looking accompaniment to grilled meat or fish.)

Vegetable soup

Wash, peel (if necessary) and roughly chop whatever combination of veg takes your fancy

T

Tip: If you are a grazer or like to snack while watching TV or at your desk, prepare yourself with boxes of healthy snacks such as carrot or celery sticks or dried fruit. The trick is to anticipate your snack attacks and have the healthy alternatives pre-prepared and ready to be grabbed, because if you have to peel a carrot or trim a piece of fruit, you'd probably reach past it for something instant such as a bag of crisps.

– but it's usually a good idea to put some onion and garlic in there; place in a saucepan that has a lid; season with salt and pepper; add enough water for about two centimetres on the bottom; fit the lid; then cook gently on a low heat for about fifteen minutes, until the veg is soft. Tip it all into a blender, cover with water and liquidize; return the purée to the saucepan and add water to make it whatever consistency you prefer; bring to the boil and stir until smooth.

T

Tip: The ideal daily water consumption for a man has gone up in the last decade, from between one-and-a-half and two to between two and two-and-a-half litres. This is because of the big increases in air conditioned environments and time spent in front of VDUs, both of which serve to dry out your body.

The healthiest shopping trolley

Dairy

Non-fat yoghurt – iodine, calcium, vitamins B2 and B12, phosphorus, protein
Olive oil spread – as a substitute for butter it will reduce the risks of heart disease, diabetes, obesity and colon cancer
Skimmed milk – vitamins B2, D and K, calcium, iodine (protects the thyroid), potassium
Low-fat feta cheese – vitamins B6 and B12 calcium, protein
Eggs – protein, tryptophan (an essential amino acid), choline (a brain-boosting nutrient), vitamin B2

Meat and poultry

Skinless chicken – vitamins B3 and B6, tryptophan, protein, selenium (an important metabolic catalyst)
Turkey pieces/slices – vitamins B3 and B6, tryptophan, protein, selenium
Lean beef – tryptophan, protein, iron, zinc, selenium, phosphorus, vitamins B12, B6, B3 and B2
Lean pork – vitamins B1, B2, B3 and B6, phosphorus, selenium, zinc
Calves' liver – vitamins A, B2, B3, B5, B6, B12 and C, copper, folate, selenium, tryptophan, zinc, iron, protein, phosphorus

Fruit

Apricots – Beta-carotene
Avocados – cholesterol-lowering oleic acid
Ruby grapefruit – vitamin C, soluble fibre, lycopene (an antioxidant), cancer-inhibiting limonene
Kiwi fruit – vitamin C
Pineapple – vitamins C and B1, bromelain (a digestive aid and an anti-inflammatory)
Figs – vitamin B6, potassium, fibre
Blueberries – cell-protecting flavenoids, polyphenols (flush toxins and protect the heart)
Raisins – iron
Raspberries – fibre, vitamin C, cancer-inhibiting ellagic acid
Cantaloupe melon – potassium, vitamin C
Bananas – potassium, carbohydrate
Lemons & limes – vitamin C, cancer-inhibiting limonene
Mangoes – alpha- and beta-carotene

Pulses, nuts and grains

Lentils – fibre, protein, iron, folate, vitamin B1, manganese, iron, potassium, tryptophan
Soy beans – protein, iron, omega-3 fatty acids, fibre, vitamins B2 and K, magnesium, potassium
Kidney beans – protein, iron, tryptophan, fibre, vitamins B1 and K, magnesium, potassium, folate
Whole oats – manganese, selenium, fibre, tryptophan, protein, vitamin B1
Brown rice – manganese, selenium, magnesium, tryptophan
Wholewheat pasta – complex carbohydrate, fibre, protein
Walnuts – omega-3 fatty acids, manganese, copper, tryptophan
Almonds – manganese, vitamins B2 and E, magnesium, tryptophan
Peanuts – manganese, tryptophan, vitamin B3, protein, folate
Sunflower seeds – vitamins E, B1 and B5, manganese, magnesium, tryptophan, selenium, magnesium

Vegetables

Broccoli – vitamin C, beta-carotene, cancer-inhibiting sulphoraphane, immune system-boosting indoles
Onions – flavenoids (a natural plant antioxidant)
Cabbage/spring greens – vitamins K and C, antioxidants
Artichokes – fibre, silymarin (a powerful antioxidant)
Squash – vitamin C, beta-carotene
Sweet potatoes – vitamins A and C, manganese, antioxidants
Garlic – sulphur compounds that reduce LDL cholesterol, protect against cancer and lower blood-clotting risks

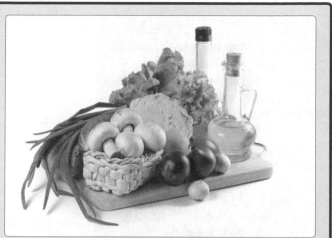

Chinese cabbage – calcium
Watercress – vitamins A and C, iron, folic acid, calcium, sulphoraphanes (anitoxidant and cancer-inhibiting)
Spinach – iron, carotenoid antioxidants (immune system-boosters)
Tomatoes – lycopene (an antioxidant), coumarins (an anti-inflammatory, blood clot inhibitor)
Aubergines – fibre, chlorogenic acid (an antioxidant and LDL cholesterol inhibitor), nasunin (protects the brain cell membranes)
Green (or red or yellow) peppers – vitamins A, C and B6

Fish and seafood

Salmon – omega-3 fatty acids, vitamins D, B3, B6 and B12, selenium, protein
Crab – protein, phosphorous, vitamins B3, B12 and C, zinc and copper
Sardines – calcium, iron, protein
Mackerel – omega-3 fatty acids, protein, vitamin D
Tuna – omega-3 fatty acids, vitamins B1, B3 and B6, selenium, protein, tryptophan
Clams and mussels – vitamin B12, magnesium, potassium

Drinks

Cranberry juice – vitamins C and K, fibre
Green tea – flavenoids; regular green tea drinkers have lower rates of bacterial infection, heart disease, cancer and osteoporosis
Don't buy orange or grapefruit juice – squeeze your own

Herbs and spices

Root ginger – magnesium, potassium, vitamin C, and is proven to aid digestion and circulation and work as an anti-inflamatory
Black pepper – vitamin K, iron, manganese, fibre, antioxidants, improves digestion
Rosemary – fibre, iron, calcium, improves blood flow to the brain, boosts immune system, is an anti-inflamatory
Thyme – flavenoids, vitamin K, boosts cell membranes of the heart, brain and kidneys
Parsley – flavenoids, vitamins C and A, iron, polyacetylenes (inhibits cancer), freshens breath
Cinnamon – manganese, fibre, cinnamaldehyde (prevents bacterial infection, inhibits blood clotting)

F

Fact: Type 2 diabetes used to be known as Adult Onset Diabetes because it was rarely found in anybody under the age of 35 – it is triggered by the cumulative effects of bad diet and lack of exercise. However, during the last twenty years the eating/exercise habits of British and American children have become so poor type 2 is now regularly being diagnosed in children as young as thirteen.

Eating out

There is no reason at all why you can't carry on enjoying restaurants and still eat healthily, provided you follow the same guidelines as you would when eating at home. Make the same informed choices from the menu as you would from the supermarket shelves, to pick

T

Tip: If you are going to eat sandwiches most days, invest in a breadmaker. Priced between £50 ($100) and £100 ($200) they are remarkably simple to use – you can put a loaf of bread on in less time than it takes to make a piece of toast. You choose what flour you use and can add fruit, walnuts, olives or practically anything. The finished product works out to cost around twenty pence (forty cents) per loaf. As a bonus, home-baked bread is more substantial and requires more chewing, meaning you will eat less of it.

a balanced meal. Even if the establishment doesn't flag up its healthy options, there should be plenty of choice that isn't boiled beyond its nutritional life or swimming in fat – if there isn't you should consider eating somewhere else.

Importantly, don't be afraid to ask what's in dishes, and if they are reluctant to tell you find another restaurant. Also, if you want something cooked in a certain way or served without dressing or sauce most decent places should be happy to oblige; even if you just want an unadorned salad or plain grilled skinless chicken they should treat it with the same culinary care and presentational flair as anything else. If they won't adapt their dishes on their menu it probably means their food isn't being cooked to order but simply reheated instead – another good reason not to give that establishment your money.

Fast food

You pretty much know what you're getting when you go to McDonald's or KFC or Subway, and you shouldn't be too shocked at the apparent calorie and fat/nutritional value imbalance. This doesn't mean giving burger or pizza joints the swerve as a little bit of what you fancy does you good. Just don't try and live on the stuff – you won't if you've seen Morgan Thurlock's movie *Supersize Me*. Try and follow these guidelines: stay away from anything breadcrumbed and fried – even if it is the healthier-sounding chicken or fish it will still be a fat bomb; ask yourself if you really need cheese and bacon; and avoid the sauces and dressings as they will be minefields of salt and sugar. The good news is that many burger joints are now offering a choice as to how your sandwich is constructed, allowing you to avoid particular ingredients, which is far more relevant to your healthy-eating plan than supplementing a fatburger with a handful of McCarrots.

Exactly what it says on the tin

What the label says	What it means
Organic	The food has come from a grower, farmer, processor or importer registered with a DEFRA-approved certification body. Pre-packed meals or dishes labelled organic must contain at least 95 percent organic ingredients. Organic ingredients are those grown or raised without the routine use of chemicals or hormones.
Free range	Only usually relevant to chickens, it means the hens have had continuous access to outside space. In the EU this has to be four square metres per hen; in the US there are no size restrictions.
Natural	This has no legal definition and therefore could mean anything, but the Food Standards Agency maintain it has to fulfil the basic requirements of the Trades Descriptions Act, therefore something calling itself "natural" is unlikely to have been knocked up in a laboratory.
Fat/sugar/cholesterol/sodium-free	The product contains less than 0.5g of fat or sugar per 100g/less than 2mg of cholesterol and below 2g of saturated fat per 100g/less than 5mg of sodium per 100g.
Low-fat/cholesterol/sodium	The product has no more than 3g of fat per 100g/less than 20mg of cholesterol and 2g of saturated fat/or less than 35mg of sodium.
No added sugar	This refers to regular refined sugar such as you'd put on the table; the product may still be sweetened with corn syrup or one of the other sugars such as dextrose, fructose or glucose.
Reduced-fat/sugar/sodium/cholesterol	This is a relative term, and can only be used to compare the reduced item with its regular equivalent in the same range. Then it has to have at least fifty percent less of whatever ingredient it claims is reduced.

Sandwiches

Opting for wholemeal when it comes to the bread or pitta or wrap, ditching the butter in favour of olive oil spread and going easy on the mayo ought to be second nature for anybody on a healthy eating plan, which means your sandwiches will be all about what's inside them. And that can be as nutritious as you want to make it. Homemade sandwiches are a great option for a healthy lunch if there is little choice locally or decent restaurants are prohibitively expensive, but you must remember to counter-balance the bread with a relative amount of mixed filling. Look upon building a butty in the same way as preparing a nutritionally balanced meal – your only

A

Expert advice: "Give in to your cravings. Your body has a metabolic memory that tells you what you need by stimulating your desire for foods you've had in the past that contain the nutrients you're now short of."
Dr Sarah Schenker

T

Tip: When ordering a sandwich, opt for Swiss cheese, as it contains less than one third of the sodium found in cheddar, and therefore will be much kinder to your heart and kidneys.

limit should be your imagination – then put it between two pieces of (wholemeal) bread.

Buying sandwiches almost offers the same choice these days. The big chains selling pre-packed sandwiches usually offer a healthy option as part of their range, and give detailed nutritional information on the labels, allowing you to make your own informed choices. It is worth remembering that the bread used for the majority of pre-packed sandwiches – whatever colour it might be – will not be nearly as nutritious as the bread you could buy to make your own sandwiches, so be aware that you probably won't be getting a great deal of fibre out of it.

Sandwich shops offer even greater scope for healthy eating, as you should be able to choose exactly what goes in. Like the pre-packed variety, though, don't expect to gain much other than carbohydrate from the bread, and always be wary of the pre-mixed fillings, as what is used to bind the tuna or the eggs or whatever together is liable to be inexpensive and bursting with fat, salt and sugar.

T

Tip: Many of the fast food chains now offer a healthy option, but this isn't why they exist, and therefore not what they do best. You'll get better and higher value salads elsewhere.

The best of the web

food.gov.uk
The Food Standards Agency is an independent organization set up to represent the public's interests as regards food safety. They are the force behind easily understood labelling on food.

nutrition.gov
The official US government nutrition-dedicated site, packed with detailed, regularly updated information and healthy eating related reports and research.

nutrition.org.uk
The website of the British Nutrition Foundation, which although seeming more aimed at healthcare and nutrition professionals offers some very interesting reading. More suitable for those who already have a basic knowledge.

soilassociation.org
The body who certify organic producers and will tell you everything you need to know about organic farming, growing and eating.

healthyeating.net
A comprehensive and thoroughly enjoyable healthy eating site, with an emphasis on cooking and fantastic food.

nutritiondata.com
You need to register, but once you have this site will calculate the nutrition content of practically any food you care to name; it also offers dietary advice.

Ten top tips for healthy eating

▶ **Read food labels carefully**
You may be taking on far less nutrition than you realize.

▶ **Change your diet gradually**
Don't revamp your habits too radically as that will lead to confusion and the likelihood of resentment, greatly reducing your chances of sticking to it.

▶ **Spread your nutrition across your whole diet**
Don't attempt to include half-a-dozen superfoods and not worry about the rest; look at getting some sort of benefit from every part of your diet, then vary it to incorporate as many different things as possible.

▶ **Treat restaurants much like you would your home**
Follow the same guidelines you would in your own kitchen and don't be afraid to ask questions or make off-menu requests. But don't take your trousers off, obviously.

▶ **A little bit of what you fancy does you good** Allow yourself a day off a week from your healthy eating plan: you've earned it.

▶ **Eat regular meals, especially breakfast** This will give you far more control over what you are eating as it will cut down the likelihood of your grazing during the day.

▶ **Keep healthy snacks ready**
If you are going to snack keep a healthy alternative to hand – carrot sticks, dried fruit, satsumas and so on – at work as well as at home.

▶ **A little change goes a long way** Small things like having that quarter pounder without the cheese or holding the mayo on a sandwich will add up to huge long-term benefits for your health.

▶ **Eat more raw food** It will not have lost the nutrients that get destroyed during cooking and the extra chewing involved will make you feel full, faster.

▶ **Keep the cookery simple**
Nothing is more likely to put you off eating fresh food than elaborate recipes and unusual ingredients – dishes such as roasted vegetables, blended soups and grilled lean meat take minutes to prepare and offer the food's unadulterated flavour.

At night

(2)

Ideally you should go to sleep when you feel tired and wake up naturally when your physical and mental systems have had enough sleep to completely refresh themselves. At least that's how it used to work when we lived in an agricultural society and the only clock anybody needed was their body clock. But while this was clearly much better for us it's unlikely that too many modern men are going to want to do anything as medieval as going to bed at sundown.

Are you getting enough?

Probably not.

Sleep requirements vary from person to person, but most adult men need between seven and nine hours' good-quality sleep per night. A small percentage can get by on as little as five or six hours', but very few will be able to function efficiently on less than that. However, although these sleep requirements are one of the fundamental, unchanging building blocks of being a human, some sixty percent of men in the UK and the US say they don't get anything like that much.

Then there's the question of sleep quality. A considerable proportion of those who are sleeping for the optimum eight hours per night clearly aren't experiencing sleep that's good enough to be effectively restorative. According to a recent survey, 75 percent of men between the ages of 25 and 50 experience difficulties sleeping that leave them waking up unrefreshed at least two mornings a week. And around half of that number felt

so tired during the following days that they believed it affected their mental and physical performance.

These figures shouldn't come as a shock, either, as modern society has evolved to put such pressures on men that the importance of a good night's sleep has been marginalized in a trade-off to wring more "productive" hours out of every day. Everybody works longer hours than ever before – in the UK people spend longer at work than any other nation in Europe, and in the US the average working week has increased by twenty percent in the last two decades. Men also have far more hands-on involvement in child-rearing

F

Fact: Twelve percent of all serious road accidents in the UK are caused by tiredness; this figure rises to twenty percent for motorway accidents. That is far more than the amount caused by drunkenness.

How it all works: sleep

The strangest thing about sleep is that, in spite of how vital it is to keeping us functioning, science doesn't actually know that much about it. What happens if you don't get enough is well known (see box on p.42), as is the fact that sleep restores you to how you were before the day took its physical and mental toll. But how it actually achieves this is much less straightforward.

Growth hormones are secreted during sleep, which aid the repair and renewal of tissue. This is why babies, growing children and adolescents going through puberty need considerably more sleep as that is when their growth and bodily development happens. The notion of "beauty sleep" is because of the cell repair that sleep promotes. The immune system is recharged as we sleep, as the melatonin secreted acts as a strong antioxidant, and neurons within the cerebral cortex are regenerated, effectively refreshing the brain. Also, particularly during the Rapid Eye Movement (REM) periods of the sleep cycle, the brain reorganizes itself by sorting out what has made an impression that day through new connections within the synapse. These fresh pathways generate new, easily accessed memories, and it's believed that these apparently random thoughts being classified forms the sometimes bizarre basis for our dreams.

Not all sleep is the same sleep, and during each undisturbed eight hours we will go through up to six sleep cycles consisting of four separate stages. Stage one, light sleep, is when the body gets itself into sleep mode by regulating and lowering cardiovascular rates and decreasing body temperature. Stage two is intermediate sleep, when blood pressure is lowered, allowing the body to totally relax, and it's during this period that the brain will be refreshed. Stage three, deep sleep, usually occurs after about twenty minutes and is the most difficult to wake up from. It's during this time that tissue growth and repair happens and our physical energy levels will be restored. Stage four, REM sleep, won't happen until you've been asleep for at least an hour. This is when you dream, as there is brain activity and the eyes dart about behind the lids – hence the name. It's during these periods that the hormone cortisol is secreted, which promotes alertness. As each REM stage gets longer as the night continues, after sufficient sleep we wake up raring to go.

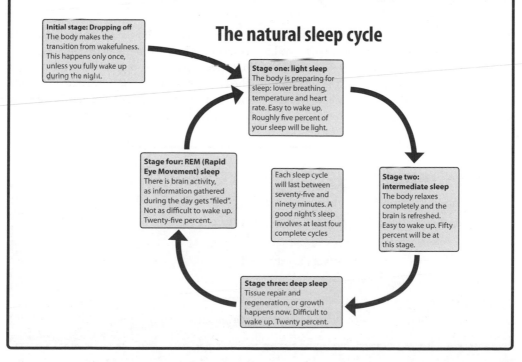

The natural sleep cycle

Initial stage: Dropping off
The body makes the transition from wakefulness. This happens only once, unless you fully wake up during the night.

Stage one: light sleep
The body is preparing for sleep: lower breathing, temperature and heart rate. Easy to wake up. Roughly five percent of your sleep will be light.

Stage two: intermediate sleep
The body relaxes completely and the brain is refreshed. Easy to wake up. Fifty percent will be at this stage.

Stage three: deep sleep
Tissue repair and regeneration, or growth happens now. Difficult to wake up. Twenty percent.

Stage four: REM (Rapid Eye Movement) sleep
There is brain activity, as information gathered during the day gets "filed". Not as difficult to wake up. Twenty-five percent.

Each sleep cycle will last between seventy-five and ninety minutes. A good night's sleep involves at least four complete cycles

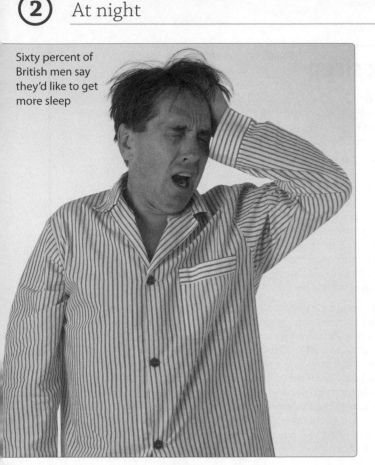

Sixty percent of British men say they'd like to get more sleep

surprising that, in some circles, not wasting your time sleeping is seen as some sort of macho badge of courage.

Although total sleep deprivation can, fairly quickly, have a devastating effect on the body (see box on p.42), of far greater concern is the creeping results of getting a couple of hours less than you need most nights of the week. It's this continual sacrificing of proper sleep that is one of the biggest contributors to the general stress levels and the low-grade maladies that are part of everyday life for so many twenty-first-century men.

What sleep deprivation does

and domestic duties than their fathers did. Then, as members of the post-rock'n'roll generation, we're expected to continue with an exciting social life into middle age and beyond. It's a wonder we find time to get any sleep at all, and at the same time it's hardly

There are three levels of sleep deficit to consider. The first is the occasional night of bad sleep, usually brought on by a night on the lash, by travelling or by an extraordinary situation at work. Most of us can survive even a couple of such nights in the same week

You should be getting more sleep if...

You seem to catch every bug that's going around, particularly in winter

You sleep through the alarm or turn it off without waking up

You suffer crashing late-afternoon fatigue

Even a small amount of exercise leaves you exhausted

Your daily coffee intake is creeping up

Forgetfulness has become noticeable

You feel generally lethargic and lack concentration for even short periods of time with only the mild discomforts of irritability, slightly impaired focus and afternoon fatigue the next day. Provided such nights don't become too regular, they'll do little lasting damage to your health as you can "catch up" the lost sleep by following it with a couple of early nights.

The next level is short-term sleep-deprivation, or acute insomnia. This is usually the result of something clearly identifiable, which can be isolated and ought to have a finite impact on your peace of mind and physical well-being. Among the most common causes are specific stresses such as a death in the family or a divorce, discomfort brought on by an injury or illness, or a problem that needs solving.

If you know you have a situation that may impair your sleeping patterns, make it as easy as you can for yourself by creating the ideal sleeping conditions (see box on p.57), and try to go to bed earlier, preferably after a relaxing warm (but not too hot) bath. Only resort to medication under extreme circumstances, and then for as short a period of time as possible. If, as is common with this type of sleep disorder, you wake in the night and cannot get back to sleep, don't just lie there willing yourself into the land of nod. You will need to completely relax and

B

Best investment: pillows, £30 ($55)
A peaceful sleep is a restorative sleep, but that can only happen if your head and neck are properly supported, thus your pillow has to be on the case as well as merely in it. Yet where you lay your head is likely to be the most neglected aspect of your bed. The right pillow for you must offer sufficient support for your head, so that the top of the spine remains on the vertical axis, but the neck is allowed to droop forward slightly, as it would if you were standing up. Yet it should be soft enough to provide that psychological comfort factor. If you sleep on your side a firmer pillow is recommended as your head will need the most support to stop it from sagging sideways, if you sleep on your back it should be medium-firm, while a front sleeper should go for the softest options so the head isn't pushed higher than the shoulders. The strain on neck muscles resulting from positioning your head too high or too low could be enough to disrupt your sleep without causing noticeable physical pain. Natural pillows mix different blends of down and feathers for, respectively, softness and firmness, while synthetic fillings offer a range of levels of support.

Choose your pillow in relation to your mattress, because the two will have to work in harmony with each other.

Your partner and you may want hugely different things out of a pillow, but as long as you match their cases what's inside can suit your personal needs.

Don't wait until you renew your duvet or mattress to buy new pillows. Because they have to take the concentrated weight of your head they will wear out far more quickly – two to three years is what you can expect out of a good pillow.

Wash your pillow a couple of times a year – you'll be amazed at how it'll plump back up.

Buy pillows from a specialist bedding store or department, and don't be afraid to try out different types.

this may mean getting out of bed (see box on p.44).

This level of sleep loss will be uncomfortable and will interfere to some degree with your moods and abilities. Your powers of concentration and judgement will be greatly impaired and you will be far more susceptible to whatever bugs are going around as your immune system will start to suffer. But providing you are aware of your reduced capacities and are appropriately careful it shouldn't have too many long-term consequences. Also, as the causes of this type of impairment are finite the effects on your sleep should be too.

Where real problems are occurring,

A week without sleep

Days without sleep	What happens to you
One	Not much. The next day you'll be a bit grumpy and probably feel very tired from about four o'clock in the afternoon, but most of us can cope with missing one night's sleep.
Two	The early morning will be particularly difficult as, thanks to how your body clock is set, the urge to sleep will be strongest. You will be constantly irritable and concentration will be difficult. Physical fatigue becomes persistent.
Three	Mundane, automatic or repetitive tasks – driving, typing, operating machinery at work, etc – become very erratic, whereas anything that needs to be thought about actually "wakes the brain up" and gets done, albeit much more slowly than usual.
Four	Reasoning and rational reactions become less likely as the brain loses the ability to inhibit your emotions. Very short-term memory loss will occur – that is the inability to remember events since sleep deprivation began. Physical fatigue is, by now, acute and very uncomfortable.
Five	Speech is slurred, sentences don't flow and problem-solving abilities are falling apart as the brain's neurotransmitters become altered, meaning it is working harder and harder to accomplish less and less. Joints and muscles ache and your immune system will be severely compromised.
Six	The ability of neurotransmitters to function is now so reduced that dizziness and blurred vision will occur, while your sense of who you are – your personality – is becoming rapidly reduced.
Seven	The deterioration of your brain's ability to process thoughts will now be such that you will experience hallucinations and instances of paranoia and delusion.
Long term	You will be at increased risk of disease and infection as your immune system will be suffering; there is a much greater chance of your becoming obese; your long- and short-term memories stop working efficiently; and there is a much greater likelihood of depression.

especially among men, is with chronic insomnia. This needn't be as dramatic as it might sound, that is not sleeping at all, as the term covers any form of sleep impairment that lasts for longer than a few weeks. The effects of this condition are similar to those of acute insomnia, but are indefinite and will become progressively worse over time. Then, because the fatigue, the lack of focus and the irritability become constants, they, and the insufficient levels of sleep that led to them, become accepted as a new norm which in turn is encroached upon when circumstance dictates…

While chronic insomnia is often brought on by an underlying physical or mental problem, these days it is as likely to be self-inflicted, with the ill-effects being all but ignored, to the degree that the sufferer believes nothing is actually wrong. If you feel you may be depriving yourself of sleep – that is you regularly get less than seven hours, need an alarm to wake you and don't feel particularly refreshed in the morning – spend a week going to bed early every night (at least eight hours before you get up), not drinking in the evening and following our Ten Top Tips (see p.57). If you feel much better after those seven nights, alter your sleeping habits accordingly; if it's made no difference then there may be something else wrong. Go and see your doctor and talk as frankly as possible, and let him or her suggest a course of action.

T *Tip: Apparently unexplained weight gain may be down to a lack of sleep. Sleep balances levels of the hormones ghrelin and leptin in our brains, which serve to regulate appetite by helping to control when we feel full or hungry.*

part of the cycle in a number of ways. This applies to more than just nightcaps, and is why, after a night on the booze, you may go out like a light but not feel at all refreshed in the morning.

Alcohol impedes the flow of tryptophan to the brain, which is the source of the neurotransmitter serotonin that is vital to maintaining deep sleep. It then triggers the release and production of adrenalin, which stimulates the brain towards wakefulness. Also – and this is particularly important for diabetics who enjoy a drink – it can lead to a drastic lowering of blood sugar known as night-time hypoglycemia. Under normal circumstances, when blood sugar levels drop the liver converts carbohydrate reserves into glucose, which it releases into the bloodstream as replenishment (see p.20). However, once the liver detects a quantity of alcohol in the bloodstream, it shuts down

Knock the nightcap on the head

Because alcohol is a sedative it will help you fall asleep quickly, but it will actively work against you staying that way for longer than a couple of hours. Once metabolized into your system, alcohol disrupts the deep sleep

A *Expert advice: "Eating properly and at regular times will greatly help to stabilize sleep patterns and make sleep more restful, as the digestive system will not be working against the body as it tries to relax."*
Dr Sarah Schenker

Getting back to sleep

Don't lie there trying too hard to get back to sleep. This conscious attempt to force yourself back to sleep will, in itself, wake you up, then the frustration of not actually managing it will start to stress you out, further contributing to your wakefulness. Get up and read, have a warm drink or do something relaxing until you start to nod off.

Whatever you do, don't have a smoke (in bed or anywhere else). Nicotine is a powerful stimulant, while the almost immediately ensuing withdrawal pangs will further serve to keep you awake.

Have a turkey and lettuce sandwich. Turkey meat is naturally rich in tryptophan which is metabolized into the sleep-aiding serotonin (this contributes enormously to so many of us nodding off after Christmas dinner), while lettuce has been prized for its sleep-inducing properties since the days of the Ancient Greeks. It contains the calming folic acid and an opium relative called lactucarium. The carbohydrates in wholemeal bread will also help.

any glucose provision while it works to rid the body of this toxin, which can leave blood sugar levels plummeting. This in turn sparks the release of hormones that misguidedly attempt to address the situation by bringing on hunger, which stimulates the brain, disrupting deep sleep.

The drugs don't work either

Sleep medication – either prescription drugs or, as is the case in the US, powerful over-the-counter pharmaceuticals – will never be a long-term answer to sleeping disorders. The majority of sleep medications on the market either go to work on the chemical balance of your brain or slow down your central nervous system to bring on extreme drowsiness, but all any of them will do is relieve the symptoms of whatever type of insomnia is affecting you rather than addressing the underlying causes. And their prolonged use – anything more than three or four weeks – can do you a considerable amount of harm.

It is relatively easy to get hooked on sleep medication, physiologically or psychologically (or both), meaning you will suffer withdrawal when you do give it up. Extended use can lead to a kind of hangover effect, in which a residue of the chemicals stays on in your system during the day, causing a continual feeling of drowsiness

Mythbuster: the older you are the less sleep you need

It should read the older you are the less sleep you'll *get*, which is very different. Once a man is fully grown – reached his twenties – he will need the same amount of sleep for the rest of his life. However, by the time he's reached his sixties he'll be getting less restorative sleep each night for a number of reasons: the body produces less of the sleep hormone melatonin; he will be more likely to feel twinges of pain from joints or muscles; older people are more susceptible to changes in the sleeping environment; and calls of nature are liable to have an increasingly disruptive effect.

This is why so many older people get up so early, and may take naps during the day.

and a reduced ability to concentrate that feels not unlike chronic fatigue. Drug-induced sleep is never quite as restorative as natural sleep, and this gets more so as medication use continues. Eventually the rhythms of your deep sleep become altered and REM sleep is disrupted, meaning that what you've been taking to help you sleep is, ironically, preventing you from sleeping properly.

That said, sleep medication can be effective in the short term, provided the causes of the sleeping problems are external and finite – jet lag, shift change, death in the family, etc. However, if your sleeping

Power napping

A few years ago the notion of "power napping" was introduced and widely derided as nothing more than a cover for sleeping off a three-bottles-of-wine business lunch. The reality is, however, that taking a couple of short naps – and we do mean short – during the course of the day will go a long way towards reducing stress and keeping your creativity and cognitive powers sharp and focused. Power napping allows the brain to switch off for the duration, and to take advantage of the first two parts of the four-stage sleep cycle (see box on p.39) without sinking into deep sleep or REM sleep. As stage-two sleep re-powers electrical impulses in your nervous system, you will feel mentally regenerated, but without any of the sleep inertia and attendant wooziness on waking that comes with the later stages.

It's something that cats and old people have known for ages; now all you've got to do is get your boss to see it that way.

The secrets to productive power napping

Sleep for between ten and thirty minutes only – much more than that and you will tip over into deep sleep and awake groggy rather than refreshed.

Set the alarm.

Don't even attempt it If you have been drinking coffee all morning, as the caffeine will keep you awake.

Do it in the dark – either close the blinds or, if you've no sense of shame, wear a sleepmask.

Don't try to power nap after a high-fat/high-sugar meal: the energy involved in breaking that down will stop you dropping off.

Avoid power napping in the late afternoon, as you will be far more likely to drop into a deep sleep and not wake up for a while.

Don't get cold. As your body temperature drops when you are asleep and wrapping yourself in a blanket at your desk might be somewhat indiscreet, make sure the room remains warm enough.

Convince yourself, and your co-workers, that you're not just being lazy and that this will ultimately aid your productivity.

problems are anything other than temporary, consult your doctor and make sure that together you concentrate on curing the insomnia rather than merely treating the symptoms with medication.

Types of sleep medication

Over-the-counter

Almost all the available brands contain antihistamine as their main active ingredient, and these products are in no way intended for prolonged use. Using them over an extended period can lead to constipation, forgetfulness, inability to concentrate and problems with your vision.

Prescription

The three most widely used types of prescription sleep medication are:

Benzodiazepines

These are tranquilizers, and work by slowing down the central nervous system. Side effects include continual drowsiness, reduced physical coordination and memory lapses.

Non-benzodiazepines

These increase the effects of gamma-aminobutyric acid (GABA), a brain chemical that inhibits the transmission of electrical impulses within the nervous system. They assist with creating restful sleep patterns rather than putting the user to sleep, and although safer than the benzodiazepines can become addictive. They are also used as anti-depressants and as blood pressure regulators.

Melatonin receptor agonists

These hypnotics, such as ramelteon, increase the effects of the sleep chemical melatonin on the brain, thus bringing on drowsiness. Side effects can include nausea, headaches and dizzy spells; these are sleep onset drugs and have little effect on staying asleep.

Herbal helpers

There have been various herbal sleep potions in use since at least the days of the Ancient Egyptians, and many of them still prove popular today. They work by calming nerves and settling anxiety to ensure the taker is as relaxed as possible when trying to sleep. They should be used only as directed. The most effective and widely available are:

Valerian

A natural sedative that reduces cardiovascular rates to ease muscle tension and nervous stress, valerian is taken either in capsule form or brewed as tea. Because it slows the heart rate, you should be very careful not to take too much, and it can become psychologically addictive if you take it for too long.

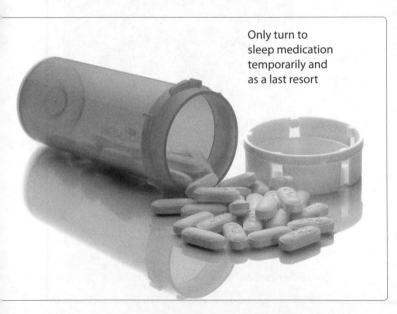

Only turn to sleep medication temporarily and as a last resort

How it all works: circadian rhythms

Better known as the body clock, circadian rhythms are the 24-hour sequences that human beings' lives operate on, evolved to coincide with the day/night cycle of the Earth's rotation. Circadian comes from the Latin words *circa* meaning "about" and *diem* meaning "day". The most basic of these cycles is the one that controls our feelings of sleepiness and wakefulness, coordinating them to it getting dark in the evening and light in the morning.

Although the body's circadian rhythms can be influenced by outside stimuli such as artificial light, noise or temperature, they are endogenously generated – that is they originate inside the brain. They are triggered by the suprachiasmatic nucleus (SCN), which prompts the pineal and the adrenal glands to release the hormones that bring you in and out of the sleep cycle.

The SCN works on light-sensitive neurological signals originating in the optic nerve, and as the day starts to get dark it activates the pineal gland into production of melatonin, the hormone that promotes drowsiness. As the night progresses it will make sure that melatonin levels within the brain drop. Then when dawn breaks – the brain takes in a great deal of information about light levels through closed eyelids – production is stopped and cortisol is released from the adrenal glands. Also known as the "stress hormone", cortisol increases blood pressure and blood sugar levels and, thanks to the circadian rhythms, will be at its highest in your body early in the morning, when it serves to wake you up.

Signals from the SCN will have caused your heart rate and blood pressure to fall during the night. It will also control other aspects of the sleep/wake cycle such as appetite suppression during the night, and dropping of body temperature.

It is the disruption of a person's circadian rhythms that brings on jet lag as, for instance, somebody travelling from the UK to New York will "lose" five hours on the real clock but their body clock is still set as it was, meaning an advanced circadian cycle. Thus they will feel tired early in the evening and wake up very early in the morning for two or three days, until the circadian rhythms reset themselves.

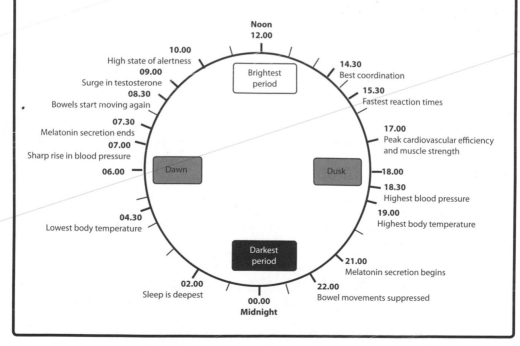

F

Fact: Over the last thirty years, the average height and weight of British men has increased significantly, yet the size of a standard bed hasn't. You may need a king- or queensize for you and your partner to get a decent night's sleep.

Passion flower

A very effective calming herb, passion flower is particularly useful if you suffer from periodic limb movement or restless leg syndrome (see p.54) as it will prevent muscle spasms. It is taken as tea.

St John's Wort

This herbal anti-depressant will improve the quality of your sleep rather than send you off, as it boosts the nervous system and calms anxiety. It is taken as tablets or capsules, but you should consult your healthcare professional before use if you are on other medication.

Camomile

Camomile tea has a thoroughly deserved reputation for calming the nerves and so aiding falling asleep, but as it also settles the stomach it will ease any indigestion that may be keeping you awake.

Reishi mushroom

Often found in Chinese cooking, this wild-looking mushroom has been used in China to combat insomnia for centuries as it lowers blood pressure and has an all-round calming effect. Taken in capsules.

Going to the mattresses

As you ought to be spending nearly one-third of your life asleep, your bed will be the most used piece of furniture in your house. Thus attention to the mattress is a must.

The most important rule when buying a bed is to buy the biggest that is practical, but what type of mattress you choose (see box opposite) will be a matter of whatever feels best. A good mattress should last between seven and ten years, and will cost from around £200 ($380) up to £700 ($1350) for a double or from £300 ($575) to £2000 ($3800) for a kingsize. That may sound like a great deal of money, but £500 ($950) for a mattress that lasts seven years puts the cost of a good night's sleep at just under twenty pence (35 cents). And that's split between you and your other half.

The smell of sleep

If you want to make use of your olfactory sense – and your other half will truly appreciate you introducing some aromatherapy to your bed – the essential oils lavender, orange blossom, spearmint, bergamot and sandalwood are renowned for their soothing, sleep-inducing properties. To help you relax before you go to bed, add a dozen or so drops of any one of them to a warm bath and soak for at least fifteen minutes – be careful not to get bath water in your eyes. Or, when you go to bed, put a couple of drops of an essential oil on your pillow.

Never put neat essential oils on your skin, but first blend them with almond or vegetable oil – fifteen drops in one fluid ounce of almond oil. Massage the oil into the back of your neck, throat and forehead.

Type	Internal construction	Properties	Expect to pay
Open-sprung	Rows of hourglass-style coil springs, each connected to those it adjoins	The most commonly used mattress, but provides the least independent support as each spring's movement affects those adjoining, meaning couples tend to roll together	Around £250 ($480) for a standard double
Pocket-sprung	Rows of hourglass-style coil springs, each self-contained in a fabric pocket	Encasing the springs allows them to move independently, meaning a sleeper's movement will have far less effect on their partner	Around £500 ($950)
Latex	High-density latex foam	Moulds to the shape of the body as it moves, to provide pressure-relieving support; will also be hypoallergenic	Around £650 ($1200)
Memory foam	NASA-developed viscoelastic	Softens in response to body heat and weight, moulding to your body shape and then holding that impression after you've shifted to allow you to settle back into it, minimizing disruption. This will provide total support while allowing natural movement. Will also be hypoallergenic	Upwards of £750 ($1350)

However, more for the sake of your back than your wallet, make sure you and whoever else will be sleeping on it try out a mattress thoroughly and at the same time before you buy. Lie down on it together in all your regular sleeping positions, maintaining each one for several minutes. You should feel comfortable and supported and not roll towards each other, and there should be no noticeable sag as you move around or just continue to lie there.

Many mattress suppliers talk about "medium firm" as being the ideal degree of support. What that means is that the mattress holds your spine in the same position it would be in if you were standing up. The lack of support in too soft a mattress means the body bends and its weight forces the spine to sag and curve unnaturally. This leads to interrupted sleep as the body is not able to

Turn it around

A mattress will last longer and provide better support if it is turned over or rotated every six months. This will stop it wearing unevenly, as it goes a long way to preventing any permanent internal contouring brought about by having the same shapes on it in essentially the same positions night after night. For sprung mattresses, alternate between rotating the mattress (spinning it so the foot becomes the head) and flipping it over (so the top face becomes the underneath). With latex and memory foam mattresses, do not flip over, merely rotate twice a year.

move or reposition itself so easily, as well as back ache upon getting up because the spine has been allowed to fall out of line, and fatigue in the muscles of the trunk because they will have been working to support you. Too hard a mattress means the only points supported are the heavier ones, and the resistance it gives to the body's weight puts too much pressure on the back as it will not be fully supported. This usually results in lower back pain and over time can lead to chronic back ache.

Measurements of mattress support are given in spring gauge and spring count for open- and pocket-sprung mattresses. The lower the spring gauge figure the stronger the springs, thus offering greater support, and the higher the count the firmer the mattress will be. Latex mattresses should be at least nine inches thick; those with a sprung core offer a more responsive support, though you will find them to be more expensive.

Sleep like a warthog

About one-third of all men habitually snore loudly enough to disturb their partner's sleep.

This figure is much higher among older or overweight men, and it compares with about twelve percent of all women.

Snoring occurs at the back of the mouth, where the soft palate, the base of the tongue, the top of the throat and the uvula come together. When you are asleep, and the muscles in the jaw and mouth are fully relaxed, it is easy for this area to collapse to some extent, partially blocking the airway and causing the tissue to vibrate as air passes over it in either direction, creating the snoring sounds. The more the inside of the back of your mouth relaxes, the more it collapses, meaning an even smaller opening and considerably louder snoring.

B

Best investment: mattress topper, £100 ($190) These have been very popular in the US for a long time, and are now starting to make headway in the UK. They are mattress-sized pads, quilted and down- or polyester-filled, that hook on to the top of the mattress, giving an extra layer underneath you. They will provide all-round extra support and, as you sink into it very slightly, give your bed an increased feeling of cosiness. A mattress topper will also extend the life of your mattress as they offer a degree of protection.

Don't buy a mattress topper online; go to a shop where you can physically handle or lie on one.

Wash or dry clean your mattress topper every time you turn your mattress.

Drinking, smoking and snoring

The two most efficient causes of heavy snoring are alcohol and tobacco enjoyed that evening. The lasting effect of a large amount of drink will be to relax the throat muscles, pretty much guaranteeing some obstruction to the airways. Smoking will greatly increase the likelihood of airway blockage as it causes both catarrh and a swelling of the inside of the throat. The chances of airway blockage will escalate in relation to the amount smoked and passive smokers will be similarly, if not quite so acutely, affected. To greatly reduce your chances of snoring, there should be a gap of at least four hours between your last alcoholic drink/smoke and going to sleep.

Mouth anatomy is a major contributing factor to snoring, with a long uvula, a long or low soft palate and enlarged tonsils or adenoids all working to narrow the airway and promote vibration. Boozing, smoking or taking drugs during the evening can have an adverse effect on the throat muscles (see box above), and the overweight are much more likely to snore loudly as layers of fat around the throat will push the sides of the airway in as the muscles relax. Nasal congestion can also cause snoring: partial obstruction will mean you have to pull harder to take in air, thus the tissues at the top of the throat are pulled closer together, increasing the likelihood of vibration. A complete blockage will mean you breathe with an open mouth,

a cause of snoring in itself. Nasal obstruction could be temporary, because of a cold, or a more permanent condition resulting from an inflamed or misaligned septum (the divide between your nostrils), in which case you should see your doctor.

Prevention, not cure

You can't really "cure" snoring, in the same way that you can, say, a sore throat, because it's caused by a set of circumstances creating a particular physical condition, that is your obstructed airway. All you can do is remove as many of the contributing circumstances as possible and work to keep the condition from occurring.

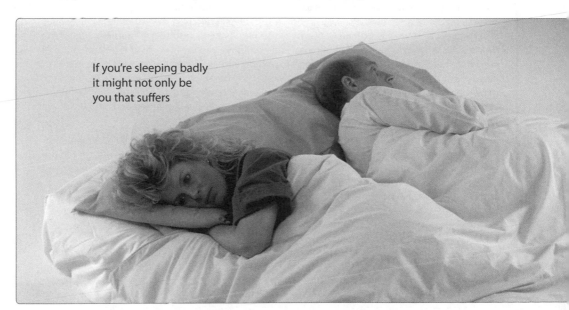

If you're sleeping badly it might not only be you that suffers

Many people snore simply because their mouth has come open as they sleep on their back, and a widespread remedy for this is to sew a tennis ball or golf ball into a pocket attached to the back of a tee shirt. The discomfort it causes when the snorer rolls on to his back makes it virtually impossible to settle, thus he will shift out of that position. Purpose-built chinstraps – or simply tying a headscarf around your chin with the knot on top of your head – will keep your mouth closed, while nasal strips are a popular option to keep the nose open.

Mandibular Advancement Devices (MADs) are gumshield-like plastic contraptions, worn at night, that fit over both sets of teeth to push the lower jaw and base of the tongue forward, creating a bigger airway opening and avoiding tissue vibration. These are softened in hot water then placed over the teeth and bitten down on to mould to a perfect fit. They are then left to harden on cooling. The upper and lower plates are hinged, and a screw adjustment is made to push the lower half up to twelve millimetres forward, holding the jaw in that position while you are asleep. These devices can cost between £50 and £100 ($95 to $190), and might not be necessary for every snorer, so seek professional advice before laying out for one.

A more drastic method is surgery, either with the knife or, as is becoming increasingly popular, with a laser. The traditional method involves a general anaesthetic and the soft palate and tissue surrounding the airway inlet being trimmed and tightened to prevent

Obstructive sleep apnoea

Obstructive sleep apnoea (OSA) is the most common form of sleep disorder, affecting five percent of men over the age of thirty, although far fewer below that age. It is an extreme result of the same conditions that lead to snoring. OSA occurs when the airway becomes completely or significantly blocked and breathing stops for a short amount of time, usually between ten and twenty seconds (the word apnoea is Greek in origin and means temporarily without breath). As the sleeper misses breaths they will reposition themselves to open the airway, which can lead to stirring out of a deep sleep phase and into shallow sleep to start the sleep cycle again. Because this can occur several times an hour, it is extremely disruptive to a night's sleep, resulting in tiredness during the day. It also sees the possibility of dangerously raised blood pressure at night as the deprivation of oxygen to the bloodstream causes the heart to pump harder. It can also have a considerable effect on your partner, as the reopening of the airway is usually heralded by a loud explosive snort, and many claim that the person lying next to them regularly stopping breathing is such an alarming situation they are unable to relax enough to get a good night's sleep themselves. The OSA sufferer, of course, has no idea he's doing it.

The OSA sufferer is very likely to be a heavy snorer and, as with snoring, the likelihood increases relative to weight gain. Although the same methods of preventing snoring can be effective in the treatment of OSA, stopping your snoring may not prevent OSA. An increasingly common remedy, especially in the US, is the fitting of a Continuous Positive Airway Pressure (CPAP) device. This is a mask worn over the nose, or nose and mouth, through the night, which is connected to an oxygen cylinder that blows pressurized air into the airway with sufficient force to keep the soft tissue from collapsing and blocking the opening. The obvious drawback with this is that many people feel unable to sleep wearing the mask, but research has shown that those who do find it very successful. CPAPs should only be recommended for people with serious OSA – incidents occurring over twelve times an hour or lasting for more than twenty seconds – and should always be bought and fitted under the advice of a sleep disorder specialist.

Allergy alert

One of the most common causes of snoring is an allergy the snorer didn't know they had. The feathers in a pillow are a very likely candidate, as is the mattress filling or house dust mites in the bedroom. Try different combinations of a new foam-filled model; the mattress with a couple more sheets; and the bedroom made dust free by hoovering on a daily basis and wiping all surfaces down with a damp cloth – not forgetting picture rails, door frames and skirting boards. Have your partner keep a snoring diary to find out what works.

vibration. Laser surgery is an outpatient procedure during which the soft palate and uvula are trimmed – this may require more than one session, as the doctor will go on shaving off tissue until the snoring stops.

A very straightforward prevention method, and one that might have an all-round beneficial effect, is a lifestyle change. Lose weight, as the more obese you are the more likely you are to snore; give up smoking, or at least cut down on the cigs; and don't go to bed half-cut.

Try and take it seriously. Please.

The thing about snoring is unless you have to sleep with a snorer, it's funny. Snoring has been a comedy staple since before movies had sound, and we seem to have been programmed from childhood to snigger at the sight and sound of somebody "sawing logs". Add to that the fact that most snorers

– quite naturally – have no idea they're doing it, and it's often difficult to get them to fully appreciate how seriously disruptive it can be to domestic life. So if your partner tells you you've got a snoring problem, take their word for it and do something about it.

Sleepwalking guy

Somnambulism is another comedy failsafe, but in real life sleepwalking is seldom as consistent or as disruptive as snoring. Most is fairly trivial, a matter of getting up and walking around for a bit – often not leaving the room – then returning to bed. Occasionally, sleepwalkers will perform complex tasks or negotiate involved journeys – it's not unheard of for sleepwalkers to be found behind the wheel of a car. Although a sleepwalker's eyes will be open they will be unseeing, and this trance-like state is actually REM sleep. This is why sleepwalking is far more common among children, as their

M

Mythbuster: waking a sleepwalker will give him a heart attack

Because sleepwalking usually occurs in the deepest phases of the sleep cycle, sleepwalkers will often start or jump quite violently (which is where this notion comes

from) and be confused or disoriented. Should you wake one, be prepared for them not to know who you are or where they are. However, it isn't by any means necessary to wake a sleepwalker, as many will get back into bed and remain unaware of their night-time excursion. You may want to gently, but firmly, guide them back into bed.

sleep cycle involves a greater proportion of deep sleep than adults'. It has never been scientifically established that sleepwalkers are acting out dreams.

Much sleepwalking in adults is stress-related, which means you are possibly already having shallower, less-restful sleep. Other major contributors are a chaotic sleep pattern or irregular sleep habits. Excessive alcohol can be a factor too, and a drunkard's disrupted sleep cycle can promote sleepwalking – a big problem with drunk sleepwalkers is urination

Common sleep disorders

Disorder	Symptoms	Causes	Self-help
Restless leg syndrome	Uncomfortable twinges within the legs, creating the urge to move them; involuntary leg movement. RLS can occur before you fall asleep	Stimulants before going to bed; smoking; very sedentary lifestyle	Stretch or massage your leg muscles; take a warm (but not too hot) bath; take regular, leg-related exercise like walking, running or cycling
Sleep paralysis	Inability to move experienced upon waking up or as you fall asleep; attacks usually last less than a minute. About fifty percent of all adults are believed to have been affected by it at some point	A momentary disconnect between the brain and the body	Although it can be frightening, sleep paralysis is harmless, but it cannot be prevented as it occurs randomly; nothing can be done about it other than to keep calm
Narcolepsy	Drowsiness or even falling asleep during the day; disrupted and non-restful night-time sleep	Science is unsure of what causes narcolepsy, but the most popular theory involves a chromosome disorder leading to a deficiency in sleep-controlling hormones	Sufferers should seek professional help, and will most likely be prescribed a stimulant to keep them awake during the day, and thus promote deeper sleep at night
Periodic limb movement	Cramping or rapid, involuntary movement of the limbs. (Not the same as restless leg syndrome, as PLM occurs only when the sufferer is asleep.)	There is primary or secondary PLM – the former occurs randomly, the latter is liable to be the result of an underlying condition – commonly diabetes or anaemia; it can also be a symptom of OSA or narcolepsy	Most primary PLM sufferers require no treatment as it is widespread and harmless; if it is a symptom of another problem, that should be treated

in inappropriate locations.

Habitual sleepwalkers (more than once or twice within a couple of weeks) should make sure they are as relaxed as possible and totally prepared for a good night's sleep before going to bed (see box on p.57). Regular sleeping schedules and patterns will help to organize your sleep cycle more effectively. You should only need to seek medical help if, after bringing in these corrective measures, the night-time excursions persist.

A

Expert advice: "Men should take a more proactive approach towards sleep and make proper time for it. Sleeping well is as important as eating well, it's not something that happens when there is nothing else to do."
Dr Liliana Risi

Dream a scary dream

Nightmares occur only during REM stage sleep and will often invoke such a state of fear, panic or anxiety within the sleeper they will usually wake him or her up. Whether the sleeper remembers all or some of what scared them so much in the dream is as likely as it is not, but they will be aware of something wrong and therefore could wake in a state of panic. While nightmares are really little more than the brain rooting out some upsetting memories, as they are being dreamed they will be very real, and should be addressed if they start to occur too often.

Nightmares are very prevalent among children, when they are considered a normal aspect of development, but in adults frequent – more than once a week – or recurring nightmares are a sign that all is not what it should be. Because you have no control over your dreams, the most immediate way to treat nightmares is to work out what is causing them and try and deal with that. The reasons behind them usually fall into one of two categories.

Inner stresses

The majority of nightmares occur around a stressful event in your life, and as that situation recedes in prominence so the

M

Mythbuster: cheese gives you nightmares

On the contrary, a small amount of cheese as a late-evening snack might actually help you sleep. As a dairy product, cheese is rich in calcium which will promote a feeling of calm. It is also a fairly good source of the amino acid tryptophan, which serves to calm the brain itself and so reduce stress levels to aid falling asleep.

The idea that eating cheese late at night

causes nightmares is thought to date back to a 1950s health scare when it was believed – but never unequivocally proved – that the tyramine (another amino acid) in cheese was reacting with a popularly prescribed anti-depressant to cause mild hallucinations, which manifested themselves as particularly vivid dreams. Or maybe it goes back even further, to the nineteenth century, when Dickens' Ebenezer Scrooge blamed his *A Christmas Carol* adventures on, among other things, "a crumb of cheese".

dreams should stop. Such an event could be bereavement, or a problem at work, or the breakdown of a relationship, but reacting with the occasional nightmare is not a sign of any acute problems. Talking to friends and family about your anxieties will help, as will any of the methods for getting a good night's sleep, as explained in this chapter.

More serious are the nightmares associated with post-traumatic stress, as the same situation can recur in a dream as the sleeper relives whatever awful events they were caught up in. This will need to be addressed with counselling and psychotherapy, therefore professional advice must be sought. Recurring nightmares can also be a result of undiagnosed depression, and if you think this might be the case, you should talk to your GP about it.

Extraneous influences

Regular heavy drinking is a prime suspect for causing frequent nightmares, as alcohol is a depressant and thus is very likely to have a negative effect on dreaming. An abrupt withdrawal from alcohol can lead to nightmares too, simply because that process results in anxiety, jumpiness, mood swings and poor sleep patterns. Suddenly giving up drugs – street drugs as well as prescription drugs – can have the same results, as it will throw the system in much the same way.

It could also be that side-effects from drugs prescribed for another condition are behind your nightmares – beta blockers, antihistamines and appetite suppressants are the most likely culprits. If your nightmares coincide with a course of prescription drugs, see your doctor immediately.

T

Tip: Anti-snoring nasal strips are useless for those of African or African-Caribbean descent.

The best of the web

sleepfoundation.org
A US site discussing all aspects of sleep and with an e-newsletter and listings of specialist sleep centres and units within hospitals.

sleepnet.com
Another US site, with a lively sleep-related forum, and comprehensive links to sleep specialists both online and in person.

britishsnoring.co.uk
The website of the British Snoring & Sleep Apnoea Association, offering instant diagnosis and help, plus a wide range of anti-snoring products and personal consultation at their Surrey HQ.

sleepdisorders.about.com
A good starting point for investigating a wide range of sleep disorders in much more depth than most websites.

sleeping.org.uk
The membership website for the British Sleep Society, a registered charity aimed at healthcare professionals and dedicated to improving their understanding of sleep-related matters.

sleepcouncil.com
A British organization seeking to raise awareness of the importance of sleep. The website has many useful tips and a link to the Insomnia Helpline (020 8994 9874).

Ten top tips for sleeping better

▶ **Keep your bedroom exclusively for sleeping. And sex, obviously** It contributes hugely to your sense of relaxation if in your mind your bedroom has no other associations than rest and sleep. And sex, obviously.

▶ **Sort out your bed** It's no wonder the most cited reason as to why a man prefers staying at his girlfriend's rather than her coming to his place is because "her bed smells so nice". Crisp, fresh bed linen, calming aromas and a general sense of sanctuary will let your body know you are serious about sleep.

▶ **Maintain your bedroom at a slightly lower temperature than the rest of the house...** Ideally, you should aim for 15–18°C (60–65°F), as your body temperature will drop, and if the room is too warm it can work against you.

▶ **...and as dark as possible** Your body is programmed to sleep when it's dark and be awake when it's light. As light can seep through the eyelids you should eliminate all light sources from the room – this includes LED clocks.

▶ **Don't watch TV in bed** If you do so until you fall asleep your brain will be overstimulated, and this will delay your dropping off and make deep sleep harder to come by. Do something relaxing like reading or listening to soothing music instead.

▶ **Don't drink just before bedtime** Although alcohol's sedative powers will relax you, it will also disrupt your sleep in a few hours' time.

and if you still can't drop off...

▶ **Keep to as regular a routine as possible** It's recommended you go to bed and wake up at the same time every day, or as near as possible, because to drastically change those hours, even over the two days of the weekend, could be enough to reset your body clock.

▶ **Avoid a large or, worse still, spicy meal within two hours of bedtime** It will bring with it the likelihood of indigestion which will play havoc with your sleep patterns, and a full stomach is likely to increase pressure on the bladder.

▶ **Take regular exercise** Being physically tired at bedtime will always help you fall asleep, but don't exercise just before turning in as the increased blood flow will make you more alert, adrenalin will still be pumping around your system and your body temperature will be much higher than is conducive to dropping off.

▶ **Stay away from late-night stimulants** This isn't just cocaine and speed or tea and coffee; nicotine too is a powerful pick-me-up. Then don't forget that chocolate contains small amounts of theobromine, a stimulant in the same chemical family as caffeine.

In the mirror

(3)

Looking good, feeling good. It's always easier to be more confident about the world in general when you like what you see in the mirror. These days, though, not only is there a great deal riding on looking young, but there is so much on offer to help you stay that way. It helps to have a head start.

The skin you're in

It was only twenty years ago that the notion of a man with a skincare regime would've led to all manner of sniggering about his sexuality. These days, although it's still far from the norm for men to cleanse and moisturize with the same enthusiasm as their female partners, an increasing number are recognizing the benefits of skincare. Which isn't really surprising. Once you realize that flawlessly fresh-faced individual looking at you out of the mirror is the same man the rest of the world sees, it can be quite a boost to your self-esteem.

Healthy on the outside starts from the inside

The best thing you can do to achieve healthy, glowing skin is to drink at least two litres of water per day. It's as simple as that.

Sufficient water intake should be the basis of all good skincare routines, as it keeps your entire system hydrated. This allows nutrients to be absorbed, helps blood to circulate, flushes out toxins and prevents constipation (see below). But most importantly, as human skin is around ninety percent water, it will make sure yours will remain at its optimum, leaving it soft and radiant-looking.

M

Mythbuster: eating chocolate gives you acne

Diet has very little effect on acne, as its causes are mostly hormonal (see opposite) and its likelihood hereditary. Although eating huge amounts of oily or greasy food can manifest itself in extra oil on your skin and hair, even this isn't enough to cause acne, so a few bars of chocolate definitely won't make a difference.

How it all works: spots

Blackheads are not caused by dirt from outside getting under the skin, but a mixture of the naturally produced oil called sebum and the protein keratin getting trapped within a hair follicle to form a blockage. This will then get its colour from skin pigment (melanin) dissolved in the oil, which rises to the surface of the blocked opening. Whiteheads are the same accumulation of sebum and keratin without the dissolved melanin, and are formed at the surface of an already closed follicle.

Spots are a side effect of being rundown or constipated, as your system will not be functioning properly or toxins are not being shipped out. Although keeping your skin cleansed and exfoliated will help keep spots at bay by removing potential pore-plugging dirt and dead skin, the prime causes of pimples come from within.

Acne is an outbreak of blackheads and whiteheads caused by the excess of sebum oil produced in the hair follicles creating blockages and eruptions under the top layer of skin. It happens in adolescent boys as during puberty a surge in the male sex hormone androgen causes the production of sebum to go into overdrive, meaning the hair follicles can't get rid of it all via their usual natural processes. The problem usually clears up in your twenties, and the chances of full-blown acne lessen as we get older, but it can be triggered by high stress levels or continued use of anabolic steroids, as in each situation the adrenal gland will increase androgen production.

Although popping a zit is one of the most satisfying of cosmetic procedures known to man, it is also one of the worst for your overall complexion. Squeezing a spot will open up the follicle and push sebum and melanin out towards the mirror, but the same action will also push a percentage of it back into the adjacent tissue, resulting in a bigger, more painful spot. Instead, release blackheads and whiteheads by gently stretching and manipulating the skin around them to create an opening big enough for the oil to flow out.

An excess of oil can build up to form a blockage at the outer layer of skin

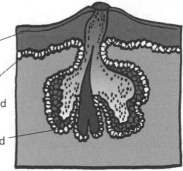

Outer layer of skin, mostly dead cells

Layer of new skin, where cells are formed

Sebum oil is produced in the hair follicle

Broadly speaking, the best diet for healthy skin is the same as it would be for overall health – cut out the junk food and excessive fat; maintain a good balance of vitamins, minerals and protein. To concentrate on healthy skin, however, vitamins C and E protect from sun damage, and thus inhibit premature ageing; vitamin A contributes particularly to keeping skin moist and also promotes quick healing; while the B vitamins

F

Fact: If you wash your face with soap, make sure it's a gentle soap recommended for the job rather than the same bar you'd wash your body with. General purpose soap is too strong for your face and will dry it out by stripping away its natural oils.

F

Fact: Constipation will show up on your face in the form of spotty or blotchy skin, as toxins usually removed through the digestive tract remain floating about in your body.

T

Tip: When shopping for an exfoliating scrub go for those with the finest grains – the more expensive brands – as they will be the most gentle. The large grains in cheaper scrubs can damage lower layers of skin and leave it feeling raw.

form the basis of skin cells and help with circulation. Iron will give you a healthy, even skin tone; omega-3 fatty acids, found in fish and some seeds, will help you regulate your skin's moisture; and fibre moves toxins, that will otherwise show up in your complexion, out through the digestive tract.

Real men exfoliate

Men's skin is about fifteen percent more oily than women's, therefore it attracts more dirt;

A

Expert advice: "Having plenty of sex can work as a bit of a beauty treatment, as it does wonders for your complexion in terms of keeping you looking younger. Because, during orgasm, you're in heightened sensitivity, there is a rush of blood, which means the blood vessels near the skin's surface are receiving more oxygen, which speeds up repairs to the cells in the skin. Research was done recently at the University of Caerphilly and over time among a thousand men and women, the ones that had sex at least three times a week looked ten years younger than those who didn't."
Sarah Hedley

men also have bigger pores than women, so the dirt gets deeper into their skin more quickly. All of which conspires to mean that men have a far greater need to do a bit more than splash on the soap and water a couple of times a day. To keep your face looking fresh, the basic and most effective step is simply to expose the healthy skin by removing what is covering it up. This has to be done sympathetically, though.

Cleanse your face on a daily basis – last thing at night is ideal – with a cleanser recommended for your skin type. You may need to experiment before you find the right one – importantly, it should be formulated for men as that means it will be a little stronger. Soak a piece of cotton wool with the cleanser and rub gently over your face, then be amazed at the amount of dirt that comes off. Getting rid of this gunk removes the smaller particles that may clog your pores, and will take off the fine layer of grime that was dulling your complexion. In the morning, wash with warm water – not too hot or it may damage your capillaries – and facial soap.

Exfoliating needs to be done once a week, and it involves rubbing your face over with a mix of a grainy scrub and water, allowing the mild abrasion to lift off the layer of dead skin cells. This is an incredibly effective procedure, as to regularly remove this complexion-clouding layer will give your face an even, flawless appearance, probably knocking a few years off your age. After you have exfoliated there is no need to cleanse.

Following either cleansing or exfoliating, always moisturize your skin to replace natural oils removed by these processes. You will need to experiment to find what moisturizer will be best for you, and how much you need to apply, but, like the cleanser, go for those formulated for male skin. Many moisturizers contain subtle bronzing agents, representing a safe way to get a suntan (see box on p.62).

Smokers' skin is a terrible thing. Would you believe he's only nineteen?

Smoker's skin and other self-inflictions

A sure-fire way for the skin on your face to look older than your years is a forty-a-day cigarette habit. Smoking activates the enzymes that break down collagen, the protein that provides elasticity to allow skin to remain taut as it moves. Without this it becomes loose and starts sagging, losing any natural glow to appear lifeless and prematurely aged.

Boozing won't help your complexion either, as the dehydrating effects of alcohol when drinking heavily will undermine the good work done by all that water you've been taking in. The result will be that your skin will dry out; it can also leave you with a permanently red face, as alcohol dilates the capillaries in the cheeks and nose to leave that angry-looking flush – a prime example being that sported by W.C. Fields. Excessive tiredness – another side effect of heavy drinking – can adversely affect your complexion, too. The skin cells repair themselves most efficiently while you sleep, and if you're not getting enough proper sleep then cell damage will start to show in the form of blotchiness and dry patches.

Ironically, although a decent tan is seen as a sign of good health, there's nothing particularly desirable about exposing your skin to intense sunlight. Ultraviolet radiation – UVA and UVB – is the main cause of premature ageing of the skin and skin

Sunbeds: a safe option?

In the UK 25 percent of all men admit to having used a sunbed at some point and, now that the dangers of ultraviolet rays have been acknowledged, responsible tanning salons will limit the length of sessions to around five minutes. However, while it is claimed that sunbeds are much less risky than open-air sunbathing, because the doses of UV rays are regulated in terms of intensity and duration, a recent BBC report maintained that frequent sunbed users were 75 percent more liable to develop skin cancer and display signs of premature ageing. These findings support the view held by the majority of dermatologists: that any extra UVA and UVB radiation is an unnecessary risk, and that people who use sunbeds still go out in the sun. To this end, the only relatively safe tan will be the one you can buy in a bottle.

cancer, because it breaks down collagen to reduce elasticity and cause wrinkles, while promoting the formation of free radicals that can cause cancer by changing the genetic make-up of the skin's cells.

Shaving

Probably the most chore-like of our morning rituals, but also probably the most important. Looking unshaven is one of the few things we can't cover up and has been voted the first thing job interviewers have noticed about a candidate. It's also reckoned to be a turn-off in the bedroom and will be a cause of growing irritation throughout the day.

The closest shave

Use each razor blade or cartridge no more than four times and throw away throwaways after one use, as they will no longer be sufficiently sharp. Rinse your face with hot water before lathering up, as this will soften your beard and make it easier to cut, but wash with cold water after shaving, as it will close your pores and move blood away from the skin surface to minimize any post-shave swelling or tenderness. Take your time, and leave the gel or cream on your face for at least two minutes before starting in with the razor, as it will take that long to fully soften your beard.

Once you get the razor going, go over your face twice, first time lightly and with the grain; second time against it and slightly firmer, but don't press so hard it feels like it's dragging. Shave by feel rather than look, as your fingertips are the best judge of whether your face is smooth or not, and don't use a razor with a lubricating strip, as

T *Tip: Shave after you've showered, as your beard will have been softened by the water and the steam in the bathroom. If the mirror is steamed up, there are products you can apply to it to keep it clear available at most pharmacies.*

T *Tip: If your aftershave stings your skin with more than a mild tingling, it is too strong for you and is irritating your skin into tiny swellings. Switch to something without either alcohol, peppermint or citrus, or, better still, use a soothing, moisturizing cream.*

To remove an ingrowing hair

Carefully release it from below the surface using fine tweezers and a magnifying mirror, then once the end is free, do not pluck it out as it will grow back under the skin. Instead leave it and shave as recommended above. Once a hair has been released, dab the area with witch hazel to treat any swelling or irritation.

it will give a false impression of what your face feels like.

Getting the bumps

Shaving or razor bumps occur when the shaved end of a hairshaft gets trapped inside a hair follicle and as it continues growing it presses up against the underside of the skin. This can cause painful "bumps" and a rash-like reddening of lighter skin. Men of African and African-Caribbean descent are far more liable to shaving bumps than Caucasians, as their hair will not grow straight, and therefore is more likely to turn inwards or sideways; also it is generally stronger, thus will push harder against the skin.

If you suffer from razor bumps, guard against them by following these steps:

Keep your skin in tip-top condition by exfoliating every day, using a soft facial brush rather than your fingers. A circular motion with the brush will remove dead skin cells, and clear away any dirt or grease blocking follicles, allowing hairs to grow beyond the skin's surface. Do not use a scrub that contains abrasive particles, though, as these can actually impede follicles. Opt for one with salicylic acid, a powerful dermabrasive.

When shaving use gel or cream with a large amount of moisturizer in it; avoid shaving foam as it tends to dry out the skin.

Moisturize after shaving, and do not use post-shave products that contain alcohol as these will close the follicles and dry the skin.

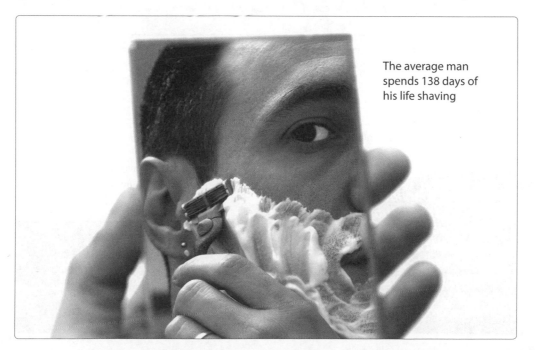

The average man spends 138 days of his life shaving

Get your hair right

Hair type	Particular problems	Remedies
Dry	Frequent breakage due to the lack of natural oils making it brittle	Change hair care regime to use milder products and less frequently; avoid blow-drying or alcohol-based treatments; use products containing vitamin B; increase essential oils in diet
Oily	Hair looks lank and wet; oil gets on clothes and skin	Wash daily with a mild shampoo; cut down on combing or brushing; reduce oil in diet (fried foods!); rinse with products that have lemon juice or vinegar bases to restore natural balance
Curly	Gets very dirty; becomes dry and brittle	Wash it daily; air dry, combing backwards with a large tooth comb; do not brush; apply a light oil daily
Fine	Looks limp; is difficult to style	Use products with a protein or vitamin B base; wash and rinse in hot water to stimulate follicles; use a heavier gel for styling
Thick	Tangles; has a hard feel to it; has a mind of its own	Wash three times a week, with a shampoo with no vitamin B or protein; pat semi-dry with towel, then apply low heat – from a distance – while brushing in the direction you want it; avoid gels or mousse as they will increase its body
African/African-Caribbean	Tendency to dryness; brittle and breaks under the stress of combing	Wash frequently; air dry, combing out gently; use products containing B vitamins; apply specialist oil daily; be prepared to work at it

Don't shave extra-close; if the hair is so short it momentarily pulls back beneath the skin after it has been cut, there is an increased chance it will get trapped. For this reason, only shave with the grain of your beard and don't stretch your skin as the razor passes over it.

Heads up

It's said that, unlike women, once men get past their twenties they settle on a haircut

T *Tip: Once your hair is thoroughly wet, rub the dollop of shampoo in between your palms and then apply them to your head – if you whack it straight on to your hair, the chances are it won't distribute evenly across your scalp.*

T *Tip: After swimming in a chlorinated pool, always wash your hair with shampoo and then rinse thoroughly before applying conditioner.*

T

Tip: Don't wash your hair while sitting in the bath because you will be rinsing it off in the dirt you've just washed out of it. This will make it very difficult to achieve any sort of shine.

T

Tip: If you have normal or oily hair and, during the summer, the sun is drying it out, treat it as dry hair for that period.

and stick with it, more or less, until either death or male pattern baldness intervenes. But whether this is true or not, most men will feel more confident about life in general if what's going on above their eyebrows is the absolute best it can be.

Hair health

Healthy hair is, essentially, a contradiction in terms, as by the time a hair shaft has poked its way above your scalp it's already dead. What sort of shape it's in, however, represents a pretty accurate reflection of your general state of health. If you are in fine fettle, taking on a good balance of vitamins and minerals and drinking the requisite two litres of water each day, your hair will display this fact to the world; but if you are run-

down or deficient in nutrients, you locks will bear witness to that too.

Of course, what you do to your hair will have a huge effect on what it looks like and how long it lasts, but it will always have a much better chance if you are healthy to start off with.

Hair dos and hair don'ts

A simple approach to hair care will always be the best. Adding gel or styling mousse will be a matter of choice, but one that should only be taken once the hair itself is in tip-top condition.

How often you should wash your hair depends on your daily routine, the environment your hair is in and how much styling product you use. It may need washing every day – if you work out daily, get filthy at work, or use a lot of styling products

Making a stink

Sweat doesn't actually smell. Body odour comes about when sweat hangs about on the skin allowing bacteria to feed on it, causing it to break down into the aromatic fatty acids which produce that unpleasant odour. The groin and armpits will be the main culprits, as the glands in those areas produce the oils and proteins the bacteria thrive on, as opposed to the rest of the body which will, largely, sweat salty water. Your feet will have their own unique ripeness because although they produce the bacteria-friendly oils and proteins, being shut away in warm, dark, unventilated socks and shoes breeds fungus that will add to the stench.

Stopping the stink is a matter of inhibiting sweat production in those areas so that the bacteria has less to feed on and regularly washing with antibacterial soap – this will not be the same soap you should be using on your face – to remove old sweat and any developing cultures. Dirty clothes are a breeding ground for bacteria, which feed on the sweat that has dried into the fabric. Feet should be dried thoroughly after washing and dusted with antifungal powder; take your socks and shoes off as often as is politely possible, to allow them to air.

F

Fact: The life of the average male hair is between three and five years, growing between one and two centimetres per month. It grows faster at night than during the day and accelerates when the weather gets warm.

T

Tip: Always keep the blow-drier moving as it is very easy to damage your hair or burn your scalp without realizing – a burnt scalp may not hurt but the hair follicles will be damaged and dried out, thus more oil will be released in that patch to compensate.

– or it may not warrant it more than once a week, but the more it gets washed the milder the shampoo you should be using. Stronger shampoos will strip the hair of its natural proteins and oils; if this is happening too regularly the hair won't regenerate these elements and will become lacklustre and brittle. Conditioning after each wash – or using a shampoo with a built-in conditioner – replaces these natural oils, and will form a protective barrier against the hair drying out or getting damaged by its environment.

When washing, pay particular attention to the hairline at the front of your head, the nape of your neck and the area just above your ears, as these areas tend to attract the most dirt yet get the least attention during shampooing. Work the shampoo in gently with your fingertips, remembering that your hair is most vulnerable when its wet, leave it for a minute or two, then rinse under clean, warm (not hot) running water. After this, rinse once more and rinse again – the most

M

Mythbusters: baldness balderdash

Hanging upside down cures it. This theory assumes that increasing the blood flow to the scalp and the hair follicles will stimulate hair growth, but there is no scientific evidence whatsoever that you will experience anything other than dizziness.

Stress makes your hair fall out. It won't, but it may make it vanish faster if you were going that way anyway. This is because of the general low physical condition you'll be in because you are are stressed.

Baldness skips a generation. This is based on the disproved idea that you inherit the baldness gene solely from your mother, who can only have got it from her father.

Masturbation as a boy will cause baldness as a man. It won't make you go blind, either.

Bald men are more intelligent. A myth perpetuated by the film and TV industry which, for a long time, has used the image of a balding, bespectacled "egghead" as visual shorthand for intellectual.

Bald men are more virile. This idea is due to the baldness gene being linked to the male sex hormone, but there is no proof of this whatsoever. However, if it's what women believe then it's little wonder slapheads aren't arguing with it.

Eat your hair healthy

Complaint	Dietary cause	Remedy
Dry hair	Lack of essential fatty acids	Oily fish; seeds – particularly flaxseeds and pumpkin seeds; olives; nuts; avocados
Greasy lank hair	Lack of vitamin B; much too much oily food	Wholegrain products; dairy; eggs; leafy green vegetables; cut down on fried food
Thinning hair	Iron deficiency; low protein levels	Red meat; liver; leafy green vegetables; wholegrain products; beans; eggs; dairy; soya products; fish
Weak, easily broken hair or split ends	Lack of silica (it promotes hair strength); low protein levels; deficiency in vitamins A, B, C, E, K	Silica is found in strawberries, rice, leafy green vegetables, onions, cucumber, celery and cabbage; protein is in dairy, milk, eggs and fish; vitamin A in carrots and broccoli; B in green vegetables and seeds; C in citrus fruits; E in avocados, whole grains and green vegetables; K in seafood, dairy, green vegetables and yoghurt

common reason for people having lifeless-looking hair is that all the shampoo, and thus all the dirt, hasn't rinsed away.

If you are only washing your hair once or twice a week, it's probably best to repeat the shampooing stage.

If you are applying conditioner, dilute it in a cup instead of putting it directly on your hair, as this will allow for a more even application and make complete rinsing out much easier. Make sure the conditioner is massaged into the ends of your hair, as that is where it will be needed most. Leave it on for four or five minutes before rinsing off with the same thoroughness as for the shampoo.

The best way to dry your hair is to allow it to air dry without you touching it but, as that is not always practical, towel dry by patting and blotting rather than rubbing. If you have to use a hot-air drier, make sure you keep it moving, keep the heat setting down as low as possible and don't use it every day.

The bald truth

Approximately 37 percent of all men will suffer male pattern baldness (MPB) of varying

Wiggy wiggy wiggy

Unless you've got the finance and the 24-hour maintenance crew to be able to sport a syrup as completely convincing as Sean Connery's in *The Hunt For Red October*, don't even think about the hairpiece as a viable option. A cheapie toupee, which means anything costing less than four figures – and you'll need two of them for when one's being cleaned – will fool nobody, and may even get you pointed at in the street. Just because nobody will actually talk about your dodgy looking wig, will not mean nobody's noticed it.

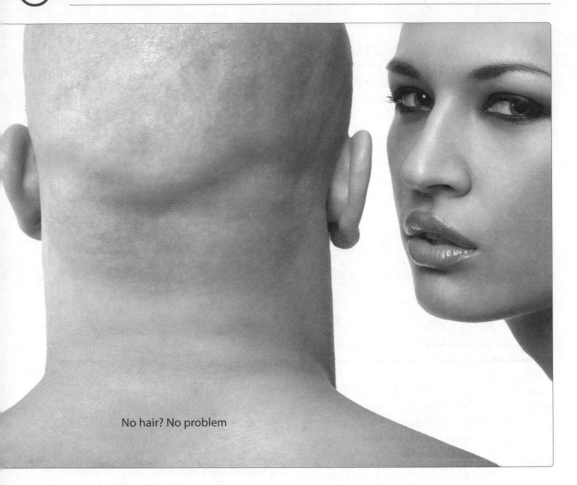

No hair? No problem

degrees – 95 percent of male hair loss is due to MPB rather than any secondary cause. It can start happening at any point beyond puberty, but the most common age range for it to kick in is between thirty and forty-five. Although it appears to be random in how it

> **T**
>
> *Tip: The best time for that initial headshave – or even a new hair cut – is Friday evening, because you'll have at least two days to get used to what you look like before you have to turn up at work with it. This will hugely help your confidence.*

causes hair loss, it will almost always start at the crown and/or the temples and progress from there, hence the term "pattern".

Will you go bald?

As seemingly arbitrary as how it affects you, is who it will affect. Every day, thanks to combing, washing and other frictions, we lose between seventy and two hundred hairs from our scalps – a fraction of the 120,000 that will be on a healthy head of hair – and baldness occurs because the hairs we lose are not being replaced. This will be due to the effects of the hormone dihydrotestosterone (DHT), a by-product of the male sex hormone testosterone. DHT attacks groups of hair follicles, leaving them alive but shrinking them to cause the production of weaker and finer hair until they become so narrow they can no longer produce hair at all.

Because MPB is hormonal you will be genetically predisposed to it, but, as yet, science has not found a way of determining who will go bald and to what degree. It was long believed that because MPB is linked to genes that are part of the X chromosome, which is handed down from your mother, baldness on your mother's father's side is a reliable indicator. However, recent research has shown there are more genes involved, some of which come from your father, meaning you could inherit it from anywhere in your family tree.

Miracle cures

Google "cures for baldness" and you'll come up with more potential, and potentially expensive, miracle cures than you could shake a stick at. For years there has been a largely unscrupulous quasi-scientific industry circling around men with receding hairlines and deep pockets, who are desperate to recapture their former glories. And the combination of Internet opportunities and today's obsession with youth and looks has made this considerably more lucrative. The truth is, because it is genetic there is no real "cure" for male pattern baldness, although there are a couple of options to slow it down a little by promoting vigorous hair growth.

Minoxidil was originally used as an oral medication to lower high blood pressure, but when a hair-growth side effect was discovered it was developed into a scalp application – it is the principal ingredient of Regaine (Rogaine

A

Expert advice: "If you want to look your best for your partner, be malleable – allow your woman to style your clothes and hair. It will leave you looking better in a way that women will appreciate – guaranteed – as so many men, even the stylish ones, dress for their mates rather than for women. Also, if you ask her, 'I'm going shopping, would you come with me and give me a bit of advice?' then follow that advice. It will let her know you are really confident and comfortable in your own skin. There are few things that are more impressive about a man than his being comfortable in his own skin. You'll make her feel better about you, it will save you a lot of shopping headaches and at the end of it you'll be dressed, according to her, the sexiest you can be. A win win win situation."
Sarah Hedley

in the US) hair treatments. Quite why it encourages hair growth is not known, but it is believed that as it dilates blood vessels so it stimulates the hair follicles. It works most effectively on the hairline at the front of your head, but any added hair growth will cease when you stop the treatment.

Traction alopecia… pull the other one!

Traction alopecia is the process by which hair follicles are killed off by having their hairs pulled at so hard that they come out with the root. It's common among those of African or African-Caribbean descent with cane row or braided hairstyles, or men with tightly stretched ponytails.

F

Fact: The scalp contains an enormous number of blood vessels, so cuts to it while shaving can bleed profusely and may take a long time to clot, so be extra careful.

T

Tip: If you're unsure about whether to shave your head or not, spend a day in a swimming cap as close to your skin colour as possible, taking frequent looks in the mirror. Obviously, this should be a day when you don't have to leave the house.

Finasteride is a drug that was developed as a treatment for prostate problems, and has been marketed as a remedy for hair loss under the brand name Propecia for about ten years. It works by inhibiting production of the enzyme that creates DHT from testosterone, therefore slowing down the damage to hair follicles and preventing further hair loss rather than initiating new growth. Once again, the effects only last as long as the treatment continues.

If Elton can do it...

Hair transplanting involves tiny pieces of hair-growing scalp being removed from a "donor site" at the back or the sides of the head, and relocated into openings cut into the bald or thinning areas. The number of hairs in each "plug" varies from ten to fifteen, down to one or two, and most transplant operations will involve a mixture of different-sized pieces. To achieve the most pleasing – and convincing – results, multiple surgery sessions will be required, with several weeks' healing between each, meaning it might take a year before you are able to appreciate the end result.

While hair transplanting has been shown to work, it has also left as many transplantees with weeping scalps, scars and mad-looking tufts of hair sprouting apparently randomly

B

Best investments: specifically designed headshaver
£10 ($12)

There are many razors and electric shavers on the market ergonomically designed to be used on the head, and with specially shaped blades. These will save you time, discomfort and the potentially humiliating experience of having to go to work with squares of tissue stuck to the cuts on your otherwise gleaming pate. The Gillette Fusion Power Stealth (right) was designed with headshaving in mind and has blades that flex to fit the contours of your skull as you apply light pressure.

Is your hair loss illness-related?

Hair loss can happen as a result of an underlying condition or a course of treatment you are taking for something. In these cases it will be more immediately noticeable as large amounts of hair will come out when you wash it or comb it, or will be appearing on your pillow or clothes' collars. If it is related to another complaint it will be accompanied by other symptoms, and the primary cause should be treated on advice from your doctor. As a rule, once the primary problem clears up so will the hair loss. If it appears to have come about as a side effect of a treatment you are undergoing, once again, take advice from your doctor.

Conditions that might cause hair loss

Thyroid and pituitary complaints
Lupus
Diabetes
Radiotherapy or chemotherapy
Anything that brings on fever and high temperatures, such as flu or viral infections
Steroid treatments
Fungal infections of the scalp
Post-surgical trauma
Iron or protein deficiency

from their heads. The starting point for anybody considering a hair transplant should be personal recommendation, or, because the skill of the surgeon is paramount, you should at least be able to see an example of his work in the flesh rather than in a photograph. After that, the rule of thumb is that you get what you pay for – which is likely to be anything between £1500 ($3000) and £6000 ($12,000). The price differs so wildly because the number of sessions can vary, as can the number of plugs transplanted.

It's not for everybody, though. Those with fine or thin hair should not consider it as an option, and you should wait until your male pattern baldness has reached its conclusion – a hairline that continues to recede after bald bits have been filled in will leave some very odd-looking gaps.

Headshaving

The huge advantage of approaching a rapidly receding hairline by shaving the rest of it off is that you will no longer be "that bloke who's losing his hair" but "that fella with the shaved head". The crucial difference being

Go grey gracefully

Grey hair is the result of a lack of melanin in the hair follicle, meaning there is no pigmentation in the new growth of hair and it will be white – grey hairs are actually white, it's simply that mixed in with coloured ones the effect is grey. Forty percent of men will have some grey hair by the time they reach their fortieth birthday, with many of them getting it well before then.

There is nothing you can do about it. No food supplements or dietary changes will reverse this process or stop it happening, so just go with it. And if you decide on a dye job then get it done professionally. DIY results are seldom very subtle.

that it now looks like your idea: you could have a luxuriant head of hair and be merely following a fashion.

Be warned, though: much as a clean pate will always look more dynamic than well-established male pattern baldness or – horror of horrors – a comb-over, it's not a look that will suit everybody. Small round heads will be best suited to this style, while pointy heads, uneven skulls or big bulges at the back are less so. However it's worth remembering your head will look enormous first time you see it without hair – everybody's does.

Strong features can be both a blessing and a curse, as while a clean head will accentuate a firm line of the jawbone or the sort of eyes that women find irresistible, a big nose or ears will look even bigger. Also, if you have the shape of face that can't wear hats, or you simply feel uncomfortable in them, it's probably not a good idea to shave your head as you will need to go hat shopping fairly quickly – in summer the sun will scorch your scalp, and in winter you will lose a huge amount of heat through your head.

Smoothing it off

It is advisable to get your first headshave done professionally. This is because people will put your freshly shaved scalp under enormous scrutiny during those first few days and the last thing you want is any nicks or cuts or patches of stubble spoiling that vista of gleaming, oiled scalp. Besides, you're about to shave all your hair off, so you've got enough to worry about at this point. Any old-school barber who does wet shaves will do it, as will the more modern practitioners who have the required electric equipment. After that, you'll need to start flying solo because you'll need to redo it every few days. Although the DIY approach isn't particularly difficult, the skin on your scalp is far more sensitive than on your face, thus shaving it requires more care and patience.

First-timers, whatever method of shaving will be used, should cut hair down to a Number One or, at most, 3mm (an eighth of an inch). Then, and each time after that you shave it, take a hot shower first, as that will soften the hair, relax the scalp and open the hair follicles as much as possible. After that, while the hair is still damp, gently massage tea tree oil into your scalp with your fingertips and follow these simple steps:

If wet shaving:

1. Apply a well-lubricated shaving gel or cream – not foam – massage in well, and allow to stand for at least five minutes.
2. Using a new blade each time, shave with light, long strokes – there will be no obvious grain to follow as, unlike your face, the hair on your head grows in many different directions.
3. Don't go over shaved patches again, as this will only irritate the scalp.
4. Change the blade immediately if you feel it's no longer cutting smoothly.
5. With a hand-held mirror go over any bits still lathered up, then check by feel that the shave is clean.
6. When attending to any still-stubbly spots, be careful not to redo any shaved bits.
7. Rinse off head with cold water.
8. Pat dry with a towel, as rubbing your freshly shaved head will scrape your scalp.
9. Gently rub over with witch hazel to close pores and treat any tiny nicks.
10. Massage scalp with a tea tree oil-based moisturizer to prevent infection and bring up a healthy sheen – tea tree moisturizer should be applied to the scalp every morning, whether you have shaved it or not.

If electric shaving:

1. Gently and lightly pass the shaver over the head in long orderly strokes – don't use the rotary rubbing technique as this will greatly aggravate or even cut your scalp.
2. Using the mirror and fingertips, check for missed patches and go over them carefully.
3. Be patient! Because you have to be more

careful, electric shaving your head will take proportionately longer than electric shaving your face, and, even including the lathering up, longer than wet shaving it.

4. Gently rub over with witch hazel to close pores and treat any nicks.

5. Massage scalp with a tea tree oil-based moisturizer to prevent infection and bring up a healthy sheen – tea tree moisturizer should be applied to the scalp every morning, whether you have shaved it or not.

As part of your routine

In each case, you'll need to shave your head at least once every three days – the best practice is to fall into the same routine as shaving your face – but make sure you follow a daily scalp care routine. It should be cleansed with cotton wool and facial cleanser every day, as without hair to cover it up it will be a magnet for airborne dirt, but never exfoliate, as that will dry it out and leave it sore.

After cleansing, apply a moisturizer, preferably containing tea tree or another natural oil, and in the summer be careful to use sunscreen. Moisturizing the scalp is particularly important for those of African or African-Caribbean descent as black skin tends to be naturally drier, and the sunscreen element should not be ignored. It is also recommended that you shampoo your scalp a couple of times a week, with a product containing tea tree or another scalp conditioner.

That gleaming smile

Everybody's teeth are different, and the natural shades can vary quite dramatically from person to person – fewer than fifty percent of us have perfectly white teeth. Add

T

> *Tip: The most reliable natural tooth whitener is a mixture of baking soda and salt, which will also kill the bacteria that causes plaque.*

Dress to impress

Suits are sexy, according to our resident sex and relationships expert Sarah Hedley. To wear a suit in a situation in which you didn't have to wear one, and to wear it in such a way that it is immediately obvious that you are dressed that way through choice and not because you've been told to, can repay enormously when it comes to impressing women. It makes you look like a) you're making a bit of effort; b) you're self-assured enough to be dressing how you want to; and c) which is the clincher, you've given careful consideration to what other people might like to look at on you.

According to Sarah, "Women have been dressing for men for years and know exactly how to get attention and exactly how much attention they are going to get by showing a particular amount of cleavage or a certain length of skirt. Guys, however, don't seem to be aware of it and, single guys especially, are more likely just to dress for themselves or so as not to stand out from their mates. That's why when a guy wears a suit in a situation where others might not, it looks like he is dressing because he understands how it's going to work for him and that's pretty impressive.

"That said though, it's got to be the right suit, not one that says 'I work in a bank so my mum bought me this suit' and it has to fit properly because that will mean you'll be much more relaxed in it."

to this the degree of staining that can occur from smoking or black coffee, red wine and tea, and the reality is that our teeth get more discoloured with age, and it's no wonder keeping them pearly white requires effort beyond brushing twice a day.

Whitening or smokers' toothpastes can be effective, and there are two main types: abrasives and bleaches. The former contains tiny abrasive particles that will destain your teeth by friction, and are not recommended for older men as this action will also wear away tooth enamel that will be naturally

T

Tip: If you get a tooth knocked clean out, wrap it in plastic to keep it as hygienic as possible and take it, immediately, to an emergency dental hospital. It may be possible to put it back in.

thinner. Toothpastes containing peroxide are reliable tooth whiteners, but to be effective the active ingredient needs to be in contact with the surface of the tooth for an extended period, thus at least five minutes brushing each session is required. Even then it will take several weeks of daily brushing for either type of toothpaste to show significant results.

Professional bleaching is probably the best way to remove stains from your teeth, and most dentists will carry it out. The gums and soft tissue will be protected by gel or a rubber shield, and hydrogen peroxide will be applied to the teeth by encasing them in a custom-fitted, gumshield-like device that is filled with the chemical. Your dentist will fit the mouth pieces, and conduct the first couple of sessions – the teeth need to stay in the solution for between thirty minutes and an hour – then you will carry on at home for two or three sessions a week for about a month. There are several home tooth-bleaching kits

Don't get tucked up for a nip and a tuck

How much it will cost will vary enormously from surgeon to surgeon, and even the same procedure can cost different amounts for different people, as each will involve a unique amount of work. However, ball park figures for the more popular operations are:

Rhinoplasty (nose job) £2000 (In the US $4000)

Liposuction £1500 ($3000)

Ear surgery £2000 ($4000)

Botox £170 ($340)

Facelift £4000 ($8000)

Pectoral implants £2000 ($4000)

on the market, but it is always advisable to get it started by a dentist.

Laser whitening, or power whitening, is a much quicker procedure and can be finished in the same day. Your dentist will fit a protective rubber shield around your gums and then brush a chemical solution on to your teeth that will be activated by firing a laser on it. This treatment can turn teeth several shades lighter in under an hour, but not everybody's teeth will be strong enough to withstand it and your dentist should advise you on that.

Home bleaching kits cost around £50 ($100), professional bleaching will be upwards of £500 ($1000) for your whole mouth, while for laser whitening expect to pay at least £700 ($1400) per session.

F

Fact: Lemon juice is an effective natural tooth whitener, but it will also destroy your teeth by dissolving the enamel, and neutralizing the calcium needed to rebuild it.

Cosmetic surgery for beginners

With society's emphasis being so far skewed towards youth, and constraints on time

You're going to put what *where*?

When you go for your first consultation with a cosmetic surgeon make sure you ask the following:

What *exactly* does the procedure involve?

What are the risks?

Will the results impede my life in any way?

What should I do to make sure everything goes as smoothly as possible?

What is the recovery time?

What steps will be taken if something goes wrong?

making quick fixes increasingly desirable, it's no surprise that more and more men are undergoing cosmetic surgery procedures. In the US it's a multi-billion dollar industry – in 2006 twenty percent of all nose jobs and fifteen percent of all liposuction was performed on men – while in the UK the number of men opting to go under the knife has risen by three hundred percent over the last five years. And as techniques get ever more sophisticated, so the range of procedures on offer gets ever wider. As well as the long-established nose jobs and botox injections, popular ops now include pectoral and buttock implants to become instantly ripped, cheekbone augmentation and jawline reshaping for that full-on chiselled look and penis enlargement for obvious reasons. Should you be one of the millions of men apparently thinking about getting a nip or a tuck or a bit put in, there are certain aspects you should first consider.

Before you take even the first step towards the scalpel, think long and hard about why you want this particular operation. It's very dangerous to assume that instantly altering your appearance will solve your problems or improve your life just as quickly. Difficulties you had in life pre-surgery will still be there post-op. After you've thought that one through, choose a surgeon that is registered either with (in the UK) the General Medical Council's Specialist Register of Plastic Surgeons, or (in the US) the American Society of Plastic Surgeons, and even then it's ideal to go on personal recommendation, from somebody whose results you can inspect.

Once you meet your surgeon, he or she should be able to use digital technology to show you what you will look like after the procedure. They should also never try to talk you into anything you're not sure about. Don't commit yourself to anything too hastily, as there are plenty out there to choose from.

The best of the web

dentalhealth.org.uk (UK)
The British Dental Health Foundation, offering advice about all things dental, including tooth whitening.

naaf.org
The website for the National Alopecia Areata Foundation, which offers support and practical advice as it seeks to raise awareness about the hair loss conditions.

grooming-health.com
A comprehensive male grooming site, offering tips, advice and questions answered service, and up-to-the-minute product reviews.

dh.gov.uk/en/Publichealth/CosmeticSurgery/index
The Department of Health's website has the most comprehensive advice and information section for those considering cosmetic surgery.

headshave.baldlygo.com
Virtual headshaving online. Check out what several celebrities might look like with clean heads, then post your own picture and try it out for yourself.

Ten top tips for looking better

▶ **Don't even think about a comb-over** The only way you'll get away with it is if you have the same size bank account as Donald Trump. And even that won't stop people sniggering behind their hands.

▶ **Drink more water** Your skin is ninety percent water, thus keeping well hydrated will keep it looking fresh.

▶ **When towel-drying your hair pat and blot only** It is very fragile when it is wet and rubbing it will cause excessive breakage.

▶ **Go easy on the smoking and drinking and whatever** Why people who burn the candle at both ends tend to look the part is because it dries your skin out – seen Keith Richards lately?

▶ **Invest in an ergonomically designed razor** If you are going to shave your head, it will save a great deal of general grief.

▶ **Don't wash your face with regular soap** It will dry out your skin's natural oils. Use specially formulated facial soap or face wash.

▶ **Never clean your teeth with lemon juice** It may get them white, but it will also strip them of their enamel.

▶ **After every dip in a chlorinated swimming pool,** you should shampoo your hair and rinse off thoroughly, as lingering pool chemicals will dry out your hair.

▶ **Never squeeze a spot** This could push the excess oil back under your skin. Stretch and manipulate the skin around it to release the oil.

▶ **Buy your own skincare products** Men's brands will be specially formulated for male skin and the chances are hers won't be strong enough for you.

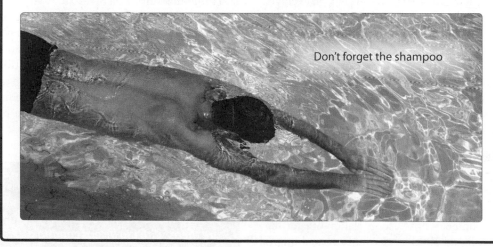

Don't forget the shampoo

In the middle

The old spare tyre ... a bit of a pot ... the beer gut ... love handles ... all coy euphemisms that give the impression men have an almost affectionate relationship with the activity of putting on weight. Or maybe it's a grimly ironic acceptance of what seems to be something of a default setting these days, as huge portions of bad food and less day-to-day exercise (as discussed elsewhere) conspire to pile on the pounds. However, in order to do something permanent about putting it on – or keeping it off – you'll need to understand exactly what fat is and how much damage it can do to you.

Apples and pears

You won't just get up one morning, look down and not be able to see your feet – it's a far more insidious process than that. Due to the decreasing speed of their metabolism, if men carried on eating and exercising at exactly the same levels from their twenties into their fifties, they would gain, on average, nearly two kilograms of fat a year.

Of course, genetic differences mean this is far from an exact science, and there is no way of predicting who would put on how much weight. What is pretty much a certainty is that you will put it on around your waist in the form of a big belly.

Belly belly bad

As a man, you will be naturally predisposed to putting centimetres on the waistline as the years roll by. This contrasts with the situation for women, whose accumulation of later-life fat will pad out the hips, buttocks and thighs before it starts to settle on the belly.

Science is baffled as to why you will

be apple-shaped whereas she will be pear-shaped, but one thing doctors are sure about is that your belly fat will be very bad news. If left to its own devices, there's a very good chance your belly will turn round and murder you.

Surrendering to a "middle-aged spread" is one of the worst things you can do. Belly fat is the most unabashedly toxic type of fat there is, and piling on the pounds around your waist will threaten your coronary health to a far greater degree than a big backside. Also, by virtue of where you're carrying this heavy weight, your belly can affect several other aspects of your physical well-being such as your energy levels and the state of your back.

F

Fact: The vast majority of young male gym goers see a "ripped" six-pack as the foremost reason they are there, with big biceps coming a pretty close second.

78

How it all works: putting on and shedding fat

Body fat is excess muscle fuel – fat or carbohydrate – stored in fat cells, also known as adipose cells, to make sure we have a reserve of energy if times get hard. An adult man will have between seventy and two hundred million fat cells, which expand in size rather than increase in number to accommodate extra fat, and are located either just below the skin (subcutaneous fat) or within the abdominal cavity (visceral fat). A certain degree of fat is vital to our systems, with up to sixteen percent of the body's weight being healthy for men, and around twenty percent for women.

Carbohydrate digested in stomach

↓

Sent to liver in bloodstream

↓

Processed into glucose

↘

Sent to muscles for fuel, via bloodstream

↘

Any surplus is stored in adipose tissue as

Our bodies move when fat, glucose or glycogen are delivered to the muscles through the bloodstream, where it is combined with the oxygen, also arriving via the bloodstream, to form adenosine triphosphate, or ATP, the energy that powers the muscle cells.

Inevitably, taking on board more fuel than is being used causes an excess, which the body puts into storage as fat. When a large number of calories have been consumed, the fat cells produce enzymes that capture any unburned fatty acids and glucose, drawing it into the cells where it will be converted to fat and kept as a fuel reserve. Hence an inactive overeater puts on weight. However, increased activity or a low-calorie eating plan causes a loss of fat because, as more energy is required than has been consumed, the body draws on these loaded cells and breaks the stored fat down into glycerol and fatty acid – the same components the digestive system reduces the fat we eat to – which allows it to be released into the bloodstream. Once there, the fatty acid goes directly to the muscles to be turned into ATP, while the glycerol is taken to the liver to be stored and converted into glycogen for future fuel.

Unsurprisingly, the quickest way to accumulate fat is to eat a great deal of food that is high in fat. This is because glucose burns far more efficiently in the muscles than fat, and is thus the body's fuel of choice, while the fat cells can process fatty acids into fat almost ten times as easily – it takes 23 calories of internal energy to convert a hundred calories of glucose into fat for storage, but only 2.5 to convert the same amount of fat.

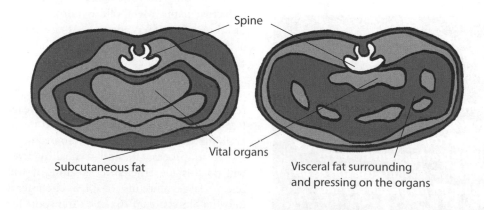

Spine

Subcutaneous fat

Vital organs

Visceral fat surrounding and pressing on the organs

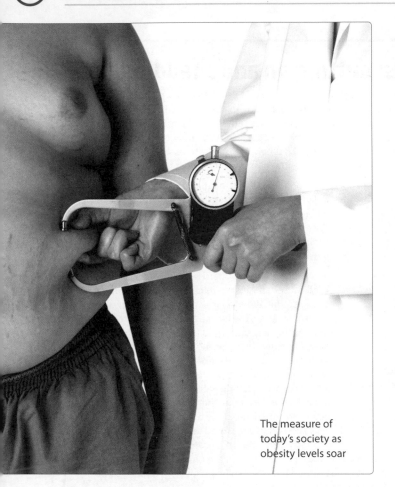

The measure of today's society as obesity levels soar

(it sits on the surface just below the skin or within the muscles). Although you need a degree of visceral fat to surround and protect your organs, it shouldn't be so much that it starts to show in the form of a belly. It will pack tightly around the vital organs – it is far denser than subcutaneous fat – and attack your heart by playing havoc with your insulin control mechanisms, thus sending your cholesterol levels soaring. This is why, historically, men are more susceptible to heart disease than women, and anybody with a higher than thirty percent concentration of visceral fat is a prime candidate for type 2 diabetes, strokes, heart disease and high blood pressure. They will be much more at risk than the unfit or those with all-over fat.

The fat going on your waist will have a high concentration of visceral (or intra-abdominal) fat, whereas fat being accumulated elsewhere will be subcutaneous

T

Tip: Eat less more often as, ideally, your digestive system should be given five smaller meals a day to deal with rather than three large ones. If you can do that you increase the chances of everything you've eaten being utilized rather than stored as fat. However, don't use this as an excuse for perpetual grazing.

Metabolic mayhem

There are so many adverse conditions occurring in the body as a result of excess belly fat that they have been given the collective name Metabolic Syndrome – or Insulin Resistance Syndrome. At the centre of these conditions is the system's inability to efficiently metabolize visceral fat.

Primarily, visceral fat affects the liver, which is responsible for regulating the release of cholesterol into the bloodstream (see box on p.23). When there is too much fat in the system the liver goes into overdrive trying to process it, and a healthy liver will do this *too* efficiently, meaning it will release large amounts of LDL cholesterol into the bloodstream to act as transport for the fat cells. The increased amount of LDL cholesterol creates waxy deposits, known as plaques, that attach themselves to the artery walls to narrow and eventually block them. There will also be too much glycerol being taken into the liver for processing into glucose.

Eventually, the liver becomes overworked and functions far less efficiently. When that happens the fat starts to build up in it, swelling the organ and causing a condition known as non-alcoholic fatty liver disease. This, in extreme forms, can be a precursor to cirrhosis.

Visceral fat also releases a chemical known as angiotensinogen, which combines

F

Fact: Visceral fat causes so many problems within the body and has such a proactive effect on the vital organs it surrounds that scientists are starting to view it as an organ in its own right, rather than a digestive by-product.

with renin, by itself a harmless secretion from the kidneys, to cause the narrowing of blood vessels. The fatty acids produced

Seven habits of highly overweight people

Food shopping when hungry
You are guaranteed to buy more than you need, then will be obliged to eat it. Incidentally, the same rules apply if you've had a couple of lunchtime drinks before heading towards the supermarket.

Being bored in proximity to convenience food
Hanging about at airports, waiting for colleagues in coffee shops, watching mindless television, stopping at a motorway service station on a long drive… all these are situations that will drive you to reach for the snacks or sandwiches, whether you're hungry or not. Keep a healthy alternative to hand.

Not eating breakfast
After eight hours' sleep you need to fuel up almost as soon as you get up, and to skip breakfast will trick your body into starvation mode, meaning it hordes reserve calories as body fat, plus late morning hunger will find you snacking before lunch.

Drinking too much
This isn't just beer or wine, but giant fizzy drinks or orange juice or tea and coffee with sugar. Opt for cold water.

Not getting enough sleep
Sleep deprivation means a reduction in cortisol secretion, the hormone that controls your appetite, and that can end up with you experiencing increased fat storage.

Not planning meals in advance
Too often this results in grabbing whatever is to hand and easy to prepare, which usually means fast food or convenience food. Spend some time at the weekend sorting out what you're going to eat during the days ahead.

I've started so I'll finish
It is deeply ingrained in so many of us to finish what is on our plates – the problem is it's liable to be a great deal more than it used to be. Too much, in fact. Leave some behind.

Body Mass Index

A widely used method of determining how fit or fat you are is the Body Mass Index, or BMI. It is a 150-year-old calculation designed to assess how overweight a person might be relative to their height, and display the result as a single figure.

To calculate your BMI divide your weight in kilograms by the square of your height, as measured in metres, then apply the resultant figure to the chart below. But do so with a healthy-sized pinch of salt: the Body Mass Index may be the definition of choice when it comes to formalizing the current obesity crisis but it is a notoriously rudimentary system and doesn't make any allowances for race, gender, age or muscle mass.

Body Mass Index	Weight status
Below 17	Possible malnutrition
17.1–18.5	Underweight
18.6–25	Normal
25.1–30	Overweight
30.1–40	Obese
Over 40	Morbidly obese

BMI Calculator $\dfrac{\text{Weight (kg)}}{\text{Height (m) x Height (m)}}$

Or, if you prefer, click on **nhlbisupport.com/bmi**, feed your figures in and let the online calculator do the hard work.

A

Expert advice: "Keeping your weight down is a whole lifestyle approach, so you can't eat what you like and then come down to the gym and assume a good workout every once in a while is going to take care of it. To get fit and stay fit and make sure your body's operating at full capacity you have to have a combined exercise and diet programme. The two go hand in hand."
Gideon Remfry

by the belly fat also release molecules that adhere to and roughen the interior artery walls, making it easier for the plaques to take hold. All of this conspires to vastly increase your chances of high blood pressure, strokes or cardiovascular disease.

A big, hard belly will raise the likelihood of type 2 diabetes as well. The presence of visceral fat will create a condition in the system known as insulin resistance, in which the body's cells no longer respond to insulin as a regulator of blood sugar levels. With glucose levels running unchecked in the bloodstream the pancreas ramps up insulin production to try to clear things out and that serves to make things worse as the body's metabolic balance is further tilted off centre. Such a state of affairs is a fairly certain precursor to diabetes.

M

Mythbuster: the ladies love the love handles

In a survey of women carried out by an American dating website, in the "He should have" checklist a flat stomach was the third most important factor when it came to first impressions of a man – after well-cared-for hair and good teeth, but slightly ahead of clean shoes. However, a big belly also came second in the "Instant turn-off" category, just behind being badly dressed. With the men in the same survey, "Lose some weight" was far and away the top answer to "How would you want to change your appearance?"

Likely lads

Genetics plays a huge role in how you will accumulate fat, but there are several environmental causes that are entirely within your realm to control. Saturated fats are a major contributor to visceral fat, so men with diets high in animal fats or dairy should change their ways. Excessive alcohol consumption is another trigger – hence the "beer belly" notion – and will damage the liver and further contribute to its malfunctioning. Interestingly, though, there has been some recent research to suggest that moderate drinking – a glass of wine a night, say – will actually work to prevent visceral fat. Smokers, too, have a much higher chance of developing a big belly – a recent study in Japan showed men who smoked accumulated visceral fat at a much higher rate than non-smokers, although scientists have yet to fully understand why.

The other prime candidates are the perpetually stressed. Although it's frequently assumed that stressed people burn off fat

T

Tip: Be careful with the sauces and dressings, especially the mayonnaise-based concoctions, as they can contain massive amounts of fat and sugar.

You should be worried about the killer in front of you if…

You have a waist measurement of more than 100 cms or 39 inches Measure your waist by standing up straight, lifting your clothes and running the tape around your body halfway between your hip bone and lowest rib; keep the tape level all the way around and don't let it cut into your flesh.

Your belly is hard Because visceral fat accumulates so densely within the abdominal cavity, so many big bellies will feel hard when other fat areas on the same body are wobbly. To assess what sort of fat you are carrying in front of you try to shake your belly to see if it flops about; if it stays still you have a high proportion of visceral fat.

You get more than thirty percent of your calorific intake from saturated fats (dairy, meat, eggs) or trans fats (hydrogenated fats found in processed foods, commercial fried food, hard margarine). These fats are far more likely to manifest themselves in the body as visceral fat than the unsaturated varieties are.

Fat sex probably isn't the best sex

That extra poundage could seriously affect your sexual performance. The obese are twice as likely to suffer from erectile dysfunction because the blood supply needed to inflate the spongy tissue in the penis is impeded by narrower arteries and blood vessels, plus there's the fact that the blood has further to travel.

with nervous energy, belly fat actually occurs as the direct result of stress. When you are under strain a hormone called cortisol is produced by the adrenal gland and released into the system to raise blood pressure and blood sugar. Research at Yale University has shown that sustained high levels of cortisol in men of all ages and older women promote the accumulation of fat around the belly. And the test subjects' girths went up in direct relation – the greater the stress, the more cortisol produced, the more visceral fat, the bigger the belly.

Don't think this doesn't apply to you

It is possible to be of slim build, with no visible signs of a belly, but still have a dangerous level of visceral fat in your body, because it's all about percentages. Between ten and fifteen percent of visceral fat (as a percentage of you total body fat) is fine and normal; if it is approaching thirty percent you are heading for trouble, and if it is over that, do something about it right now.

On the other hand, it's possible to be vastly overweight but with pretty healthy visceral/subcutaneous fat ratios – recently in Japan, a team of Sumo wrestlers were tested for fat make-up and were found, in spite of their size, to have lower levels of visceral fat and blood cholesterol than apparently healthy non-athletes. This endorses the theory that exercise keeps visceral levels low.

Or are you just fat?

The type of fat that most of us have, and quite a few of us have too much of, is subcutaneous fat, the soft, loose, expandable

F

Fact: An average-sized and averagely active man with 25 percent body fat, is storing approximately enough energy to last him a month.

Doctor, doctor...

Any of the warning signs in the box on page 83 ought to be enough to convince you to do something about your belly; however the only accurate measurement of how much visceral fat you have in your belly is with a CAT scan. To get one of these you will have to visit your doctor, but it is highly unlikely he or she will send you for a test as pricey as that. What they are certain to do, though, is measure your waist, then your blood sugar, blood pressure and blood cholesterol and talk to you about your lifestyle, to ascertain how much of a risk you are running.

Fat planet

The percentage of adults who are obese in the following countries:

United States: 33 percent

Australia: 23 percent

United Kingdom: 22 percent

Germany: 13 percent

France: 12 percent

Japan: 3 percent

Source: World Health Organization

layer of connective tissue – known as adipose tissue – that exists just below the skin. On men it is far more likely to be on their upper body, whereas women tend to accumulate it lower down.

Subcutaneous fat forms a protective layer that exists to cushion and insulate the body, and is where excess nutrients are stored to provide energy in lean times. The reason the body converts excess carbohydrate to fat is because it represents a far more compact way of storing it, as fat contains very little water, and in terms of providing energy per gram, it takes up less than half the space of carbohydrate or protein. However, the problem lies with the fat that isn't being burned and is fuelling little other than the present obesity crisis.

This is the kind of low level, casual fat that has crept up on such a large percentage of the population, and although it isn't necessarily the stone killer visceral fat might be, at worst it will contribute to all of the same problems and at best it's not a particularly good look. Then there are the difficulties its sheer physical volume can cause. Every extra 10kg (22lb) of body fat a man puts on will require an added 29km (18 miles) of blood vessels to serve the extra tissue, yet he will only have the same-sized heart to pump blood through them. This puts a considerable strain on your ticker.

Also, when you do anything in the upright position, the extra weight will have to be supported by your hips, knees and

A

Expert advice: "There has to be a happy medium, and the rule of thumb is eighty/twenty: if you have good food going into your body eighty percent of the time then you'll be able to handle twenty percent of your diet being not so healthy with very few ill effects."
Gideon Remfry

F Fact: A recent survey in the UK business magazine Personnel Today showed that, if the choice came down to two equally qualified candidates, a staggering 93 percent of HR executives would opt against the fat candidate purely on the basis of size.

F Fact: A tiny amount of body fat can make quite a difference: if you had a 1mm covering of subcutaneous fat you would start to feel cold at a temperature of 13°C (55.5°F); if you had a 2mm layer, you wouldn't start shivering until it got down to 12°C (53.5°F).

ankles, creating a great deal of cumulative wear and tear on your joints. Carrying all that unnecessary poundage also increases the amount of effort you'll have to put in to perform just about any regular task, which is why overweight people are so frequently out of breath. Then it will affect how you sleep – see Chapter 2. Once you start getting jowly, the airway in your throat becomes restricted, leading to the snoring and apnoea that will disrupt your sleep patterns and so contribute to a lower feeling of general well-being.

The runaway weight train

One of the biggest reasons for doing whatever it takes to avoid piling on the pounds is that the weight you're starting to accumulate will very quickly assume a momentum that will become progressively difficult to stop. This is why it's such a relatively short step from overweight to obese, and the causes of this unhealthy spiral can be psychological as well as physiological.

Top of the list is a vicious circle of inertia. Although an overweight person will use more energy performing exactly the same action as a less-heavy individual, the chances are the former will perform far fewer movements. This can be as a result of the physical problems resulting from weight gain – stressed joints, breathlessness, tiredness and so on – restricting movement, or simply because the brain is subconsciously aware of the extra effort involved and so will demand as little movement as possible. Either way, it means less exercise of any kind, thus fewer calories burned off, and this state of affairs will spiral as your weight goes up.

Society's attitude towards the overweight doesn't help either. Many in the UK feel it is the unseen "ism" that doesn't get the acknowledgement given to, say, racism or sexism, yet can lead to widespread discrimination and such psychological problems as low self-esteem, anxiety and

Calories counted

A calorie is the unit of measurement for the energy needed to raise the temperature of one gram of water by ten degrees Celsius. A kilo calorie (kcal or C) is equivalent to 1000 calories. This is what's used on packaging to denote the amount of energy provided by a particular food.

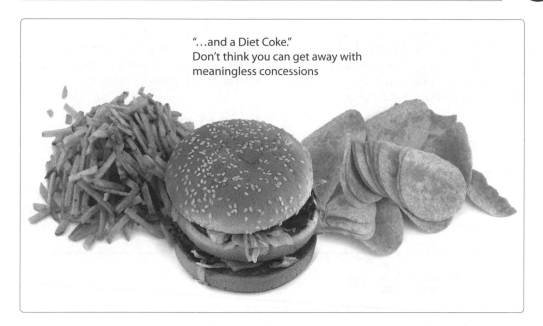

"…and a Diet Coke."
Don't think you can get away with
meaningless concessions

even depression. This in turn ramps up a weight gain cycle by precipitating such fat–friendly situations as increased alcohol intake, comfort eating, binge eating and reduced physical activity.

Then there's the possibility that dieting itself will contribute to continuing weight gain. Many weight-loss eating plans are simply too drastic, and the system's reaction to a sudden and sustained fall in calorific intake is one of metabolic panic – assuming starvation is imminent, the body starts storing fat to cope with this and so weight actually goes up. This can prompt the "diets just don't work for me" syndrome, which won't do any dieter's motivation much good

and can set off the psychological problems discussed above.

"Yo-yo" dieting, periodic crash dieting alternated with unhealthy or binge eating can be a problem too, as the reaction to the confusion caused within the metabolism is

T

Tip: Taking the skin off a piece of chicken before you cook it will reduce the fat content by over 75 percent. Even if your chosen method of cooking is frying.

Check your calorie intake

It's very easy to take on far more calories than you need without actually realizing it – an averagely active man will need about 2800 kcal per day, compared with a woman's 2000 or a pre-adolescent child's 1750. Now consider that the average slice of pizza contains around 300 calories, a pint of lager around 200, a quarter pounder with cheese 500, a tuna baguette with mayo 530, a bag of crisps 175 and a 100g bar of Cadbury's Dairy Milk chocolate 530. There are many interactive calorie counter websites that will allow you to calculate what it is you're taking on board and how you might need to address it.

one of playing it safe, which means storing fat. In this case, the dieting often becomes more extreme to achieve the same results, which can lead to health problems beyond those associated with weight gain.

A pain in the back

Having to carry that belly out in front of you all the time can do more than simply wear you out. It can affect your spine, alter your posture and become the major factor in the chronic lower back pain that affects so many men as they approach middle age.

Spinal trap

A healthy human spine has three gentle curves running along its length, which provide the strength and resilience needed to keep us upright, and enable the body to have a correctly balanced centre of gravity. The spine is made up of 33 connected

Spoilt by choice

As a society we're so far developed that we've got to a point that what's on offer has evolved way beyond what's necessary for survival. And faced with such a selection, we are far too often choosing beyond our needs.

Dr Sarah Schenker explains, "In the twenty-first century, we've got greater spending power, there's greater availability of foods and we have greater choice, but it's far more multifactoral than that. There's the way society is now: we're eating on the run, we're eating alone, we're substituting different meals for different times in order to fit them in with our lives, and how much time people spend out of the home eating their meals is important – younger people, especially young men, are probably eating the majority of their meals away from the home, except at weekends.

"All of this has led to the breakdown of the traditional three meals a day, and that is a very big change in how we eat because of the choices it puts in front of people. Before, when there was much less choice, we ate fairly instinctively. Now with anything you like on offer, faced with the choice of an apple or a bag of crisps or a bar of chocolate, most people will go for the crisps or chocolate because they're much more available and they taste nicer.

"When there was only a limited choice of local produce, or food that was in season, or you had to assemble, prepare and cook the food yourself, there was a far greater chance you would go for something like fish or chicken or something nutritious. Largely because that was what was there, and there wasn't any particular convenience factor to be considered because you were going to have to cook it yourself anyway – you simply made time in your day. Now, although those choices are still available, you're also faced with the choice that means you have everything done for you and you can eat anything at any time, anywhere. While it's not necessarily human nature to choose what's bad for you, it becomes very difficult to avoid what is convenient and being presented to you so attractively. Immediate gratification is very hard to fight.

"Also, the move away from previous traditional meal times has meant nobody is hungry any more – or not hungry in the traditional sense, just slightly unsatisfied. When people were sitting down to three meals a day, they hadn't eaten for maybe six hours so they were ready for a nutritious meal – a large meal. Their bodies wanted it and would be letting them know, because that's what hunger is, your body telling you it's low on nutrients. People graze all day long now, so they're seldom hungry enough to want a proper meal, and to make it worse they're not grazing on particularly nutritious food, because the choice of grazing food these days is immense and very attractively presented. You could eat cakes all day long."

T

Tip: Eat more slowly and you'll eat less. It takes the brain approximately twenty minutes from when you started eating to register if your stomach is full, and because, these days, we tend to eat much faster often we pass the point of being full without realizing it and continue, eating too much.

resting. This lower segment of the spine will be principally supported by the core muscles of the abdomen and the lower back, in combination with those around the hips, buttocks and pelvic area. It's in this area that lower back pain occurs, and because a large belly can radically affect its delicate balance any man carrying that sort of load will greatly increase his chances of persistent lower back pain.

It's why fat guys waddle

Gaining a large, solid belly will alter your posture, which will contribute to more than just lower back pain. Having to support that excess weight just in front of your lumbar vertebrae will start to pull them forward, extending the natural curve of the spine

vertebrae, 24 of which are moveable, to provide the necessary flexibility. They are divided into three groups: cervical, the top seven, which support the head; thoracic, the next twelve down, to which the ribs are connected; and the lumbar, the five largest and lowest of the flexible vertebrae, which bear most of the weight of the trunk. The remaining nine vertebrae are the pelvic vertebrae, which are fused together into two groups – the sacrum, the five directly below the lumbar, and the coccyx, the four at the base of the spine.

The lumbar section of the spine is absolutely crucial to maintaining your comfort as it effectively holds up everything above the hips, distributing the load while you are either active or

How many sugars?

Added sugar in the modern diet is one of the most dangerous sources of empty calories, as they often lurk under confusing pseudonyms, and are far more prevalent than you might imagine and will play merry hell with your blood glucose levels, hence the type 2 diabetes problem.

The most popular aliases for added sugar are:
Dextrose, fructose, glucose, corn syrup, lactose, maltose, sucrose, high-fructose corn syrup, molasses, fruit juice concentrate, malt syrup and corn sweetener.

You are most likely to find the highest proportion of added sugar in:
Soft drinks (not diet soft drinks), cakes, biscuits, commercial fruit juice, fruit squash, dairy-based desserts including some yoghurts, bread and other baked goods.

which, in turn, will cause the pelvis to tilt too far forward. This means the legs have to move out from under the hips as you walk, kicking forward and spending a much greater part of the stride cycle in front of the body than is natural. Hence the waddle, which will add to the strain on the knees, which are already supporting excess poundage.

In this situation, the chances are that the muscles around the pelvis, buttocks and lower back are not well developed – likely a result of a lack of exercise – and therefore cannot provide extra support. This altered posture means the head has to adjust itself to stay level, and the pulling forward involved will put extra strain on the neck and the shoulders.

Within the lower back itself, the distortion of the vertebrae puts enormous strain on the discs – these are the spongy slices of tissue that allow the vertebrae to move against each other in comfort. Once the spine starts to be pulled out of line like this, the discs themselves can become damaged. These discs, and the out-of-position spine, can also create pressure on nerves leading from the spinal column. Any of these situations will lead to sharp lower back pains or even sciatica.

Dragging you down

The extra weight also puts added stress on the ligaments and tendons surrounding the spine – this can result in painful tears and strains, which may cause the surrounding muscle to spasm, producing powerful pain waves. This occurs because the core muscles that surround the spine have a duty to protect it, and when a joint or ligament is stressed the

T

Tip: Don't feel obliged to finish what's on your plate – in spite of what your mum taught you! Over the last decade the size of portions in restaurants and takeaways has risen dramatically, meaning it's very easy to overeat without being aware of it.

A

Expert advice: "The fruit and veg message is so strong because it works – people who are eating the five fruit and vegetables a day are healthier, are less likely to be obese and have less illness: that is well documented."
Dr Sarah Schenker

brain instructs the muscle to contract tightly around it to provide a solid defence. These muscles themselves will already be subject to added strain through simply having to support this belly's extra weight and, like those mentioned above, will probably be underdeveloped to start off with.

Get rid of it

Losing that belly might not be rocket science – eat less, do more, is pretty much all it takes – but to do it efficiently, effectively and with minimum risk to your health there are a few guidelines that should be followed. Your ideal combination of exercise and diet will be a matter of taking elements from Chapters 2 and 3 of this book, then applying them to a weight loss conclusion – one that rebalances your calories in/calories out equation.

No need to give up everything

Crash diets might work in the short term and mean you drop a few kilograms during the first few weeks, but in the long term they will not be sustainable without damaging your health. Likewise, such extreme diets as the Grapefruit Plan, or the Cabbage Soup Diet, or the Beyonce-endorsed maple-syrup-and-cayenne-pepper menu, are not recommended for any length of time. Low carb, or worse still no carb, diets are not a good idea either, as they tend to involve compensations in other areas – specifically loading up the meat and dairy – which can seriously bump up your cholesterol levels.

The basis of any sensible weight loss eating plan is simply to cut out fats, refined sugar and simple carbohydrates, but retain sufficient protein, nutrients, natural sugars and complex carbohydrates. Although cutting the carbs on plans like Atkins or South Beach will show spectacular early results, complex carbs, as are found in whole grains, are vital to give you the energy to start the exercise programme that will form the other side of your weight loss schedule.

Put some effort in

Exercise is vital to healthily managed long-term weight loss, if for no other reason than that raising your calorific expenditure will allow you to offset some of your intake, meaning you can enjoy the odd pizza or a couple of beers without feeling guilty. Also, while it improves your cardiovascular levels

"I'll bet you didn't recognize me from the previous page!"

and generally makes you feel better, exercise will stimulate your metabolism into burning calories far more efficiently. Then, every kilogram of muscle you put on will require more calories burned to maintain the same weight in fat.

Perhaps as importantly, exercise will give you something positive to be doing rather than simply feeling like you are giving things up, and help you focus on becoming fitter and healthier, rather than merely thinner. Men who adopt an exercise programme to go along with their eating plan are more than twice as likely to keep the weight off than those who don't. This is believed to be because keeping fit becomes a habit.

Keep a food diary

Before you start a new eating plan, keep a food diary for a couple of weeks, logging everything you eat, an estimation of its calorific content, at what time and with whom you ate, and leave space for comments. That way you can accurately access what needs to be changed on your personal menu – nutrition-wise as well as from the weight loss point of view – and look at the situations and the company in which you are eating what, as that can have a serious impact on your weight management.

Beware of diet pills

Thanks to Internet shopping the slimming pill business has boomed during the last few years, and the sort of weight-loss drugs that would need a prescription in the UK or the US are being bought as "diet supplements"

F

Fact: Over the past 25 years the number of calories Americans consume through drinks – soda, fruit juice, alcohol, milk – has more than doubled. The average daily intake coming purely from beverages has gone up from 260 to 560 calories with no corresponding reduction on the food side.

Lose that gut (Part 1)

"The first thing to do is look at how the high fat and high added sugar foods are getting into your diet and you'll probably find that at least one is cropping up in each meal or each eating opportunity. You might have a Danish pastry for breakfast; then at break time pick up a can of Coke; lunchtime might involve a packet of crisps; then mid-afternoon you have a chocolate bar. Come the evening, perhaps it's a takeaway or maybe burger and chips, or perhaps if you've eaten something healthy for dinner you might then finish it off with a few cans of lager. Then what do you cut first? How do you take those initial steps to change your eating habits, because they're going to be the most difficult?

"One of the best things to think about in the beginning is what you have in between the main meals, because as they are secondary they will be easier to change. Think what would be the healthy alternative to that can of Coke? Maybe pick out something from another food group, like a banana, to get you through to lunchtime. Then in the afternoon instead of the chocolate try a yoghurt from the calcium-based group. That's how you can start changing the balance of things, then carry on going forward from there. It's pretty simple."

Dr Sarah Schenker

in unregulated overseas marketplaces. Although these pills will usually prove successful for a quick weight loss fix, they should never be contemplated on a long-term basis, as they are powerful, dangerous and potentially addictive drugs. Which is why they are so tightly monitored in the first place.

Slimming pills mostly fall into three categories: appetite suppressants, metabolism accelerants or fat blockers, or combinations thereof, and each has its own set of potential dangers. The former boost the levels of the hormones such as serotonin in the brain, to bring about feelings of fullness or satisfaction. They can quickly become addictive, as when the body stops getting the nourishment it needs because you're simply not eating enough it starts to bypass the boosted hormones and put other hunger-recognition systems in place. This often leads to increased dosages, because the feelings of satisfaction the drugs bring on represent something of a high, so psychological addiction isn't far behind. And with it comes all the personality changes and anxieties associated with mood-altering drugs. Recent US studies have also shown

Yes, you will have to give up something

Bypass, banding or balloons?

Of course not every weight loss method involves working hard to change lifestyle, and the alternative is to go under the knife. The three most common procedures are gastric banding, gastric bypassing or the insertion of a gastric balloon, and none of them should be entered into until you've talked it over with your doctor.

Type of operation	What it involves	How it works	Pros	Cons
Gastric banding (or lap banding)	A restrictive band is placed around the stomach, to divide off a small pouch at the top and leave a small opening into the main chamber	The small pouch fills up quickly, food then passes slowly through the opening to be digested as normal. It leaves you feeling full almost immediately, and greatly limits the amount of food that can be eaten	Recovery time of around two weeks; a less complicated operation than bypass, therefore shorter stay in hospital; less expensive (by around 30 percent); reversible	Lower, slower weight loss than gastric bypass; not suitable for the hugely obese (BMI over 45)
Gastric bypass	The stomach is stapled across near the top, to create a small closed pouch; a section of small intestine is run from this directly into the lower intestine	Food passes straight from the pouch into the lower intestine, bypassing most of the stomach and small intestine. It also hugely reduces the number of calories that can be absorbed	Suitable for the very obese; results in greater, quicker weight loss than banding.	It is a major procedure, therefore expensive; carries more risks; much longer recovery time; difficult to reverse
Gastric balloon	A 500cc balloon is inserted into your stomach through your mouth.	The balloon is inflated by filling it with a sterile saline solution, meaning your stomach is partially full before you even start eating, thus you eat less	Relatively inexpensive; performed under local anaesthetic; can be done as an outpatient	Weight loss is slow; the balloon can leave you feeling constantly bloated

prolonged use of appetite suppressants damages the heart valves as well.

The metabolic accelerants contain amphetamine-like substances – ephedra or ephedrine is the most common – which can cause all the psychological problems of speed drugs, such as aggression, mood swings, paranoia, plus such physiological troubles as raised blood pressure, strain on the heart and an increased likelihood of heart attacks and strokes.

> **F**
>
> *Fact: In the US, the average daily calorific intake for grown men is 3600 per day, almost 33 percent more than they actually need. The average for the UK is not much better at 3400.*

> **T**
>
> *Tip: If you're a regular light drinker take a couple of nights off each week. A 125ml glass of wine contains around 88 calories, while a half litre of beer can contain between 180 and 220 (depending on what type of beer), so taking three glasses of wine or pints of beer out of your intake, twice a week, could save you between five hundred and twelve hundred calories per week. And help you sleep better on those two nights.*

Fat blockers inhibit the actions of the enzymes that break fat down in the intestines in order for it to be absorbed through the intestine wall, thus they prevent the actual digestion of around forty percent of all fat consumed. These drugs have to be administered and taken in precise amounts, as their major side effect is that even a small amount of variation from the correct dosage can result in a total loss of bowel control.

Change your habits

Do you always have a burger when you meet the guys on the way to the game? Will you usually pick up a bag of chips when you get off the bus late at night? Is there a beer-and-pizza ritual that is involved every time you watch a DVD at home? Losing weight

Suck it up

Liposuction, or lipoplasty, is a body-sculpting procedure that targets specific areas of fat build-up, and is becoming so popular among men that in 2006 fourteen percent of all liposuction patients in the US were male. It's relatively simple – a hollow stainless steel needle is inserted into the area concerned and the offending fat, quite literally, sucked out. This technique is only effective on subcutaneous fat – the neck and face or buttocks and "love handles" are prime candidates – and cannot be applied to visceral fat, so you're still going to have to put a bit of effort in to lose that gut.

Before you sign up for it though, it is worth bearing in mind that over fifty percent of liposuction recipients put that fat back on within five years. This is either because those particular accumulations were genetic, or because the individuals never paid any attention to the science or theories of weight loss and so never addressed the bad habits that put the fat there in the first place.

Lose that gut (Part 2)

"To get rid of that gut you've got to look at food first. Especially for younger men, the first thing to do is cut out the rubbish from the diet. This has to be done straight away, because you can't begin to address it while you're still eating badly. Then you've got to look at resistance training on a regular scale, and that means three times a week, because the more lean muscle tissue you have the more efficient you will be at burning body fat. You can do cardiovascular training; it's great and should be a part of your routine, but although you burn body fat while you're doing it. However, when you stop the burn stops and there's no after effects. But as it takes more energy for the body to support lean muscle tissue than it does fat, it will continue to burn calories while you are at rest. Thus if you create as much lean muscle as possible, the more efficient you become at burning body fat."

Gideon Remfry

is as much about altering what you do as it is about changing what you actually eat. Focusing on this idea very often reveals that it's your circumstances dictating your diet rather than the other way around.

As you start planning your new eating regime, look for patterns, places and associations within your regular life that may lead you into eating badly as a habit –keeping a daily food diary will help to make things clearer. If you can identify such regular situations, the best thing you can do, rather than avoid them completely and possibly feel resentful, is to adapt your approach to them. Get off the bus at a different stop so you avoid passing your favourite chip shop; turn up to meet the others a bit later so there's less time to eat or sink that extra pint; eat

Don't eat that, eat this!

High calorie	Low calorie
Mozzarella cheese	Feta cheese
Chicken	Skinless chicken
Draught Guinness	Bottled Guinness
Sandwiches	Wraps
Cream	Plain yoghurt
Waffles	Pancakes
Deep pan pizza	Thin crust pizza
BK Big Fish	Whopper
Streaky bacon	Back bacon
Ice cream	Sorbet
White chocolate	Plain chocolate
Bagel	Croissant
Rack of lamb	Rib of beef
Spaghetti Bolognaise	Fettuccini Alfredo
Apple crumble	Apple pie
Hamburger	Hot dog
Lager	Bitter
Sirloin steak	Pork chop
Waldorf salad	Caesar salad

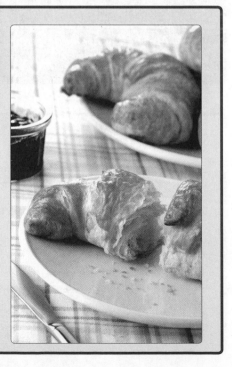

Calories burned

These are the calories burned per hour by a 76kg (168lb) man; the sports' figures err on the side of the casual participant rather than the fiercely competitive. Ideally, your exercise plan should involve burning at least 1500 calories per week, falling to 1200 once you get over the age of sixty.

Activity	Calories burned per hour
Running (ten-minute miles)	710
Skiing (general)	450
Football (US)	560
Football (soccer)	550
Badminton	350
Swimming (freestyle)	600
Squash	850
Walking (moderate-to-brisk pace)	300
Basketball	550
Cycling (on the road)	620
Golf (walking, carrying your clubs)	290
Circuit training	570
Rugby	700
Raquetball	500
Weight training	220
Tennis (singles)	570
Rollerblading	500
Rowing	600
Martial arts (judo, karate, kickboxing)	710
Boxing	850

(healthily) before you settle down to watch a film and you'll be less likely to stuff yourself with pizza.

F

Fact: One single gram of fat contains three times the calories of a single gram of protein or carbohydrate.

You'll be amazed at how many calories you'll be missing out on just by paying attention to what you are doing.

Slowly does it

Weight lost quickly is liable to be weight put back on almost as speedily. Any seemingly miraculous plan that promises ten kilograms lost in as many days is in fact going to be ridding your body of retained water and muscle mass rather than fat, and this will

Fatherhood makes you fat

It's not just new mums that put on "baby weight". Recent research in Australia found that first-time fathers put on an average of three kilograms during their baby's first year. This weight gain was repeated with every subsequent child. It's believed that this is due to a combination of life being thrown into chaos – sleep patterns and meal times severely disrupted – increased stress and an abandonment of previous activities such as playing football or going to the gym. And the most worrying part of the report was that once gained this weight was never lost.

The best thing for expectant fathers to do is prepare for this in advance. Read your partner's baby books as they will be crammed with dietary information that looks at healthy eating with one eye on weight control. Also, buy a running buggy and you'll be able to carry on keeping fit and still spend time with the new arrival – it will be very healthy for baby as well.

soon reappear as your system restabilizes. Fat falls off relatively slowly, and you should be aiming for a weight loss of between one and two pounds per week as a result of small changes in your lifestyle and eating habits. Also, the longer a weight loss plan lasts, the more likely it is to become an integral part of your life rather than something to be

endured for a specific amount of time, which means you will have a much better chance of sticking to it.

Half a kilogram of body fat is worth about 3500 calories, so to lose a kilogram

F

Fact: Restaurant portions in the US are, on average, twice the size they are in France.

T

Tip: So many foods that are high in fat are low in fibre too, meaning a double whammy of accumulating fat on our bodies while not clearing out harmful deposits.

The best of the web

weightlossforall.com
A US site dedicated to helping you lose weight, and among the eating tips and programmes it offers a comprehensive chart of the calorific content of food.

myfooddiary.com
A membership website offering a vast manner of dietary advice and assistance, including a service that will analyse your food diary and provide suggestions as to how you can get the best out of your eating plan.

thedietchannel.com
Tips to help you diet and tests to establish what sort of diet you need; plus health-oriented eating plans and regularly changing diet-related features.

menshealth.com/bellyoff
Pretty much what it says on the tin, a very successful weight loss scheme for men, detailing diets and work-outs, and keeping a running total of the pounds lost by Belly Off Club members.

in a week you'll need to rebalance your personal equation by an average of 1000 calories every day. Taking six or seven hundred calories a day out of the average Western diet isn't overly difficult – change a lunchtime sandwich to a salad, but pass on the mayonnaise; skip those two or three pints after work; switch from deep pan to crispy base pizza. Then you can see off a further 1500 to 2000 calories simply with an hour's running or playing football three times a week (see box on p.97). As long as you build on each week's achievements it won't be long before you can see the results.

Ten top tips for losing weight

This will burn over eight hundred calories an hour, so make sure you're eating enough

▶ **Take on enough carbohydrate to exercise**
Any sensible weight loss programme will involve an exercise regime as well as an eating plan, so make sure you are eating enough of what you need to work out.

▶ **Don't listen to other people** Everybody is different, so what is right for somebody else's weight loss plan may be completely wrong for you.

▶ **Listen to other people** However, the experiences of people around you may be relevant as you consider what your weight loss options might be – but only as a guideline. Also, talking to your friends and family about how you are getting on will help keep you motivated.

▶ **Only eat when you're hungry**
This may sound very obvious but one of the driving factors behind the West's obesity problem is people eating out of habit, or boredom, and not because they need to.

▶ **Drink more water** Often, when you think you are hungry, you are in fact thirsty. Water will also fill your stomach with no calorific intake whatsoever.

▶ **Drink colder water** It will cool you down internally, and your body will burn a few calories bringing itself back to its normal temperature.

▶ **Don't make your regime too spartan** Otherwise you simply won't stick to it or you'll be unhappy or, most probably, both.

▶ **Look at all your habits** There will be patterns of behaviour attached to your piling on the pounds and if you look at changing them it will be a great deal easier to eat and exercise correctly.

▶ **Give in to your cravings** As long as you do so with restraint. If you fancy a bar of chocolate or some other off-plan treat, buy it – but only eat half of it.

▶ **Sub size me** Go for the regular instead of large or small instead of regular option; have the starter-size portion as a main course. Or simply leave something on your plate other than the pattern.

In the guts

5

To get the maximum nutritional benefit from the food you eat it has to pass through your digestive system as efficiently as possible. Too often, though, this won't be the case, as lifestyle and the modern diet conspire to work against the body's natural – and most effective – ways to process food, causing various levels of discomfort. Then, as you get older, it becomes progressively more difficult to keep things moving along quite as they should.

Easy to swallow, but...

Your digestive system gets ready to swing into action well before you start eating. In fact, you don't need to be sitting at the table or even seeing or smelling food – merely thinking about food will make your mouth water. The production of saliva is the first stage of the gastric process; saliva contains the digestive enzyme amylase, which works in conjunction with chewing to break the food down into something that can be easily swallowed.

Once our food has been broken down, reflex actions, instinct and the digestive process take over – see box opposite – and

F

Fact: There are more nerve cells in the stomach and intestines than in the spinal column.

we no longer have too much control. What we can do, though, is make sure all these automatic processes function as well as is possible.

Problem is, we don't seem to be doing that very well, as far and away the number one reason for men visiting the doctor, both in the UK and the US, is gastrointestinal.

Stress

Just as relaxation promotes good digestion, stress has the opposite effect – indeed the ties between your stomach and your brain are so significant that the expression "gut feeling" is far from figurative. Excitement, stress and fear can all manifest themselves in your digestive system.

When the brain is put under pressure in stressful situations, and the fight or flight condition kicks in, one of the first things it does is to shut down the digestive system.

M

Mythbuster: Stress gives you stomach ulcers

Though stress is not the initial cause of gastric ulcers, it can definitely aggravate them – the release of extra cortisol during a "fight or flight" moment will cause a surge in stomach acid.

How it all works: digestion

Once the teeth, tongue and the introduction of saliva have mashed the food down into a swallowable mass, it passes through the throat into the oesophagus, a tube lined with muscles that push it towards the stomach with an action known as peristalsis. This involves rippling contractions and relaxations of the intestine itself, pushing the broken-down food along the tube – movements that would look like a snake swallowing its prey. As a rhythmic action – the peristalsis wave – it happens along the entire length of the digestive tract, from the oesophagus, through the small intestine and along the large intestine to the colon.

At the base of the oesophagus is a sphincter, a ring-shaped muscle that acts as a valve to permit food to pass into the stomach but not back up the other way. Once in the stomach, food will be broken down further into smaller, easily digestible particles as it mixes with the acids and enzymes produced there. Food leaves the stomach as a sludgy, semi-liquid substance called chyme; it then passes into the small intestine, where it will be further deconstructed, allowing nutrients to be transferred into the system. An adult's small intestine will be five metres (seventeen feet) from end to end; as the chyme passes through the three sections of its length – the duodenum, jejunum and ileum – the nutrient-extraction process continues and the chyme is broken down even further as a series of different chemicals go to work on it.

Once through the small intestine the chyme is moved to the large intestine, a wider tube, about one and a half metres in length and divided into three parts: the caecum, colon and rectum. It passes quickly through the caecum into the colon, where the water content is drawn off and re-absorbed into the system; the dried out chyme is packed into solid faeces which are collected in the rectum. These will then be excreted through the anus.

Food enters the stomach through the oesophagus

A protective layer of mucous lines the stomach

Three layers of muscle surround it

The small intestine is entered through the sphincter

The colon collects waste before releasing it through the anus

The time it takes

In the mouth: 1–2 minutes

In the oesophagus: 10 seconds

In the stomach: 2–4 hours

In the small intestine: 1–6 hours

In the large intestine: could be as much as several days

(M) Mythbuster: Drinking milk cures stomach acid problems

While milk will immediately soothe the painful effects of excess acid, it will go on to contribute to the problem. Milk is rich in calcium; this promotes the production of the hormone gastrin, which triggers the release of stomach acid.

The brain does this so that no further energy is used to break down food and blood can be diverted from the stomach to muscles and other organs vital to an action scenario. We have been hard-wired this way, more with a view to taking on a sabre tooth tiger than to making a presentation at a sales conference. This is what causes the sensation of "butterflies" in the stomach, as such speedy internal activity produces the fluttering feelings to a degree related to the level of stress. In extreme cases of fear, the bowels and bladder may empty themselves without warning, simply to relieve you of any surplus weight.

This is how it works in extreme and unexpected circumstances, but serious problems occur when your default setting is feeling under pressure. When suffering from such chronic stress, your body's protective systems become overburdened, with the digestion system being the autonomic nervous function (involuntary vital function) most prominently affected.

The body loses nourishment as

Processed meat, refined flour, melted hard cheese – anything but fast food as far as your bowels are concerned digestion is perpetually impaired, while the problems caused by undigested food in the gut multiply (see p.111). Constant high levels of cortisol – the stress hormone – are produced, overstimulating gastric acid production, one of the most common causes of gastritis as the excess acid attacks the linings of the stomach or the small intestine to cause inflammation. Although excess stomach acid can be countered with chewable or liquid antacids – Milk of Magnesia is the best known – this should only be a temporary measure. Over time, prolonged use of antacids will reduce the necessary levels of gastric acid, and that will seriously impede the digestive system, in turn blocking the absorption of iron and B vitamins.

Belly achin' at a glance

Condition	Symptoms	Causes	Cure
Acid reflux, a.k.a. heartburn	Burning sensation behind the breastbone	Digestive juices passing up from the stomach into the oesophagus	Avoid peppermint, coffee, fruit juice and chocolate; cut down on the drinking; stop smoking
Indigestion	Nausea, excess gas, pain deep within the abdominal cavity, churning in the stomach, acid reflux	Eating too quickly, excess stomach acid, overeating, spicy food, activity straight after eating, stress	Antacid; avoid spicy food; eat slower and relax afterwards; chew your food more
Peptic ulcers	Sharp burning pain in the stomach, nausea, bloating	Breach in the mucous lining of the intestinal tract, allowing acid to attack sensitive tissue	Acid-lowering medicine; avoid caffeine, spicy food and smoking until it is healed
Food poisoning (see box on p.107)	Vomiting, dizziness, sweating, diarrhoea, weakness	Contaminated food, unwashed hands	No solid food and plenty of water until it passes
Wind	Burping, farting	Eating too quickly, gassy carbonated drinks	Chew your food more thoroughly and don't gulp it down; avoid fizzy drinks
Trapped wind	Stabbing pain deep within abdominal cavity	As above, but the air is caught inside the intestine	A warm drink will expand the intestine and dislodge it
Gastroenteritis a.k.a. Delhi Belly or Montezuma's revenge	An extreme form of food poisoning (dysentery, cholera and typhoid are all serious forms); symptoms as for food poisoning above	Bacterial or viral infection from food or untreated water; poor hygiene	Drink plenty of water; eat bland food; rest

F

Fact: The more overweight you are the more likely you are to suffer from frequent acid reflux.

Acid overload

Gastritis is the inflammation of the protective layer of mucous that lines the stomach and intestines, and is the most common of intestinal-related complaints among adult men. It can manifest itself in a number of different ways, and has about as many causes.

Quite apart from the stress factor and the overproduction of stomach acid, this film of mucous is prone to attack from bacterial, fungal or parasitic infection, the latter most commonly transferred to your gut by undercooked shellfish. Prolonged use of the anti-inflammatory painkillers such as aspirin, ibuprofen and naproxen will inhibit the production of substances that protect and sustain the mucous layer. Excessive alcohol or coffee drinking or overly spicy food will attack the mucous, while cigarette smoking contributes to gastritis as nicotine increases the production of stomach acid. Old age is another factor, as the older a man gets the thinner the mucous lining in his stomach becomes.

Gastritis can be acute, manifesting itself in sudden burning sensations in the abdomen, indigestion or nausea; or it can be chronic, building up slowly over time with a continual dull ache, general loss of appetite and a constantly bloated feeling with the side effect of plentiful gas. The latter condition is also given to sharp twinges of pain, if the intestinal tract is further irritated by something like a boost of cortisol or a particularly lively curry. Both acute and chronic gastritis can cause vomiting, and in extreme cases the stomach lining will actually bleed, with the blood showing up in vomit or faeces.

To treat gastritis, taking antacid will counter the painful effect of the stomach's acid, but then the underlying cause needs to be addressed. Often that's a process of elimination. The immediate action should be to cut out any of the potential irritants listed above, and if that makes no difference then you probably have an infection. If you believe this to be the case, visit your doctor, who, if you test positive, will prescribe a course of antibiotics. As these infections can be stubborn, be sure to complete the course and then visit your doctor to make sure you are in the clear.

You could have a gut flora problem if...

The chances are, given today's diets and lifestyles, that keeping your gut flora in a healthy balance will not be happening by itself and you will need to introduce pro- or prebiotics. Any of the following could mean an imbalance of bacteria in your gut:

• You suddenly become allergic to things and develop food sensitivities.
• Unexplained weight gain, often accompanied by cravings for sweet foods.
• Frequent constipation or bouts of diarrhoea.
• Night sweats and disrupted sleep patterns.
• Bad breath or bleeding gums.
• Colds or low-level infections refuse to clear up.

If any of these is the case, introduce a course of pro- and prebiotics (see box opposite) to your diet. If after a couple of weeks, the symptoms persist, visit your doctor.

Biotics decoded

Antibiotics: While these clear up all manner of diseases, they will also wipe out the good bacteria in your gut as they can't tell the difference. Following a course of antibiotics, reintroduce the probiotics to your system.

Probiotics: The good bacteria that reside in your gut to protect against damaging bacteria – the good guys are stronger – forming the basis of your immune system. Found naturally in yoghurt or can be taken as supplements.

Prebiotics: The food that the gut's probiotics need to thrive and which occurs naturally in whey as well as some fruit, vegetables and whole grains.

Understanding ulcers

A gastric ulcer is a kind of premier league gastritis, and occurs when the layer of mucous is completely eaten away on a small patch of the intestinal or stomach wall, a couple of centimetres in diameter. The sensitive lining will then be exposed to the ravages of stomach acid, leading to jolts of very sharp pain if acid levels surge. Around ten percent of the population of the UK will suffer from gastric ulcers at some point in their lives, with men being twice as susceptible as women, with most sufferers being between thirty and fifty.

Although the accepted term is "stomach ulcer" it is unlikely to actually be in the stomach. The correct term is peptic ulcer, as it can occur in the oesophagus, the stomach or the duodenum section of the small intestine. The first is very rare because food is not digested in the oesophagus and doesn't stay there for very long; instead it's usually caused by frequent regurgitation of acid. The second, the stomach ulcer, is far more common in women than men.

Ulcers among men are mostly in the duodenal section of the small intestine, and the usual cause is food's liquid content arriving into it while the solid parts remain in the stomach. The arrival of the liquid triggers the release of acid in anticipation of digestion, but when no solids turn up there is nothing to absorb that acid and it attacks the inside walls. Food not chewed properly promotes this situation, as does a diet with a high proportion of hard-to-break-down food – red meat, hard cheese and processed foods. It should be noted that all externally introduced causes of gastritis also contribute to the formation of ulcers.

A

Expert advice: "Men in the UK and the US are not achieving nearly the target for fibre. They should be getting at least eighteen grams of fibre per day, but, in Britain, among men, the average is less than twelve. It means there is very poor bowel health out there, which is affecting everything else to do with our digestion and well-being. Men have to eat more fibre."
Dr Sarah Schenker

F

Fact: Fifteen percent of men will develop a peptic ulcer at some time in their life, probably between the ages of twenty-five and fifty.

T
Tip: Too much coffee or alcohol can stop your bowel movements, as they are both diuretics and therefore will greatly reduce the amount of water in your system.

The good news is that peptic ulcers are relatively easy to treat. Initially, acid will be countered with an antacid or acid blocker (also known as an H2 Blocker), then medicines containing either sucralfate or misoprostol will be prescribed. These will form a protective coating over the sore to promote swift healing. A natural way to protect against ulcers is by taking zinc, as it strengthens the epithelial cells in the layer of stomach lining below the mucous and reduces the release of acid-producing histamine.

Gut level

One of the biggest contributors to continued good health is what's going on among the bacteria in residence in your small and large intestines, your gut flora. It's in here that "friendly" bacteria – probiotics – produce B vitamins, vitamin K and amino acids, regulate digestive acid levels in the intestines and help keep your digestive system moving so your bowels remain regular. This bacteria, lactobacilli and bifidobacteria in particular, also fight off such harmful bacteria as "C. diff" (clostridium difficile), "A. Strep" (A. streptococcus) and some strains of "E. coli" (Escherichia coli) by protecting against toxins and pathogens being introduced to your system.

This is an important aspect of your immune system, as it guards against allergies, colds and flu. It is also believed that it will prevent irritable bowel syndrome, and that a healthy balance of gut flora is a reliable first line of defence against cancer of the colon.

Maintaining the balance of good/bad bacteria in the gut can easily be overlooked, and not drinking enough water, eating too much junk food, a chaotic meal pattern or a course of antibiotics can tip the scales away from good intestinal health. Live yoghurt or the fermented milk drink kefir contain a good supply of both lactobacilli and bifidobacteria or, outside of these dairy products, probiotics can be taken in the form of liquid or capsule supplements.

However, once the friendly bacteria have been introduced to the system they need to be fed, and you'll need to be taking a regular

B

Best investment: pineapples As well as being an excellent source of vitamins C and B1, pineapple is one of the most effective digestive aids there is. The fruit is rich in powerful enzymes that break down protein (proteolytic enzyme bromelain) and thus are a huge asset when it comes to digesting such stubborn foods as meat or hard cheese.

What's your poison?

Type	Causes	Effects	Prevention
Salmonella	Under-cooked meat or poultry; cross-contamination of raw and cooked meat or poultry; unpasteurized dairy products; raw eggs; cream or milk "on the turn" and the sauces or fillings it may be used in	Cramps, diarrhoea, vomiting, fever	Cook meat and poultry thoroughly; keep raw and cooked apart; wash utensils, hands and surfaces well after contact with raw meat or poultry – no matter how fleeting; avoid unpasteurized dairy; cook uninspected eggs; keep milk and cream – and any dishes they are used in – in the fridge
Listeria	Under-cooked meat or poultry; cross-contamination of raw and cooked meat or poultry; unpasteurized dairy products; under-cooked or raw seafood; unwashed fruit and vegetables	Cramps, diarrhoea, vomiting, fever, skin lesions, chills	Cook meat and poultry thoroughly; keep raw and cooked apart; wash utensils, hands and surfaces well after any contact with raw meat or poultry; avoid unpasteurized dairy; thoroughly wash fruit and vegetables you don't peel
Staphlococcus	Pre-prepared salads in which the mayonnaise may be off; cream or milk "on the turn" and sauces or fillings it may be used in	Cramps, diarrhoea, vomiting, fever, headaches, general weakness	Keep salads, milk and cream – and anything they are used in – in the fridge
E. coli	Unwashed fruit and vegetables; under-cooked meat or poultry; cross-contamination of raw and cooked meat or poultry	Cramps, diarrhoea, gas, vomiting, fever	Thoroughly wash any fruit and vegetables you don't peel; cook meat and poultry thoroughly; keep raw and cooked apart; wash utensils, hands and surfaces well after contact with raw meat or poultry – no matter how fleeting

How it all works: the kidneys

The kidneys are situated near the small of the back on either side of the spinal column; they collect waste – the unwanted by-products of internal chemical reactions – from the bloodstream, then get rid of it. They do this by filtering around 150 litres of blood (317 US pints) per day as it flows into them via the renal artery which branches off the aorta that runs directly from the heart. The kidneys remove waste by passing the blood through tiny filtering units known as nephrons, then mixing it with water to become urine and depositing this into cavities called calyces. From there it is carried away by the ureter to the bladder, where it is stored before being passed out of the body through the penis via the urethra. The kidneys will get rid of about two litres of water and waste per day from a grown man.

As well as simply disposing of waste through urine, the kidneys also control the level of water within our bodies, passing more into the bladder if there is too much, or prompting feelings of thirst if there is too little. This is why you are left still feeling thirsty after some drinks, because the kidneys are still crying out for water. Another important function of the kidneys is to regulate the levels of chemicals like salt, potassium and phosphorus in the system, and remove any harmful excesses.

Each kidney contains over a million nephrons, which act as filtration units

Renal artery carries blood to the kidneys

Renal vein carries filtered blood away from the kidneys

The ureter carries waste to the bladder via urine

Each nephron contains an intricate network of tiny tubes and channels to remove all waste products

Kidney stones occur when chemicals aren't passed out through urine and build up sufficiently to form solid chunks of matter within any part of your urinary tract. These can be incredibly painful, and are either removed surgically or treated with drugs to break them down into pieces small enough to be passed through the urethra. This can be quite an experience in itself, given that a piece can be several millimetres across and far from smooth on the outside.

Kidney stones are almost three times as common among men as women, affecting men in their twenties and thirties in particular, and Caucasians being the most susceptible racial group. Symptoms of a kidney stone are: stabbing pains in your lower back; blood in your urine; painful urination; a constant desire to go; and flu-like fever and vomiting.

Irritable bowel syndrome

This is a collective term for functional bowel disorders that do not fall into any other category. The most common symptoms of irritable bowel syndrome (IBS) are chronic constipation and/or persistent diarrhoea, and prolonged cramps and/or bloating in the lower intestine. Medical science is unsure of the internal causes of IBS, but it is believed the main culprits are oversensitive nerves that cause peristalsis to happen too often and too fiercely while eating, or nerves that may be aggravated when the bowel is full and expanded.

If you think you have IBS, visit your doctor who will conduct a physical examination and give you a blood test. They will also discuss your lifestyle with you, as stress has been linked to the condition inasmuch as it has an adverse effect on the digestive system. What your doctor won't do, however, is cure IBS, as at the time of writing there is no cure for it, merely changes that can help relieve it.

The principal change will be dietary: fatty foods, fried foods, alcohol, caffeinated drinks, fizzy drinks, chocolate and milk products have all been proved to exacerbate IBS symptoms. But as everybody's condition will be unique, it will be necessary for a sufferer to work out what it is that causes their IBS to flare up and cut that out – this is best done by keeping a food diary over a month or so to implement a process of elimination. Adding fibre to your diet can help – though not if one of your symptoms is diarrhoea – and eating smaller meals more often will help your digestive system cope more efficiently, reducing the scope for irritation.

supply of prebiotics on board. These can be found in whey (what's left of milk when the curd has been removed to make cheese) or, for the lactose intolerant, in the carbohydrate fibre oligosaccharides, found in fruit, vegetables and whole grains. Garlic, onions, tomatoes, Jerusalem artichokes and bananas are all rich in prebiotics, but the amounts contained are still tiny – it takes twenty bananas to yield a gram of oligosaccharide, around half the RDA – so taking prebiotics in the form of supplements is recommended.

A

Expert advice: "Laxatives are not a good idea in anything other than the very short term. They don't add anything to your system, and you will be missing out on all the other nutrients you'd get if you keep your bowels healthy with whole food."
Dr Sarah Schenker

Waste management

Always somewhat under-appreciated, yet getting rid of the stuff we don't want is every bit as important as making the most of what we need.

How often is regular?

How often you should move your bowels depends entirely on who you are – everybody's different and their body's digestive timetable will vary accordingly. A 24-hour cycle of solid

F

Fact: Although the kidneys are one of the hardest working organs in your body, they are seldom stretched. Many people live healthy and active lives with only one functioning kidney.

T

is called "gastrocolic reflex" and is triggered by an expanded stomach, the goal being to make more room further along the digestive tract. This reflex is strongest in children, and gets weaker as you pass into adulthood.

Take it easy

Bowel movements should happen easily and almost by gravity, with no need for squeezing or straining, and the easiest will involve soft, bulky stools that hold themselves together. This will be achieved by a diet high in fibre

waste disposal is the most common, but it's by no means universal – only sixty percent of us go every day – and that will be due to habit formed out of convenience and comfort as much as anything gastric. Anything between three times a day and three times a week is considered perfectly healthy, and these figures will start to decrease with age.

The physical act of getting up in the morning will trigger an urge to defecate as the movement itself will shift the large intestine, triggering the rectum to send signals that it wants rid of the waste it's been storing up during the night. Also it is not unusual to want to go fairly soon after a big meal; this

T

Your mum knew what she was talking about

Don't eat too fast. Otherwise you'll swallow too much air with your food, leading to wind or indigestion.

Chew every mouthful properly. The enzymes that extract the nutrients from food work on the particles' surface area only, so the more small pieces there are the greater surface area for them to react with.

Don't eat standing up. It will cause you to eat faster than if you were properly relaxed at the table, thus the points mentioned above come into play.

Don't start running around immediately after you've eaten. Apart from feeling uncomfortable, it is harder for your body to digest food properly if you are exercising right after a meal.

Don't put too much food in your mouth. Smaller mouthfuls encourage you to chew your food more thoroughly – besides, cheeks bulging out like a hamster is never a good look.

Don't talk with your mouth full. Quite apart from turning the stomach of whoever is sitting opposite you, you will take in a great deal of air, meaning gas attacks will surely follow.

Drink a glass of water during your meal and after you've finished eating. Water aids the production of digestive juices, eases the flow of food along the digestive tract and keeps faeces soft.

and with plenty of water. The indigestible fibre will hold on to water to create a stool of a soft consistency, and without the fibre, what is passed into the rectum will be low on water content and therefore can be uncomfortably hard. Somewhat obviously, the more water there is to start off with, the more the fibre will have to retain – a healthy stool should be around 75 percent water.

Faeces are the colour they are because of pigmentation formed by the bacteria in the gut reacting with bile that travels the gastric tract, and the smell is from sulphur compounds produced by the bacteria in the colon. Sulphur-rich foods such as cabbage, broccoli, brussel sprouts and beans tend to make this more acute.

Keep it moving

Constipation is second only to gastritis as the most common intestinal complaint in the US, but as Americans spend more than $700 million each year on over-the-counter laxatives – that's over two dollars for every man, woman and child – it's safe to assume there's a great deal more that doesn't get as far as the doctor. As well as infrequency or lack of bowel movements, the term also covers difficult movements, hard or uncomfortable stools and the feeling the bowels are not yet emptied after a movement.

The truth is everybody will get constipated to some degree at some point in their lives, and around two percent of us are bunged up at any one time. The good news is, as far as you're concerned, they are twice as likely to be women than men.

Constipation occurs in the large intestine, when the stool is unable to pass through the colon or the rectum and out through the anus, and is usually because the waste matter is too hard and dry or collecting in too large a mass. Functional (or mild) constipation is pretty much an expected by-product of today's diet and lifestyle (see box on p.112); it will be temporary and usually clears up by itself, or with a bit of help by switching to a fibre-rich diet and drinking plenty of water. The older you are the more attention you need to pay to this, as your digestion will be naturally slowing down, thus waste will spend longer in the colon, meaning more water will be extracted from it. Deal with constipation by adjusting your eating/drinking habits rather than resorting to laxatives, which should only be taken on advice from your doctor.

Chronic constipation is any of the above symptoms that continue for more than two weeks after you have addressed the issue with diet and exercise. You should consult your doctor if that is the case, because there may be a more serious underlying problem – chronic constipation is an early symptom of cancer of the colon, and can also be a side effect of irritable bowel syndrome (see box on p.109), diabetes or Parkinson's disease.

The enema within

Although the medical profession has yet to acknowledge there is any value in enemas or colonic irrigation – they are not available on the NHS – they are a popular recommendation among the alternative health community. They have been used by mankind for thousands of years, and it's easy to understand why.

Each involves the cleansing of the colon

F

Fact: Most constipation isn't constipation at all, merely digestive sluggishness, as to be classified as constipation it must involve fewer than three bowel movements during the course of a week.

and lower intestine by introducing a liquid – saline solution or very weak coffee are the most effective – to dislodge the build-up of fecal waste on the intestinal walls. In both cases, a tube is inserted into the anus and the liquid flowed in either by gravity or gentle pressure. An enema will involve the fluid being held in the intestine for ten minutes or so while the abdomen is gently massaged, and colonic irrigation is a continuous flow through an "in" and "out" tube. As dislodging years' worth of intestinal crud build-up will be a progressive process, both will involve several sessions, with the liquid penetrating a bit further along the intestine and stripping it closer to the actual wall each time.

The effects of colonic cleansing on a man who has, for years, been eating an indiscriminate diet of modern food can be quite astonishing. Once the liquid penetrates properly what comes out is solid, rubbery and intestine-shaped, both in continuous length and outside patterning, and often black in

F

Fact: Horses get hiccups more frequently than humans do; they just don't make any sound.

21st-century blockages

The most common causes of constipation in modern times are:

Lack of water

Diet low in fibre

Too much processed food

Side effect of taking iron or calcium supplements

Too much hard-to-digest food like hard cheese or red meat

colour. There will be a feeling of lightness and flexibility around the midsection, and a boost to general well-being as nutrients get absorbed far quicker and more efficiently through the newly exposed intestinal walls. A side effect of this last point is it won't take much to get you tipsy.

An important point to remember after either an enema or colonic irrigation is to replace the good bacteria in the gut, as the cleanse will have removed them along with all the harmful stuff.

The best of the web

alternative-healthzine.com
A site rich in tips and techniques to do with alternative health and healing. It has a huge section on digestion, the liver and colon.

Eufic.org
The European Food Information Council is packed with internal healthcare articles and diet-related tips – the section on a healthy gut is excellent.

Colonhealth.net
The Colon Therapists Network's website welcomes civilians and will supply all the information you need about colonic health.

Ten top tips for digestive health

▶ **Take zinc if you are stressed**
It will strengthen the stomach lining against any excess stomach acid.

▶ **Don't drink milk to soothe a stomach ulcer** It will ultimately make it worse – opt instead for a specially formulated antacid.

▶ **Reintroduce the good bacteria to your gut** Do this after a course of antibiotics, as the antibiotics will have killed them off as well.

▶ **Don't eat standing up** It will cause you to eat faster, chew less thoroughly and swallow more air, all of which are overtures for indigestion.

▶ **Dislodge trapped wind with a warm drink** It will expand the intestine and shift the trapped air pocket.

▶ **Don't worry if you don't "go" every day** Only sixty percent of the population have a daily bowel movement. Only if it gets less than three a week should you be alarmed.

▶ **Chew your food thoroughly**
It will stand a much better chance of being efficiently digested.

▶ **To avoid constipation drink plenty of water** Stools should be 75 percent water and lack of it in the system is the most common cause of constipation.

▶ **Get a colonic irrigation** It should be compulsory for any man over the age of thirty, as it will shift the layers of crud lining his digestive tract and allow it to function properly again.

▶ **Eat live yoghurt regularly**
It will maintain the necessary levels of friendly bacteria in your gut.

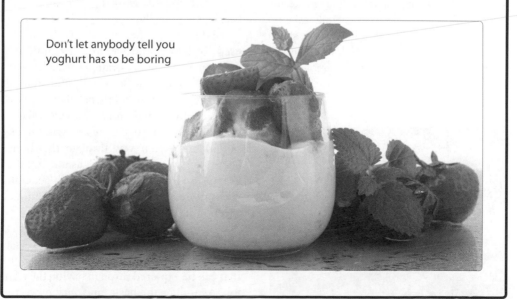

Don't let anybody tell you yoghurt has to be boring

At work

Anybody with a full-time job probably spends more of their waking hours at work than they do with their families. Therefore, what goes on there is going to have a huge impact on their overall well-being.

Why we want to work

That we need to work in order to be able to live well is pretty much a given – even worthwhile benefit fraud takes some sort of effort – and the better your job the better you can afford to live. However, perhaps more significant than work's monetary worth is its massive psychological importance, especially among men to whom the hunter-gatherer gene remains a major part of their make-up. The reason so many retired people take on part-time work, often far below the status of what they used to do, is less about the pay packet and more about the simple act of having a job. It allows a man to constantly

T

Tip: As you go through life your requirements and expectations will evolve, thus what the best job for you is will alter. One thing that won't change, however, is that wrong jobs rarely turn into right jobs over the course of time.

keep in touch with, and have a direct effect on, his own sense of self-worth.

And what do you do?

As human beings we are genetically programmed to make some sort of contribution to the advancement of the species and to the world around us, but because men can't have children this need is often expressed through work. Yet beyond whatever difference that might make to our environment, work has two important bearings on our lives.

Externally, what we do is frequently used to define who we are. In many cases this can serve to frustrate, especially when you're introduced to somebody and your job is all they use to decide what they think of you. Equally though, it can provide a handy yardstick for prestige and recognition due as you make your way through the dinner parties of the world. Indeed, as a method of keeping score with your peers, it's generally taken more seriously than how much money you might seem to have.

Internally, however, going to work is much more important than the above, as there are so many avenues vital to our psyche that can be explored through having the right job. As well as the basic, and very powerful, need to feel useful, a man's work can satisfy creative urges. This can be crucial as such unfulfilled ambitions are a massive cause of frustration among men as they approach middle age.

Then there is the problem-solving side of any level of work. This can produce immense inner satisfaction as it brings with it a feeling of being in control, and completing the series of finite tasks that comprise most jobs fulfils our subconscious desire for closure – closures that might not be as forthcoming in other areas of life. Also, progression at work will be as gratifying as advancement in your personal or family life and probably more easily quantifiable.

How to get ahead at work
(without your nose turning noticeably brown)

Take a public speaking course
It will do wonders for your confidence and presentational skills.

Don't ask questions you could have answered
Most bosses would rather you solved your own problems than bothered them.

Don't get carried away
Especially by email.

An apparently emotionally unstable worker will not get promoted
Stop and calm down, and leave that furious email in your draft folder for a few hours, then read it again.

Go beyond the call of duty (within reason, obviously)
Don't slope off home every time the office has to stay late, and take responsibility for things that need attention but might not be in your area. (While this may appear to contradict some of this book's other good health advice, it is merely a short-term thing and done occasionally for the greater good – it should never be allowed to become the norm.)

Let yourself be noticed rather than clamour for attention
Most company creeps are earmarked as such early on and toadying will only get them so far.

Be yourself
It will serve you well in the long run.

Work smart not hard
There's a commonly held notion among many bosses that if an employee is having to stay late every night they are doing something wrong – having a life outside will stand you in much better stead than burning the midnight oil.

Do training courses
If your firm runs courses take them; that's what they're there for and the people who organized them will appreciate your interest – besides, you'll be learning a new skill at somebody else's expense.

Keep up to date with your field
If you want to do well in it you'll need to know what is happening outside your firm as well as in it, and it will put you across as a Big Picture Kinda Guy.

Appear to want to progress
If you turn down two opportunities for promotion, don't expect to be given a third as you will be marked as "lacking in ambition" (but, equally, pay attention to the point above about not creeping).

T

Tip: Keeping a diary of how you feel at work can help hugely when it comes to assessing whether you should be there or not, as it will allow accurate review of your feelings over a period of time.

Is your job the right job for you?

Although simply having a job is important, anybody who has ever been in a job that is genuinely making them miserable – that's as opposed to simply not liking it very much – will appreciate the idea of having the right job as being vital. And recent evidence suggests that being in the wrong job is a far from unusual situation. The government's Skills Commission's 2008 research showed that over forty percent of the British workforce believed they had been in the wrong job at some time; twenty percent said they were currently in such a situation; and it is estimated that, of the average working life, nearly five years is spent doing something unsuitable.

This is a state of affairs that, according to the Society for Human Resource Management, is on the increase. In their 2007 survey of recruitment companies and personnel offices, they concluded there had

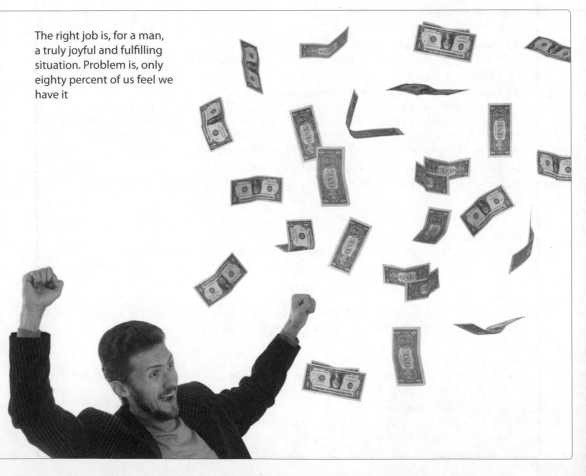

The right job is, for a man, a truly joyful and fulfilling situation. Problem is, only eighty percent of us feel we have it

been a 41 percent increase in staff turnovers, across the board, in the previous three years, and this trend looked set to continue. While the majority of reasons given for employees changing jobs were positive – promotion, more money, better environments and so on – the upsurge was being fuelled by people moving because they were dissatisfied with what they were doing. It seems that, almost as a backlash to the general reduction in job security in recent years, a growing segment of the workforce sees regularly changing employment as a natural state of affairs.

There is a modern generation of employees who see no reason to "put up" with a situation they're not entirely happy with, and as a result of the work/life balance swinging towards the former – simply because we spend more time at work these days – are likely to put personal satisfaction above financial reward or raised status. This applies to career switches too, which are becoming more and more commonplace.

Being in the wrong job, often without fully realizing it, can cause a huge amount of low- and high-level stress, because underutilization of your skills can only lead to frustration, as can being expected to perform tasks that are beyond you. And because you'll spend so much time at work,

T

Tip: Don't sweat the small stuff. Realize that a) some things simply aren't worth worrying about; b) some things you can't change, therefore stressing about them is pointless.

Is it worth it?

When clinically assessing your job's suitability, divide a blank sheet of paper into "For" and "Against" columns, and weigh it up. These are some of the points everybody should consider:

You dread Monday morning
You might not even realize you do, but if you are continually more tired than you should be on Monday mornings, it's because subtly increased stress levels mean you're not sleeping well on Sunday night.

Your firm's ambitions no longer measure up to your own
It can be damagingly frustrating to be stuck in a situation you believe will not allow you to progress to the level you aspire to.

You don't get along with your colleagues
Whether this is due to a different outlook on how the firm functions or you simply don't like each other, a lack of pleasant personal interplay at work can be wretched.

You don't feel as if you are being listened to
Everybody has ideas and some of them are good, so the people above you ought to hear you out. If your suggestions aren't being taken seriously it implies you aren't either.

"Decompression" when you leave for the day seems to be taking longer and longer
This can often lead to drinking too much, or can have an adverse effect on your domestic life if it means work-related problems come home with you.

You've hit the Glass Ceiling
They are very real, and if it seems like you've suddenly stopped progressing for no apparent reason you're probably squashed up against one.

How it all works: stress

When confronted with danger or entering a stressful situation, the senses – eyes, ears, touch etc – send sensory nerve impulses along the spinal cord and the brain stem, alerting the brain to what is happening. Once these signals have been processed within the brain stem, commands called autonomic nerve responses are sent back down the spinal cord (the central nervous system). Autonomic nerve fibres are part of the peripheral nerve system that connects the brain, via the spinal cord, to the body's internal organs and glands. The signals that run along them serve to regulate the body's internal environment. Autonomic nerve responses are not under our conscious control but operate purely on internal impulse, and fall into two categories, sympathetic and parasympathetic; the former prepares the body for action and the latter is a calming influence.

The sympathetic responses to stress cause the pupils to dilate to let in the maximum amount of light and promote clear vision, the bronchial tubes to open to allow the most air into the lungs, the stomach lining stops producing digestive enzymes and the liver releases extra glucose into the bloodstream for energy. None of this we have any control over, and is an instantaneous natural reaction. Most importantly, the sympathetic nerve impulses stimulate the adrenal gland, and its reactions form the driving force of our reaction to stress.

The adrenal gland sits on a cushion of fat on top of the kidneys, and under normal conditions plays a role in the production and deployment of energy, but in time of stress is pushed into overdrive. Its outer layer, the cortex, starts producing extra amounts of the corticosteroid hormones, one of

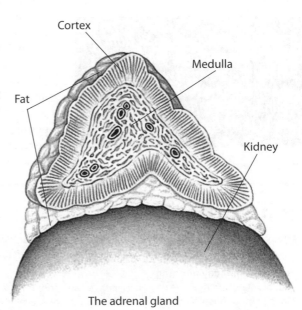

The adrenal gland

which is cortisol, also known as the "stress hormone". In normal circumstances our cortisol levels are highest in the early morning, as it helps us wake up, but now, in preparation for fight or flight, this amount will greatly raise the blood pressure, allow blood sugar levels to rise by increasing the breaking down of glycogen and has anti-inflammatory properties. The inner part of the gland, the medulla, releases the hormone epinephrine – adrenaline – which increases the heart rate and stroke volume, and boosts the supplies of oxygen and glucose to the brain and the muscles by constricting the blood vessels in the skin but dilating those in the muscles. It raises the levels of glycogen production in the liver and has a suppressive effect on the immune system, so no internal energy is being wasted.

The adrenal gland will keep these levels up as long as the brain continues to feel under threat, which is why chronic stress can be so physically damaging, but if the situation is resolved the parasympathetic responses kick in. They will constrict the pupils, contract the bronchial tubes, resume the production of stomach enzymes, reduce glucose levels and normalize activity in the adrenal gland.

having to do something you simply don't have any feel for or interest in is going to make your career path seem more like a prison sentence.

Signs can be apparent even before you start: if you don't hit it off with your prospective boss at the interview, the chances are you never will; if you are merely taking the job for the money or as a means to some other end, that is probably all you will ever get out of it; a lengthy commute certainly won't get any shorter when you're a few years older.

> **F**
>
> *Fact: Shift workers are much more likely to suffer from stress-related problems than other workers – fatigue, sleep and digestive disorders are widespread, relationships and social lives suffer, they have a much higher incidence of cardiovascular disease, and are likely to die younger.*

Feeling the pressure

During 2007, over a third of all new complaints treated by GPs were the result of work-related stress. Including depression and anxiety brought on by it, this meant a total of 13.8 million working days were lost due to stress, at a cost of almost £4 billion to the economy. In the US, it is estimated that occupational stress costs employers $200 billion per annum in terms of absenteeism, reduced productivity, frequent compensation payments, higher staff turnovers, and costlier health insurance. Sixty percent of American working days being lost are workplace stress-related, and it is reckoned that between seventy and ninety percent of all visits to healthcare providers, by men, are due to stress, though that is occupational and otherwise. The United Nations International Labor Organization is calling stress at work a "global epidemic".

These figures are set to carry on rising as we work longer hours, are expected to do more, enjoy less training and have lower

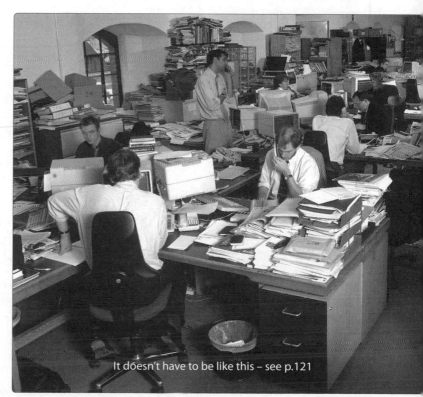

It doesn't have to be like this – see p.121

F

Fact: Work-related worries are the most common cause of chronic stress among men in both Great Britain and the US.

A

Expert advice: "Knowing if there is actually something specific wrong with you or if you are just stressed depends on how well you know your own body and psyche and their states of fitness. People need to take more interest in themselves when they are well, then they would be much more able to tell when something is not quite right – men are not very good at that. If you are worried or think something might be more than externally caused stress, you should go to your GP."
Dr Liliana Risi, GP

levels of job security. Also, work-related stress tends to have far greater effect on men than the domestic- or relationship-based varieties, as they are generally less in control of their own destiny than they are at home.

While positive pressure is a powerful motivator for either production or performance, this can easily tip over into the sort of stress that, although not actually an illness in itself, can set off both physical and mental ill health. Anxiety and depression are the two most obvious effects of stress

Eat to beat stress

Dr Sarah Schenker believes that today's convenience-food-heavy diet, especially during the working day, is a major factor in the escalating cases of work-related stress:

"People who feel they are suffering from stress or what they believe to be depression should look at their diets as the widespread state of low-level, background malnutrition can worsen the effects of fatigue which is a huge contributor to stress.

"You could just be slightly deficient in a few vitamins and minerals and you can adjust that by including a few more fruit and vegetables in your diet. It could be that you're eating a lot of energy-dense food – a lot of fatty, sugary foods – and you're beginning to put on weight which could easily have the effect of making you feel tired and stressed. So if you replace it with healthier food you'll soon start feeling more energetic.

"This is something you can't put your finger on and say it's because you're lacking this or you're lacking that, and that's why you feel fatigued and stressed; in fact you could go for all sorts of blood tests but they wouldn't show it up. It's an overall thing, which can be addressed by looking at what you're eating and working out if you are getting enough all-round nutrition to function at one hundred percent.

"Not drinking enough water is another major factor, especially with so many air-conditioned environments and people sitting in front of computer screens all day long – both of which can have a dehydrating effect. Being permanently mildly dehydrated often goes unnoticed, as it's not enough to make you feel thirsty all the time because your body has got used to it, but it's enough to make sure you're operating at maybe fifteen percent less than you could be. Then that becomes the new norm. It could be as simple as that form of chronic dehydration making you feel tired, lethargic and irritable, which will contribute greatly to your being stressed."

There's never any simple solution for work-related stress, but…

Cause of stress	An employee can	An employer should
Demands of the job	Not be afraid to ask questions or ask for help; receive and understand a detailed job description; prioritize tasks	Provide adequate training; make sure employee understands how best to carry out tasks; consider flexible working hours to relieve bottlenecks
Feelings of not being in control	Plan your working day more precisely; assume more responsibility – without treading on anybody's toes; organize your working environment; try to finish one task before starting another; resist perfectionism (but, obviously, still do the best you can)	Avoid unreasonable deadlines; provide a clear structure for career development; encourage smaller units of self-contained teamwork within a large workforce
Physical environment	Tidy up; stay fit and healthy; make whatever adjustments you can to heating, lighting or furniture; buy some plants	Listen to your employees if they say it's not right; renew worn-out equipment or furniture; decorate; buy some plants
Personal space/ workstation	Find out what their ideal working ergonomics should be and try to adhere to them (see p.127); keep it clutter-free and well organized; change positions frequently	Carry out regular workstation audits to make sure equipment is as posture-friendly as possible
Change – in routine or corporate policies	Ask questions of management rather than whisper in corners; put forward your own ideas about small changes; try and stay optimistic about change – men are actually far less keen on change than women	Improve communications; be transparent with employees about major changes; involve them in minor changes
Personal and professional relationships	Report any harassment or bullying – either experienced or witnessed; don't immediately blame others: you might be a pain to work with yourself; stay away from negative people	Take reports of harassment or bullying seriously; be prepared to intervene in personality clashes; pick your management team for people skills as much as work skills

Afternoon lows

So many of us, whatever job we're in, will experience mid-afternoon energy slumps, thanks to a combination of the body's circadian rhythm and a dip in blood sugar. It's a situation that can affect both your productivity and motivation, but one that can be addressed. To reduce the slump:

Eat less more often to even out your blood sugar levels throughout the day – huge, calorific lunches are pretty much a guarantee of afternoon drowsiness.

Mix lean protein and carbohydrate for most effective energy intake and management.

Try and get some exercise during the day – a brisk walk at lunchtime, for instance.

Don't attempt to beat the energy dip with caffeine, as any high gained will be followed by a crash later on.

Likewise, avoid sugary snacks or any empty calories.

Get a good night's sleep – every night.

and will impact on every aspect of your life, often resulting in drinking, taking drugs or eating disorders. Ongoing stress will also manifest itself in cardiovascular disease, as your system will be too pumped too often; digestive problems – irritable bowel syndrome is a favourite; back ache and other muscular complaints, because you will be physically tense much more than is good for you; and a general feeling of malaise as it will affect your immune system. If you are experiencing any of the above and the condition persists after you have taken steps to remedy it, it could be stress-related.

Get out of there

There are a number of things you can do to protect yourself as much as possible from occupational stress, among which eating healthily and making sure you are drinking enough water during the day is

Stress and the employer

As an employer you are legally obligated to treat stress like any other Health & Safety issue, and take all appropriate measures to avoid it among your workforce. Should an employee take you to court and prove the stress they suffered was preventable, there is no limit to the compensation that can be awarded. Normal sick leave rules must be applied to stress-related symptoms, and if you dismiss an employee because they have work-related stress, an employment tribunal will find you guilty of unfair dismissal unless you can irrefutably prove otherwise.

Although in the US there are no set-in-stone rules pertaining to corporate responsibilities as regards employees' work-related stress, it is an accepted condition and falls within the bounds of health and personal injury insurance. Thus legal action, taken by employees or by insurance companies against employers after they have paid out on claims resulting from occupational stress, is commonplace and usually successful. As a result, you will need to take work-related stress very seriously as regards health insurance plans, legal affairs and prevention of it. According to the US Department of Labor Bureau of Labor Statistics, nearly all companies offer access to free stress counselling for their employees, and over half of the major corporations in the US have stress counsellors on site.

Natural stressbusters

Supplement	Effect
St John's Wort	King Calm. Nature's most pacifying herb, containing hypericin which can act as an antidepressant
Ginko	Increases the blood flow through the brain to sharpen focus and improve memory
Calcium & magnesium	Helps muscles to relax
Chamomile	Soothes, calms and aids digestion
Celery juice	Lowers blood pressure and can lift the mood to alleviate anxiety
Valerian root	A mild sedative that will help you sleep and quietens the nervous system
Nutmeg	A slow-acting mild sedative that works like valerian root, but just takes longer
Kola nut	A minor stimulant, with mood-elevating properties – used to be found in Coca-Cola

where you should start (see box on p.120). Particular attention should be paid to the amount of water you are drinking, as the modern environment – centrally heated, air conditioned, often involving a computer screen – is dangerously dehydrating. And don't forget to keep an eye on the amount of coffee you are drinking, as not only is it a diuretic and therefore will speed up your drying out, but the caffeine will keep you on edge, which is never the most advisable way not to get stressed.

Beyond what you are eating is where you are eating it. The whole purpose of a lunch break was as much to do with the break as it was to do with the lunch. Although workplace culture seems to be dictating that more and more of us are wolfing down sandwiches at our workstations, the need to get a change of environment during the middle of the working day has never been greater. Getting some real, as opposed to recycled, fresh air will do wonders for your brain, and just looking at something else and interacting with different people will keep you alert. It also gives you the chance

A

Expert advice: "Lunchtimes are the ideal time to start working out. It's easy to schedule a half-hour programme three times a week, so you'll probably stick to it. Then exercising in the middle of the day will keep you from eating damaging food at lunch and because you've had your heart working hard it will boost your energy levels in the afternoon."
Gideon Remfry

F

Fact: You always know when you've had a good holiday, because you feel ready to come back to work.

to physically walk away from anything that might have been giving you a problem and either to think it through clearly (see box below) or think about something else. Then there's the physical exercise aspect of just walking about for a bit; it will get your blood flowing faster and should burn up a few calories.

Getting away from work for longer stretches than that is vital too. Holidays need to be taken for all the obvious positive benefits a vacation has to offer, but the time spent away from work gives you the chance to get it totally out of your system and reconnect with a few of the reasons you go to work in the first place – to have a good life outside it. Even if you just mooch about the house for a couple of weeks.

Try not to take your Blackberry or laptop or even your mobile phone away with you. Avoid the temptation to keep checking emails, or if for some reason you have to stay in touch, do so at predetermined times so you are not on permanent callout, possibly from another time zone. You will survive without your work, and, unless you're Mick Jagger or Jack Bauer, your work will survive without you.

Stress will affect everybody in different ways. There is no "cure" for stress as such and the only way to deal with it is to rectify the situation that is causing it (see p.121). Never be afraid to talk to somebody in a position to

T

Tip: Recent research has shown that music in the workplace increases productivity and reduces stress levels. Less straightforward though is making sure it's the right sort of music.

Learn to do nothing

One of the reasons we remain so stressed is we don't give ourselves time to think about what has happened that day. Dr Sandra Scott maintains this is a result of constantly stimulated lifestyles.

"Usually people do anything other than sit down and think, to simply be left alone with their thoughts, and it's removed a very important aspect of our lives.

"Downtime, when you come home at the end of a day, is very, very important, because you can come in wound as tight as a spring after the day from hell, and just sit on the sofa and go through it. Think about it, run through every bit of it, try and understand it, and while you may relive some of the pain that will still feel uncomfortable, and it will take a while to get to where you want to be, in the end you will feel a good deal better and probably sleep better.

"Now, because technological progress has made our lives so much quicker, many of us have been trained to believe that the smart option in these circumstances is to close the door with one hand, open the fridge with the other. Get out a bottle of wine, turn the television on and you've got over your day in a fraction of the time. Much more time efficient! That's as may be, but much less effective, as we have just put a big, great band aid on the problem and not really dealt with it at all. Things are still unresolved and that will be a big contributor to future stress as the problem continues to lurk under the surface. That half hour is so important, and it should be claimed back."

Office affairs ought to come with some sort of health warning, yet nearly half of us have had one

help – boss, union representative, personnel officer – about whatever is worrying you and try and keep your working day as ordered as possible: that way you'll feel more in control.

Sex and the city

According to recent research, four percent of us are enjoying an office romance at the moment, forty percent claim to have had one at some point and eleven percent claim they met their partner at work. Each figure is a considerable rise on a decade ago, and given that we are spending longer and longer

at work, this is hardly surprising. But it isn't simply down to the hours we work.

Work's increasing magnitude in our work/life balance means it's assuming a greater importance in everything we do. Notably among single men it's starting to become as central to their world as school will be to a child. This will often be emphasized by more flexible, relaxed and employee-centric work environments bringing the social aspects of going to work to the fore. Many firms actively encourage socializing and run out-of-office events in the name of team building, allowing colleagues to find out more about each other. Dress down Fridays play a large part in this, as these casually attired days allow another side of people to show through.

A work environment is actually the perfect dating agency, as it throws a group of similarly minded, similarly educated and similarly statused people together, then puts them under pressure for some of that time, meaning plenty of opportunity to look impressive. Indeed, getting together with somebody you work with is a far more appropriate way of starting a relationship than, say, meeting somebody in a disco where what they look like will probably be the sole deciding factor. Prospective couples will have already got to know each other without the immediate bother of trying to "pull" or be "pulled", thus the chances are they will actually like as well as fancy each other. Then there is that enormous advantage of knowing you have plenty in common and enough to talk about on a first date to avoid any awkward silences. Is it really any wonder office friendships so often turn horizontal?

If you are an employer

In spite of office romances seeming to make such good sense for employees, employers tend not to be so keen. In 2007, fourteen percent of all UK companies had policies seeking to prevent employee relationships. Although this number is falling it is for largely pragmatic reasons. Such a policy has questionable legality as it concerns what employees do in their own time; there is a growing acceptance that as working hours get longer so the workplace assumes a greater social responsibility; and it's more or less unenforceable.

As an employer, be aware of what is going on and that in most cases it will cause no problems whatsoever. Only offer advice should what's going on have a potential bearing on the firm – adultery or chain of command relationships. If it does go horribly wrong, and if that could threaten corporate harmony, be prepared to talk to both and shift one of them if necessary. But otherwise be secure in the fact that most of these turn out fine and may well result in two very happy – therefore productive – employees.

Is your chair killing you?

If you work in an office, the chances are you'll spend at least five hours a day sitting at

---

Office affairs – some points to consider

Don't assume nobody else has noticed. Body language or space-invading has probably meant it's been a talking point for weeks.

Beware of possible sexual harassment repercussions – apparently 25 percent of office affairs end in a sexual harassment accusation.

Avoid relationships with direct subordinates or superiors. No matter how the two of you may be careful for it not to affect the working relationship, it has the potential to cause enormous resentment among others – we are talking about people who will go into a strop because somebody else gets a stationery order filled first!

A messy break-up will be that much messier if you have to share a coffee machine or ride in a lift with your ex on a daily basis.

If the affair is adulterous be aware of a reaction from a wronged party that could end up in your place of work.

How it all works: the ergonomic workstation

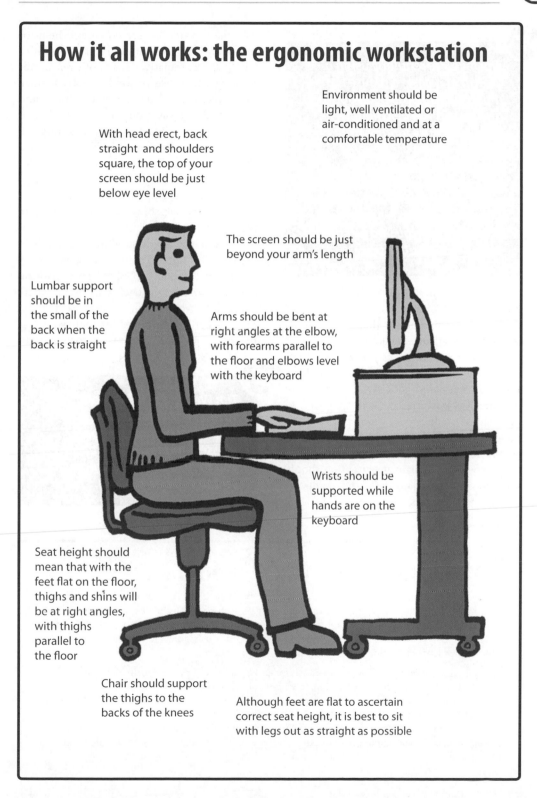

Environment should be light, well ventilated or air-conditioned and at a comfortable temperature

With head erect, back straight and shoulders square, the top of your screen should be just below eye level

The screen should be just beyond your arm's length

Lumbar support should be in the small of the back when the back is straight

Arms should be bent at right angles at the elbow, with forearms parallel to the floor and elbows level with the keyboard

Wrists should be supported while hands are on the keyboard

Seat height should mean that with the feet flat on the floor, thighs and shins will be at right angles, with thighs parallel to the floor

Chair should support the thighs to the backs of the knees

Although feet are flat to ascertain correct seat height, it is best to sit with legs out as straight as possible

> **T**
>
> *Tip: If you're regularly using a laptop at a desk, a mouse is a must, while a proper keyboard and screen will help hugely. This is because laptops aren't designed to be used over extended periods of time – two hours is supposed to be the limit – therefore they have had little attention paid to ergonomics and will push you into all sorts of unsuitable positions.*

your desk, probably in front of a VDU. And there's a good probability that it is this that is giving you all sorts of aches and pains, as poor office ergonomics is one of the major causes of work-related malaise. Indeed, shoulder, neck and backaches as the result of unhealthy posture contribute massively to headaches, tiredness and vision problems, as they are usually symptoms of impeded blood supply to the brain. To ensure you are not doing yourself any damage, attention should be paid to your chair, desk and computer screen arrangements.

The top of your screen should be at or just below eye level, and directly in front of you as the cumulative effects of even minor twisting can cause major lower back pain. The screen should be between eighteen and thirty inches away from you – just beyond your fingertips when you are sitting up straight is a rule of thumb. Your keyboard should be directly in front of the screen, with the mouse kept close to it on your dominant side. It is best to employ a wrist support that will mean the back of your hand is parallel to the desk when operating the mouse.

Your chair needs to allow you to sit in the Ninety Degree Position with your back flat against the chair back. This position means your upright back will be at ninety degrees to your thighs, which will be at ninety degrees to your shins with your feet flat on the ground. Adjust your chair's height

> **T**
>
> *Tip: Wearers of bifocal or varifocal spectacles should invest in a pair of "computer glasses" made up, that allow you to read at the distance your screen will be from you.*

Do you know what you're doing?

Being given an accurate, hard-copy job description when you start a new job can save a huge amount of grief further down the line. Knowing precisely what responsibilities and functions your position entails will enable you to approach it with a greater degree of confidence, meaning you will adjust to it quicker, and reduce any stress levels. Also, if you've got it all written down then there will be far fewer "But that's not my job"-type conversations.

Your job description should include the basis for and frequency of your performance reviews, what the salary range is for that position, to whom you will report and who will report to you. Also, be aware of what certain terms mean, and check that they are being applied correctly within your job description: job (an overall term for everything you have to do or are responsible for); task or function (an action or set of actions with a defined outcome); responsibility (making sure certain tasks or functions achieve their outcome, whether you actually do it or not); role (a set of responsibilities within a job).

and seat back angle to achieve this.

It is absolutely vital that the lumbar support in the back of the chair is snug to your lower back to relieve pressure from the base of your spine – if it is not, augment it with a cushion or a folded towel. The seat should firmly support the backs of thighs, with between two and four inches of space between its front edge and the backs of your knees.

If the chair has arms, they should be adjusted so that your shoulders are neither slouched nor raised when resting lightly on them, and this should be just below the level of the desk so your forearms angle upwards slightly. Don't rest your hands on the keyboard or the mouse when you are not actually using them.

Get up, move around and stretch as much as possible, paying particular attention to pulling the shoulders back to counteract the forward posture needed to operate a keyboard. Try "dynamic sitting" which is to deliberately alter your posture every half hour or so, in order not to remain in the same position for too long.

Tall men have big problems

If you are above average height, and in 2007 the average height for men over sixteen in the UK was 176.7cm (5 feet 10.9 inches), so much of the world won't be designed for you, particularly your workstation. Make sure your computer monitor is raised up to your eye level on a stand or a hutch, and your chair has back and shoulder support in the right places. Don't be tempted to adjust your viewing position by hunching your neck down into your shoulders, as over time this can push your top vertebrae together and will pinch nerves and gradually cut off blood

Six signs that say it might be time to look for another job

The company has stopped hiring and no longer seems to be growing
This is a sure sign that things aren't as comfortable for the firm as they once were.

Good work gets overlooked – not just yours
Everybody deserves praise for a job well done and encouragement to do even better. If this isn't part of your company's culture you can surely do better.

There is no promotion from within
If the firm is continually making management appointments from outside, they don't appear to trust their existing workforce.

Senior management is shifty about the future or the company's finances
While you can't expect everything to be totally transparent, you should be able to get straight answers to most questions.

Your colleagues seem to have as many problems as you
When that "quick drink after work" regularly degenerates into a marathon booze-sodden moan-fest, it's very likely everybody else is as fed up as you.

Everybody around you seems to be working longer and longer hours
But nobody seems to be getting any more out of the experience in terms of financial reward. This means your firm is quietly cutting back at its workforce's expense.

supply to your brain. Also, try and avoid chairs with high backs and protruding upper support sections, as they will pitch your shoulders forward. Stretching and moving your neck and shoulders on a regular basis will be particularly important for you.

Trouble at work

Nobody goes through their working life without having a few quite serious problems.

These could be anything from a bad boss or infuriating employees, to bullying or discrimination, or an unhealthy working environment. You may not want to look for a new job – indeed, why should you? – or your problem may not be that great, but still it needs to be resolved. While every problem and the people involved will be unique, there is a general procedure to be followed:

1. Work out exactly what the problem is

Make sure you are clear about who or what is

Make sure the next job's the right job

Once you decide you shouldn't be in a job, start looking for a new one as soon as possible. Even this by itself can make your working life more bearable, because at least you'll feel in control of your situation. Once you get beyond the theoretical and start applying for jobs or going for interviews, there are a few guidelines that can steer you towards the right one.

Know what you want and don't be afraid to talk about it

If you need specific hours, or have concerns over equipment, or want a certain amount of space, ask about it. Don't be shy about asking to see your potential environment, or for a rundown of what a typical corporate day involves, because then you can make your mind up and there will be fewer surprises after you start.

Don't worry about the interviewer liking you

An interview should be a two-sided affair and they should want you as much as you want the job, so give an honest-as-you-can account of yourself (see below) and be careful not to agree to or accept less than you had in mind because you think it will increase your chances of getting the job – it probably won't.

If it seems too good to be true it probably is

Too often the money/old rope transactions will turn out to be anything other than easy, and if a job offers a seemingly huge salary, the chances are you will earn at least that much in terms of sheer hard work, grief or ridiculous hours.

Keep it real

Be yourself at any interview, because if you start playing a part or get a job because they think you're somebody you're not, you'll have to keep that up for as long as you stay at the firm.

involved in your problem. This could mean making notes or writing things down more formally. This will force you into studying whatever it is and may lead you to a straightforward resolution.

2. Can it be sorted informally?

The next step will be to talk with somebody who is in a position to help, like your foreman, line manager or personnel officer. Although such a talk will be informal, you should take notes to refer to if you have to take it further.

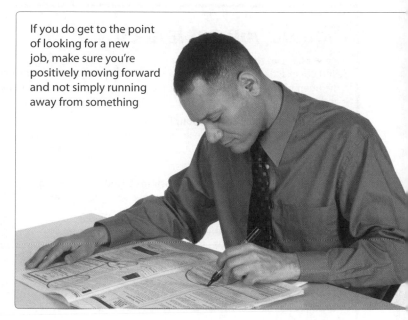

If you do get to the point of looking for a new job, make sure you're positively moving forward and not simply running away from something

3. Make a formal complaint

Should you go this far you will need to follow your company's grievance procedure – if you don't know what this is, ask for a copy. This will certainly involve making a written complaint that clearly and precisely explains your problem, and the best way to approach this is to set it out in bullet points. Once your employer has investigated the matter you should be called in for a formal hearing – it is a good idea to take somebody with you to this meeting, which is your statutory right.

4. Appeal

If you are dissatisfied with the result of this hearing it is your statutory right to appeal against it. This will usually mean having another hearing with a more senior manager.

Is everybody happy?

- 82% of men claim their jobs are adversely affecting their health.
- 30% say they have taken time off because they are stressed.
- 48% say it is adversely affecting their relationship.
- 42% describe their job as "stressful".
- 60% say their working hours are too long.
- 72% say they regularly work beyond their contracted hours for no extra reward.
- 35% say this is expected and would cause problems for them if they didn't.
- 50% of executives have left a job solely because of work-related stress.
- 93% say they work too hard.

Source: Skills Commission

Should you get laid off...

Make sure you get what's owed to you
Find out exactly what your employer should be giving you when you leave, then apply for all the unemployment benefits permissible – don't let any imagined stigma put you off: it's your entitlement.

Explain what's happened to your family
That includes the children who are old enough to understand, as they will be affected by this and dodging their questions or making excuses will only add to your stress levels.

Talk to your bank manager
The only thing banks like less than customers who never go into the red are unanswered letters. You may need extended credit facilities or rearranged payment schedules at some point, so it's best to keep your bank in the loop from Day One.

Keep to a regular schedule
Get up at a set time, do things to plan and generally try and keep as much structure to your day as possible. It will help you feel more in control of things. You'll also get a lot more done.

Stay busy
As well as job-hunting, CV-writing and contact-calling, do things around the house. You still need to work, regardless of whether you have a job or not.

Look on the bright side
Sounds trite, but it will greatly help your frame of mind if you look on this juncture as an opportunity to advance your life either by learning a new skill, getting a new job or simply reconnecting with your family.

---

5. Outside arbitration

Beyond your own company's grievance procedures, or if you have been dismissed, there are a number of impartial third parties that can be involved. Conciliation or arbitration services will be potentially less expensive than employment tribunals or civil courts, and you should consult your local Citizens Advice Bureau as to which would be most suitable for your case.

Going it alone

If you do decide you've had enough of working for The Man and opt to become your own boss you've probably already got to the point at which you've had that brilliant idea, found the gap in the market, written your business plan and got a very understanding bank manager. Now you have to embrace officialdom in the form of registering your business for tax, and any trademark/patent

registration to stop you being ripped off. The most reliable way to do this is through the services of an accountant and a solicitor specializing in these areas. Although this may seem like a(nother) unnecessary expense, a) it probably isn't what you're good at; b) a professional will cover every aspect; and c) you have far too much else to be getting on with at the moment.

During the course of your business your accountant will become your best friend, but use him sparingly and save yourself money by doing as much of the bookkeeping as you can yourself. Don't simply send him a carrier bag full of receipts and invoices. Be warned though, if you don't feel your accountant is giving you the best service, sack him. There are plenty more out there.

That was the easy bit. Now comes harder work and longer hours than you ever imagined. You'll need to be at the beck and call of customers (existing or potential)

24 hours a day and remain self-motivated at all times. There will be more grounds for divorce than you knew existed and a possible level of stress that would give the Dalai Lama pause for thought. However, all of this will be massively offset by the fact that you are as in control of your own destiny as possible, and all the rewards for your graft or ideas or innovations will come directly to you.

All work and no play

The last twenty years have been very tough on men in their working lives. During that time, in almost every area, the landscape has changed to such an extent it's unlikely our fathers would even recognize it. Short-term contracting, telecommuting, hot-desking, video-conferencing, globalization, flexi-time… these are just a few examples of what has conspired to make these changes in the name of something called "progress".

Problem is, the other thing that's been gaining ground is our stress level as we have less and less time to escape from work – either figuratively or psychologically – and so less time to relieve its pressures. Later in the chapter we'll look at what harm work-related stress can do, and how specific examples can be addressed, but the biggest contributor towards overall chronic stress is a skewed work/life balance.

This is frequently occurring in today's frantically paced world as information technology has meant we are expected to be contactable at any time. Globalization's different time zones has expanded the working day, while longer hours have become

T

Tip: If you work from home, keep regular office hours for starting and finishing your day and for lunch; it will stop you blurring the edges between your domestic and professional lives.

Are you one of life's employers or employees?

You should be an employer if you	Or an employee if you
Don't take orders very well	Can make the most of other's ideas or instructions
Assume responsibilities and leadership	Offer valuable support to the decision-making process
Are willing to be hugely flexible when it comes to dealing with problems	See things from a more tightly focused point of view, rather than taking in the big picture
Are a "people person"	Don't feel too confident telling others what to do or that they have made mistakes
Can work or make decisions on your own	Function best as an integral part of a larger unit
Don't mind being the buck's last stop	Like to go home at six o'clock, firmly closing the workplace door behind you

Self-employed pros & cons

Follow your dream	Don't give up the day job
Far more direct effort/reward ratio	Irregular income
Hours to suit	All the hours God sends
You are in charge	There is nobody else to blame
Immense self-satisfaction	Massive frustration if things don't go to plan
No good idea or innovation will go unlistened to	There is nobody to save you from yourself if you get something very wrong
Independence	Stress of shouldering total responsibility
Control over your future	Start up costs
The chance to acquire new skills	Often you'll have to do everything
Potential for vast wealth	Possibility of bankruptcy

par for practically everybody's working course. It means work is taking over the time we spend doing fun and family things and has become a double-edged sword: as the amount of time we have to devote to work-related issues goes up, we need more time away from it to recover, but that side of our lives is actually being reduced.

Retune your work/life balance

The only way to put this right again is to reorganize your approach to all aspects of your life, and, paying particular attention to how you can reduce the work-related side, regain control of how it all adds up. But to do that you've got to be aware of what's going on, so keep a diary. Yes, this seems to figure in the answer to pretty much everything, but that's because it works – to find out how to change your life you need to know exactly what's going on in it. Over the course of a month, log what you do and how and where you do it on a week-by-week basis, then examine it, maybe with

your life partner, to work out what can be redressed.

How to cut back

Better organization and time management, and clearer communications will help enormously to cut the amount of time spent on mundane tasks – being able to find things, having people understand you, not being late, prioritizing your To Do list will cut the time spent not actually achieving anything. Don't confuse working late with getting a great deal done as the more tired you get the slower you will be working, and usually it's best to pack up for the day and start again tomorrow, properly refreshed.

In your domestic life, split housework to do a little every day rather than spend half the weekend on it, invest in a few labour-saving devices and try and do errands all together instead of rushing in and out on your free days. It's best to treat housework like work – as something else that can encroach on time you could be enjoying yourself.

Delegate as much as you can in both your work life and your life-life, so you

Dress down Friday: treat or tyranny?

As your own style reveals much more about you than the standard dark suit, for many dress down Fridays have become a sartorial minefield, meaning far more stress than was ever the intention.

Stick to what you are comfortable in, but be careful about just how casual "casual" actually is. Look on it as going to a new restaurant – you don't want to get sat near the toilets for rocking up like a beach bum or pointed at from behind menus for looking too posh. Follow the lead of those who have been at the firm longer than you and dress to their level, but don't let this become a second uniform of clothes you'd never normally be seen dead in or you'll resent it more than wearing a suit. And never ever show off with expensive designer labels or people will start to resent you. Blend in and let your performance stand out.

don't do more than you need to. At work trust other people to take their share of the workload – this will improve relations with those around you, as it's fairly insulting to be saying that the only way anything will get done is if you do it. This means take a day off if you're not well, as the world won't come to a halt and you are doing nobody any favours spreading germs and bad vibes among your co-workers. On the home front, assuming you earn more than a cleaner/painter/decorator/window cleaner/gardener, it will make sense for you to farm those tasks out, freeing up valuable time to spend with

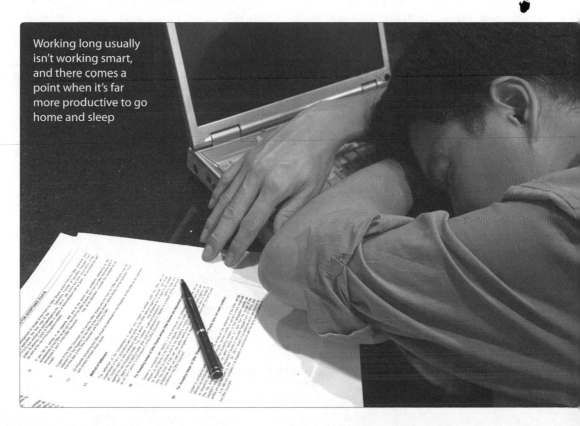

Working long usually isn't working smart, and there comes a point when it's far more productive to go home and sleep

your family or on relaxing leisure pursuits.

Explore your options and find out what your firm offers in the way of flexible hours or working from home, and if this cuts down on time spent at work or travelling to work then take advantage of it.

Rein in that ego which can so often find you refusing to quit under impossible circumstances. Men, in particular, are loath to admit they can't do something or they need help, and will often feel the need to prove they are working harder than those around them. Even in today's cut-throat corporate culture, where we are led to believe that results must be achieved at any cost, it pays enormously to work smart not hard.

What to boost up

Set aside "me time" (which could equally be Family Time) during the working week, in which the email, the mobile and the computer are all switched off and work cannot find a way through to you. At first it will feel like you're playing truant, and you might get a bit twitchy, but ride it out. This time should be reserved for something that will relax you – five-a-side football, taking the kids swimming, watching a couple of DVDs with your partner, dinner with your dad… anything – but make sure you keep that time sacred.

Learn to enjoy doing nothing, and don't spend time off looking for things to do, or, worst of all, feeling guilty about just sitting about. As regards people around you, if you start appearing unoccupied and relaxed, your family will find it much easier to approach you, meaning all sorts of fun will follow.

Do something you've always fancied doing, like learning the trumpet or playing golf or evening classes in joinery or training to run a marathon. If you thrive on challenges, which is probably why you are so involved with your job in the first place, set yourself goals that can involve family and friends, will be enjoyable, develop a new skill and only put you under as much pressure as you want. Just remember, it's supposed to be fun and you don't have to turn yourself into Miles Davis or Tiger Woods.

Make some friends, as everybody needs

The testosterone myth

Since the 1980s the popular image of striped-shirted City traders "knocking down" serious money in testosterone-fuelled dealing rooms has driven the notion that only men could function effectively in such a high-pressure environment. However, research at Cambridge University has found that men are far more likely to get it wrong under these circumstances than women, and that excessive production of the hormones testosterone and cortisol can actually play their part in market fluctuations.

The findings were that when traders go on successful runs, their testosterone soars on a level similar to a winning sportsman, leading to a feeling of invincibility and increased risk-taking – many talked of "being in the zone". This state was found to seriously impair their decision-making abilities, leading to bigger and increasingly unwise trading. Then once things started to take a downward turn, the stress hormone cortisol kicked in to counteract this recklessness and reverse the situation. The same traders would then refuse to take any chances, which would manifest itself in their opting for secure, unprofitable deals, or even not dealing at all. As a result, any downturn of the market would start to accelerate.

The conclusion was that women traders, whose behaviour would not be influenced by such hormone surges, could go a long way to creating a more stable economic climate.

How to choose a life coach

Go for one with International Coach Federation (ICF) credentials. This is the governing body of professional coaches and sets practice and ethics guidelines.

Talk to several and only consider those you have a good rapport with, as you will have to share a great deal with them.

Opt for a full-time life coach, rather than one who does it as a hobby.

Look for experience, as the more situations they have had to deal with the more knowledge they will have to bring to yours.

Make sure they are very clear about what they offer in terms of time and commitment, and how long they expect you to commit for – three months is the ideal initial period.

a support system and it might not always be your family. Making friends will also expand your take on the world in general, as you'll see other people live their lives and it may affect how you approach your own.

Get some sleep. Everything looks better and it's much easier to behave rationally when you're well rested.

Boardroom benefits

As an employer, paying attention to your employees' work/life balance and helping them keep it on track will have huge benefits.

T

Tip: Don't be a slave to your Blackberry or your iPhone or whatever. While they undoubtedly have all sorts of exciting leisure-time-related features, don't allow yours to shackle you to the office. It was only 25 years ago that cassette-loaded telephone answering machines were an optional extra and your world didn't grind to a halt if people had to phone you back later in the day, a principle that still pretty much applies.

A contented, less-stressed workforce will give you increased productivity as they will be more motivated, meaning reduced staff turnover and improved recruitment. Timekeeping will be better, absenteeism will go down and those who have to interact with customers or other companies will be more enthusiastic about what they have to get across.

Of course this won't happen by itself. You should consult with your staff on a regular basis to find out what they want, pay attention to what goes on in firms similar to yours and support your management to make sure changes are implemented as intended. If successful it will do wonders for your stress levels as well.

Life coaches: indispensable or inconsequential?

Life coaching has attracted more than its share of bad press over the last decade or so, but beneath the obvious accusations of superfluous, Californianized mumbo-jumbo, and worries about the lack of regulation, there is a lot of benefit to be had. Especially by men, as they are far more likely to engage a life coach than they are to enter psychotherapy – sixty percent of those in psychotherapy are women; seventy-five percent of life coach clients are men.

The main difference between psychotherapy and life coaching is that the former tends to focus on the past, whereas the latter looks forward to where you should be in the future. A good life coach will be far more than an expensive personal cheerleader, and should become a dedicated mentor advising you on all matters business and personal. They should help you reach decisions needed to determine and achieve your best goals and, importantly, give you somebody to talk to if things are getting a bit frustrating. It's a bit like having a best friend who actually knows what they're talking about and you don't have to worry about imposing on.

Look upon it as calling in an expert – a bit like phoning a plumber if your hot water system's on the blink.

The best of the web

berr.gov.uk
Formerly the DTi, this is the Department for Business, Enterprise and Regulatory Reform, very useful for both employers and employees as regards to rights, legislation and advice, in the UK and internationally.

cdc.gov/niosh/stresswk
The National Institute for Occupational Safety and Health offers a comprehensive online booklet to help identify, cope with and prevent work-related stress from an employee's point of view. Although an American publication, the practical advice is relevant on both side of the Atlantic.

worklifebalance.ie
Irish-based site that will answer any question you have about how work/life balance can be adjusted within your working life.

healthatwork.org.uk
An NHS-run site dedicated to promoting health and well-being in the workplace.

businesslink.gov.uk
Operating with the Business Link National Contact Centre this offers a wealth of information that will be vital to anybody considering starting up a small business.

hse.gov.uk/stress
Particularly good when offering advice on work-related stress – for both employees and employers – the government's Health & Safety Executive has much information about the working environment.

whmrc.gov.uk
The website of HM Revenue & Customs provides much more than information about tax schedules, and is packed with advice for the self-employed.

coachfederation.org
The International Coach Federation is the professional body that sets the standards and accredits life coaches. If you are considering hiring one this is the best place to start.

dol.gov
The US Department of Labor website has comprehensive advice on US labour laws and workplace ethics for both employers and employees.

Ten top tips for a less stressful working life

▶ **Tidy up your personal space**
Your life will be so much easier if you can find things quickly, and being surrounded by clutter will not help you think in an ordered way.

▶ **Don't be late** Not only will you have less time for whatever it is you have to do, you will be starting on the back foot and you will hugely irritate those around you – why should your time be more important than theirs?

▶ **Ask for help if you need it**
Everybody needs help at some point and it's certainly not a "sign of weakness" if it means you get the job done to the required standard.

▶ **Take time off if you are sick** You are not indispensable – nobody is – and those around you would much rather you stayed at home than dragged your semi-functioning, germ-ridden self into work.

▶ **Set achievable goals**
There is nothing more frustrating than a lengthy To Do list that gets moved over to the next day time after time after time, as you end up spending the evening thinking about what you didn't do rather than what you achieved.

▶ **Don't let emotions influence professional decisions** If you do they will seldom be the best ones you've ever made, and while it may have been cathartic to write that blistering email, don't actually send it until you've calmed down and read through it again.

▶ **Have a life outside work** You will physically feel better, your family will enjoy your time spent with them and it will help you keep what it is you actually do in perspective.

▶ **Don't take too much crap**
If something or somebody is making your life a misery don't suffer in silence, do something about it. Start by talking to your boss or your personnel officer.

▶ **Get out of there** Physically leaving your workplace at lunchtime, and getting a change of scenery and faces works wonders.

▶ **You can always get another job** Very few people are actually being forced to stay somewhere that's stressing them out on a daily basis and you're probably not one of them. Sometimes even the mere act of looking for another job will make you feel better.

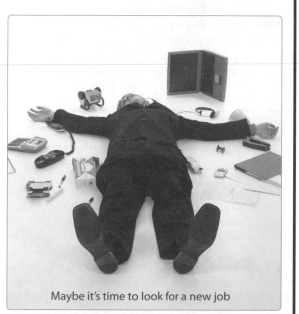

Maybe it's time to look for a new job

In the bedroom

Given the amount of time the average man is supposed to spend thinking about sex – around ten percent of his waking life if statistics are to be believed – it's surprising how little so many of us actually understand about it. However, it's all pretty straightforward and it's not at all difficult to get so much more out of it.

Sex on the brain

Within today's cultural and social climate, we are a long way removed from the notion of sex as purely a matter of procreation. Indeed it's almost become a sport – participant and spectator – but one with an apparently limitless series of arcane rules.

While this can be a great deal of fun for all involved, it also means that many of us spend a great deal of time not so much thinking about sex as worrying about it.

Am I getting enough? How do I know if she wants it? Is my technique good enough? Will I stay hard enough long enough? It's a vicious circle: the worry of it all contributes to the stresses and pressures of modern life, which in turn start affecting how you make out in the bedroom. Which in itself might give you even more to worry about.

While it's impossible to dispel all those anxieties, understanding what's going on will make everything much more relaxing. Besides, it can be that fear of the unknown that adds an enjoyable spice to your sex life.

The pleasure principle

The reason orgasms are so pleasurable – for women as well as men – is, simply, to encourage us to have more of them. It's been that way since Neanderthal times, and is a basic part of the brain's "reward pathway". This is a neurological network, hard-wired to guarantee the survival of the species and ensure that pleasurable feelings result as a consequence of us doing something beneficial. Because an orgasm is the natural conclusion of the act that's fundamental to mankind's perpetuation, the pleasure produced is on a higher level to anything else. It needs to be that good so that we want to do it again.

The orgasm achieves its goal by sending levels of dopamine – the pleasure and desire chemical – soaring in the brain, which stimulates nerves to tingle all over the body. It also communicates, via a pathway in the brain called the "limbic system", with the prefrontal cortex, allowing the sensation to be etched on to the memory.

How it all works: sex

Men can produce about 120 million sperm a day, and each takes around two and a half months to fully develop, to the point at which it contains 23 chromosomes, half the genetic material required to build a person. Sperm are made in the seminiferous tubules, about a thousand tiny tubes coiled inside the testes, which, if you laid them out end to end would measure around five hundred metres. Until they are called upon, sperm are stored in the epididymis, a large coiled duct attached to the back of the testes.

To keep all this working as efficiently as possible, the testes need to be at a temperature of around 34°C (92.2°F), slightly below body temperature. This is why, although the testes are internal organs, they need to hang outside the body in the scrotal sac, forming the testicles. The body works hard to maintain the correct scrotal temperature, shrinking the sac to draw them closer to the body if they get cold – in the swimming pool, for instance – and, when they get too warm, relaxing the surrounding muscles to allow the testicles to hang further away from the body – like when you're in the shower.

Seminal vesicle, where sperm and semen are mixed

Vas deferens, the tube that carries sperm from the testes and is cut for a vasectomy

Bladder

Rectum

Long coils of epididymis, where sperm grow

One of two testes, where sperm are produced

Spongy erectile tissue

Urethra, through which urine or semen are released

As a sex act comes to a climax, the testes expand to around twice their normal size and sperm are pushed out of the epididymis, up the vas deferens tube to the twin sacs that are the seminal vesicles. There they mix with seminal fluid to form the milky semen. Seminal fluid is produced within the vesicles and by the adjacent prostate gland. Healthy semen contains around fifty million sperm per millilitre, and around 75 percent of these should be alive, with the majority of these having normal shape and showing forward movement.

From there the semen is pushed to the ejaculatory duct, where it will be moved into the urethra – this tube will previously have been cleansed by a small emission of seminal fluid, as any traces of urine might kill the sperm. Ejaculation itself is triggered as contractions of the pubococcygeus muscle – the same one you clench to lift the erect penis – the anal sphincter and the rectum combine to push the semen through the urethra and out of the end of the penis.

The average ejaculation is between 2ml and 5ml of semen, and can contain up to 250 million sperm. In the case of unprotected sex, only about two hundred of them would make it to the egg. The rest get lost or die somewhere along the hour-long journey to the fallopian tubes.

Standing up for yourself

Given the right stimulation you'll get an erection. And although the images or sensations that brought it on in the first place will be a matter of personal preference, once it gets stirring there isn't much you can do to control it.

The hard facts

The need to reproduce is such a fundamental part of our make-up that it's really no more sophisticated than a deep-seated, undeniable urge to impregnate any fertile female we might stumble across while out hunting woolly mammoths. Of course, self-control usually gets the better of our inner caveman, but evidence of our primeval past can still, quite literally, rear up in the form of an inappropriate erection.

Erections happen because, initially, the brain has absorbed an image or sensation it perceives to be so pleasurable it can be filed away as erotic. During adolescence these associations can be pretty random and not necessarily conventionally sexy – smoking a cigarette, seeing your team score a vital goal – but the brain soon starts to filter them. As you grow older thoughts sufficient to produce an erection become almost exclusively related to sex and become a matter of refined personal taste – i.e. your "type".

Once this stimulation has been processed the brain sends messages to the nerves around the base of the penis – this is the first stage of a man's erotic auto-response – and will be registered as that tingling in the

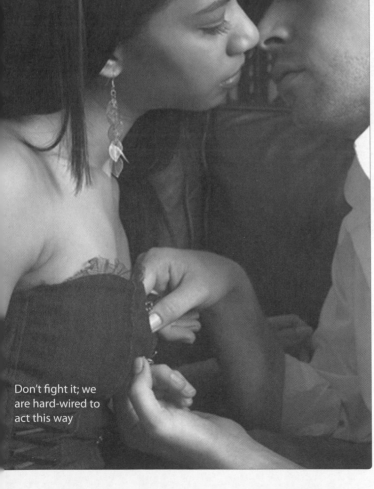

Don't fight it; we are hard-wired to act this way

loins. These impulses then relax the muscle fibres that are inside the penis, surrounding the corpora spongiosa and the two corpus cavernosum. These are tubes of spongy tissue running the entire length of the penis. The former is central and surrounds the urethra, with the latter positioned along each side. Once the muscles are sufficiently slack they allow the tissues to fill with blood, up to eight times as much as would be there when the penis is flaccid. This engorging with blood is the second stage, and what actually causes the erection.

An erection will be maintained because veins and arteries that would allow this blood to flow out of the penis have been blocked by a combination of stretched internal tissue and the contraction of pelvic floor muscles around the base of the penis. These will keep blocking the blood's return as long as the brain remains stimulated and is sending out the necessary arousal signals.

Once the stimulation is withdrawn, or you have reached orgasm, the messages from the brain change, relaxing the muscles at the base of the penis and contracting the muscle fibres within. This releases the pressure on veins and arteries, allowing the blood to flow away; the erection will immediately start to go down.

After orgasm and the deflation of your erection, the vast majority of men will not be

The most likely causes of erectile dysfunction

Diabetes
Heart disease
Obesity
High blood pressure
Smoking
Drinking
Stress
Unhappiness with your partner (either temporary or long term)
Fatigue

able to get another one immediately, as the body goes into a refractory phase. During this time it will be normalizing itself after the rigours of orgasm, and will not respond to stimulation until it has done so. This period will be at least ten to fifteen minutes, and becomes longer as you get older.

Er, that's never happened before

Every man will experience some sort of penile malfunction at some point, and as inconvenient or embarrassing as it might be it isn't really that much to fret about. There is no clinically defined line between "I couldn't get it up last night" and "You have a serious problem". However, a general rule of thumb is that if it persists, or is affecting you more than fifty percent of the time and you have ruled out the factors discussed below then you should seek professional help. From a healthcare professional that is.

However, for the majority of men who experience erectile dysfunction (ED) at some point, there are a number of factors to be considered before calling the doctor.

A

Expert advice: "Ejaculations are good to keep the prostate healthy. A recent study at the University of Edinburgh showed that men who had been ejaculating at least three times a week, whether it was having sex or masturbation, developed far fewer prostate problems."
Sarah Hedley

T

Tip: If you are in a stable relationship and are going to see your doctor to discuss erectile dysfunction, take your partner with you. It will greatly assist your doctor's assessment of the issue if both views can be considered.

Don't think about it

Back when ED was called impotence, it was reckoned to be almost exclusively a psychological problem, and although more recently it's been accepted that this is far from the case, a significant amount of it will be in your head. The series of messages and triggers to and from the brain that lie at the core of your arousal are such a complex, highly focused succession of impulses that it doesn't take much to throw them out of whack. Stresses or worries you thought you'd left on the other side of the bedroom door are a major factor, as they will be lurking somewhere in your grey matter, interfering with what you ought to be thinking about. While this can be a temporary situation, linked to equally momentary anxieties, chronic stress will bring about persistent erectile issues, and the only true remedy is to address the causes of the stress.

Erectile dysfunction can also become something of a self-fulfilling prophecy, as immediate worries about getting an erection will affect you in exactly the same way as underlying stresses about work or home life. Nervousness with a new partner or anxiety about being able to "perform" can create a vicious circle of flaccidity, whereby the worry works against the erection, causing more worry, leading to a softer penis … and nothing will disturb your internal erotic rhythms more than attempting to gain an erection by sheer force of will.

Simply relax, your partner ought to understand and help you, and, importantly, although it's always a blow to the pride, don't get so caught up in your own distress that you forget there's two of you taking part. Of course, that could be the cause of the problem: if you don't actually fancy the one you're with, or it's a long-term partner you're upset with, very often your body just won't respond.

The lowdown on brewer's droop

Even with the bottled water industry booming to a degree that your parents' generation would find bizarre, a few alcoholic drinks may well be what got you into bed with whoever in the first place. But there is a limit to how much "getting in the mood" you should be getting out of a bottle. Although it affects everybody differently, as relative to their metabolism and cardiovascular capabilities, hard drinking can mean a soft penis because alcohol increases the volume of blood in your system, depending on how much you've had of it. Although this might seem to be a good thing – the more blood in your penis the harder you'll stand, surely? – it will raise your blood pressure and widen your veins, meaning it becomes increasingly difficult to keep the veins and arteries in your penis closed during the period of arousal. Thus, blood will be allowed to flow out almost as readily as it flowed in, and any stiffness you might achieve will not be easy to maintain.

How much is too much will be a matter of personal experience, and as the only guaranteed way to avoid the droop is not to go over your limit, if you think sex is on the cards then stop drinking. Go on to water, as this will help flush your system out and, being less dehydrated, you'll feel much better in the morning.

Unsympathetic situations

Just as it seems to adversely affect practically everything else, today's lifestyle can also be detrimental to your erection. Obesity is a prime cause of dysfunction, as the extra strain on the cardiovascular system can prevent an efficient delivery of blood to the penis when required; what's more, the attendant high blood pressure will hinder your body's ability to keep blood in the penis to maintain any stiffness. Heart disease is also linked with ED, as deposits in your arteries, or blood pressure problems, can interfere with the blood flow needed to maintain an erection. Likewise, it is a common side effect

Have better sex. For longer.

Something as simple as strengthening and learning to control your pelvic floor muscles can massively increase the duration and enjoyment of your love-making. Sarah Hedley explains how an easy exercise, performed on a regular basis, can have the same effect as Viagra, but doesn't involve buying anything from dodgy websites.

"Pelvic floor exercises were always the domain of women – once you get to thirty, after childbirth and so on, the pelvic floor weakens – however, a study at the University of Bristol in 2004 showed how much benefit they can bring to men. Developing those muscles can help you control ejaculation and lead to multiple orgasms as it will be possible to achieve the sensation of orgasm without actual ejaculation. It crosses over with the Tantric theories in the sense that if you can control the pipework down there then you can control the actual ejaculation and no longer depend on it to achieve the sensation of orgasm. Then, because you haven't ejaculated, your erection won't go down and you can do it again and again. In terms of performance anxiety, premature ejaculation or not being able to get it up in the first place, this can have the same effect as Viagra without the side effects.

"You isolate the muscle that you use to stop yourself peeing midflow, but you have to make sure you genuinely isolate it – it's important that you don't clench the arse, the thighs or the abdomen, so you focus purely on the pelvic floor muscle. Then once you've isolated it you squeeze and lift the muscle – you should be able to feel your testicles pulling up. Once you've worked out how to do that – and it might take some time – then start doing the movement in sets, just like you would any other exercise. It's best to vary how you do it: ten slow ones followed by five rapid clenches, then repeat that set three times. The next time you do it, build up from that.

"You're supposed to do them every day, but I never advise anybody to do it every day because that puts pressure on them and they will be less likely to continue long term. Just as long as you build up what you are doing, it's probably a good idea to set targets of what you want to achieve."

Age and the erection

The likelihood of experiencing some degree of erectile dysfunction increases in direct relation to your age, as will the frequency and scale of the issue – from minimal through to complete. A forty-year-old man has a forty percent chance of experiencing some ED, an eighty-year-old man has a seventy-five percent chance of experiencing moderate to complete ED, and the probability travels up a sliding scale in between. Of course, extraneous factors such as circulatory problems, lower testosterone levels or taking medication are also more prevalent in an older age group and can play a significant role in the problem.

of diabetes, as the nerve and blood vessel damage that the condition can cause works against the whole erection process.

Certain medications can bring on ED too. The most common offenders are blood pressure treatments, antihistamines, antidepressants and tranquilizers. If you are experiencing difficulties since being prescribed a particular drug, talk to your doctor as soon as possible but don't stop taking the medication. Injury or surgery to the spine or pelvic area can raise the chances of erectile dysfunction too, as either could cause damage to the nerves needed to set an erection off.

Environment can also contribute, and while particular locations – pub toilet, stationery cupboard, mother-in-law's spare room – might turn some people on, they can have the opposite effect on others. And as much as impromptu, alfresco sex might seem like a good idea, if it's a bit chilly don't expect an enormous erection, because when your body gets cold, blood will be diverted away from the extremities to keep the vital organs warm. It's why your hands and feet get disproportionately cold, and why your body won't give priority to delivering the blood needed to raise an erection. This can apply to cold bedrooms as well.

Or it could be your fault

Keeping yourself fit will maximize your chances of healthy erections, as your cardiovascular system will be operating to the best of its ability. Though don't overdo it, as over-exercising can bring on fatigue which in turn can cause ED. Stay away from anabolic steroids, which can lead to erectile dysfunction, with the awkward side effect of increased sexual desire.

F

Fact: Fifteen percent of British men are infertile, yet only half of that number has sought help.

Morning glory, what's the story?

The full name for it is "nocturnal penile tumescence" and it's less to do with sexual arousal than the need to go to the toilet. During a decent night's sleep the average man will get three or four erections lasting about half an hour each, with the last one happening near the end of the sleep cycle. While that is occurring, though, the bladder becomes full enough to press against the base of the penis, preventing the blood that has flowed in (to bring on the erection) from being able to flow out again. It will stay like that until you get to the toilet, where you can watch it go down as you urinate. But if your partner thinks it's for them, there's probably no need to disillusion them about this notion.

Alcohol won't help either (see box on p.144) and the damage smoking can do to your arteries means heavy smokers are far more likely to experience ED than those who don't. Marijuana acts as a suppressant on the central nervous system, as do other opiate recreational drugs; these all interfere with the signals that trigger an erection. Apparently the effects can be cumulative, which makes you wonder how Bob Marley managed to father so many children.

Cocaine and other amphetamines will increase the user's feelings of attractiveness and potency in general, but will also cause blood vessels to constrict, limiting the volume of blood that can be pumped into the penis, and increasing blood pressure – meaning it will be more likely to flow back out again. Cocaine also delivers the double whammy of interfering with the production of enzymes that contribute to the erection process.

It doesn't have to ruin your night

If you do get yourself into a situation where it's obvious that you're not going to rise to the occasion, get creative and make foreplay last until you can perform. Or really go to town

Don't believe the hype

Sex surveys can do more harm than good, as they can put added pressure on people and, as Sarah Hedley knows, not everybody who fills them in is being scrupulously honest.

"Everybody likes to fill in these surveys and say 'Oh we do it at least three times a week', but so often that isn't the case – people's libidos, especially men, taper off as a relationship progresses or as they get older. However, because people read these surveys and take them seriously there follows a tendency for both men and women to tell each other 'Yeah, that's what I do, too' because nobody wants to be singled out as not being normal or not up to speed. And as a result, the idea that you're not actually doing it as much as everybody else can be quite intimidating."

"People need to ignore the stats and your sex life should be about an individual level that you are happy with. Then you can talk to your partner to find a level that satisfies you both. What is far more important than how many times you are doing it, is to balance that with how many times does your partner want to do it. You have to talk about that, and be honest about how much each of you wants to do it, and if you have a mis-matched libido – which 99 percent of couples do – then the issue is how you deal with that, not how many times you think you ought to be doing it. And the only way you can do that is to talk about it frankly.

"For instance, if one partner wants to masturbate because they're not getting enough sex, but that masturbation makes them feel dirty or the other partner thinks it's wrong then you have issues which are as much psychological as they are physical. You need to find a balance between you and your partner and that's far more involved than looking externally and blindly trying to keep up with what you might read about in a magazine. Sexual happiness is about not being stressed, so if anything you are doing in the bedroom is causing you stress then it isn't a good idea. If you and your partner have settled into doing it once a fortnight and you're both happy with that, then why should you care about what other people are doing?

"Part of the stress is that we – men especially – tend not to talk about anything that might cast doubt on our sex abilities so it gets swept under the carpet, even when it comes to talking to our partners. But maybe she's totally happy with just doing it once a fortnight, so trying to raise the frequency could be the cause of a potential problem. The point is to encourage communication between two people about what they want in order to achieve their sexual happiness, rather than trying to please or keep up with the rest of the world."

and turn the supporting feature into the main event; the worst thing you can do is make a big deal out of not getting an erection, as the added stress will do nothing to help.

Every sperm is sacred

It may seem remarkable that while the world's population size is spiralling out of control, sperm counts have been declining since the middle of the last century, both in quantity and quality. In the 1930s, Western men averaged around one hundred million sperm per millilitre of semen, but at the beginning of the twenty-first century this average was nearly half that (at between fifty and sixty million/ml) and continuing to fall.

According to the World Health Organization, forty million/ml is the lowest sperm count that can be considered efficient for conception, and anything below twenty million is technically infertile. In the UK the figure for men with a sperm count of

T *Tip: Although labelled as non-toxic, some commercially available sex lubricants can react with either your or your partner's bodily fluids to damage or kill your sperm. As it will be virtually impossible for you to tell if this is the case, if you are having difficulty conceiving don't use any, or do so under medical supervision.*

under thirty million/ml currently stands at 1.3 million. It's therefore little wonder that around half of the problems experienced by couples trying to conceive are the result of male infertility.

Although there is no single irrefutable scientific theory for the "Great Disappearing Sperm Mystery", the modern world takes much of the blame. Such lifestyle aspects as smoking, drinking and drug taking all play their parts, while the fatigue and stress resulting from longer working hours don't help – hoping to beat that with an increased coffee intake only exacerbates the situation. Likewise obesity, poor nutrition and a lack of physical exercise contribute to the reduction in both volume and quality of sperm produced.

Holding hands should be a big part of your love life (see box on p.151)

M

Mythbuster: cycling makes you impotent

There is as much research pointing away from this as there is towards it, yet the notion persists, largely due to numbness in the genital area experienced after a long time in the saddle. This is due to restricted blood flow, and may affect the chances of an erection at the time, but seldom lasts longer than half an hour. Also, if cycling did cause ED, why has China, with all its bicycles, got such a booming population?

A significant problem though – and one that has been growing for the last fifty years – is what's in the air we're breathing. Lengthy surveys in the US Midwest have shown an inverse correlation between levels of crop spraying and the sperm counts of men living in those areas, while the same reports found that men living in the cities with lower levels of air pollution consistently had the most and the most healthy sperm.

Fertility right

Falling sperm counts have not yet reached a point where mankind needs to put itself on the Endangered Species list, but if you are hoping to have children, it's best to do everything you can to maximize your potential.

Sort your diet out The nutrients selenium, zinc and folic acid will help the production of healthy sperm, and antioxidants (particularly vitamins C or E) make sure they stay that way.

Don't worry Although it's not known if stress directly affects the sperm-producing hormones, the effect it has on your body in general will contribute to a low sperm count and reduced sexual function.

Keep cool Your testicles will be at their most efficient if you don't let them overheat: cut down on the hot tubs and saunas, and maybe switch from Y-fronts to boxers.

Stop smoking Cigarettes not only reduce the number of sperm in your semen, but also their health and mobility and reduce the length of time they'll survive after ejaculation.

Cut down on the drinking An excessive alcohol intake will not only lead to ED, but will lower your sperm count and your testosterone levels.

Give up the drugs All recreational drugs will lower your sperm count, but cocaine and heavy marijuana use are the main offenders, causing a drop of up to fifty percent.

Exercise sensibly Your sexual well-being is just the same as your general physical well-being, and the fitter it is the better it will function.

Don't drink so much coffee Although it may make you move quicker, caffeine will make your sperm swim slower and reduce their chances of getting to the egg.

Lose a bit of weight Obesity has long been linked with low and/or damaged sperm counts, because it disrupts your hormone production and, when they are surrounded by so much fat, the testicles overheat.

Oops! Sorry about that

Premature ejaculation is the most common male sexual difficulty, and will happen to every man at some point during his life and probably more than once. However, because it is so widespread, unless it's happening on a regular basis, over a period of time, it's not worth worrying about. The causes are pretty much totally random and almost always psychological – anticipation; nervousness; over-arousal; outside stress; fear of discovery; or even fatigue – so there isn't really a "cure" as such, although worrying about it happening might actually bring it on. Your partner should be as understanding as you are about this, and often it's best not to put pressure on yourself to try again, but look for other ways to pleasure each other. If it persists, visit your GP, who may well recommend a sex therapist.

A

Expert advice: "Having more sex keeps your heart healthier. Caerphilly University did research on one thousand guys over three decades and found there was an inverse correlation between those who were having the most sex and those who were dying of heart attacks. The former group's hearts and cardiovascular systems were simply in better nick, because a very passionate twenty-minute session will burn around two hundred calories which obviously isn't as good as running, but it all helps."
Sarah Hedley

Pornography has a great deal to answer for

As well as being usually quite unpleasant and generally degrading for everybody involved, porn causes its own specific range of problems as it offers such a misleading presentation of sex and sex lives. The following are the most common:

1. I'm not either doing it or thinking about it 24/7

Few men are, and the notion that "men think

Let the Joneses be the Joneses (Pt1)

Not everybody has a more exciting sex life than you, and if they do so what? Sarah Hedley explains:

"There's a massive pressure these days for people to explore further in their sex lives, because you've got sex parties, sex shops as respectable places, and then there's the Internet which has brought forward loads of sexual options. These days people are thinking if they're not slightly kinky then maybe they're a bit yesterday, and it's becoming a bit of a burden for people not to be able to say 'Oh yeah, I did that' or 'We've tried that'. People are keeping sexual checklists of things they think they ought to have done.

"To get over that you've got to make sure you're really comfortable in what you want, and who you are and remain aware that what people are talking about doing might not be what they are actually doing. Then, remember that if people have drawn up this sexual ticklist and are powering through it, then that isn't necessarily sexual happiness. Don't worry about keeping up with the Joneses – what do the Joneses care about you? It's really not about anybody else, and should be up to you what you do."

Be sexy without being sexual

Non-sexual intimacy is an often neglected part of our love lives, Sarah Hedley says, it's important to be able to get intimate with each other without it having to lead to sex.

"Kissing, cuddling and holding hands with a partner is very important, as just the act of being close like that releases oxytocin which is a bonding chemical – it's the reaction that mothers and their kids have. You should do it as often as possible, for instance when you're sitting and watching television sit together, don't sit apart on different chairs or sofas, cuddle and hold her. It's not a substitute for sex, but as another physical expression it's quite an important thing to have. At times when you are stressed about sex, if you still have the physical outlet of holding hands and cuddling then you keep your intimacy on that very private level that only happens between lovers; you maintain that physical bond.

"Really, you should do it regardless of what your sex life is like, as it will keep your relationship strong, because she's also going to have that release of chemicals and is going to feel closer to and more intimate with you."

---

about sex every seven seconds" is a nonsense. Not unless they've really got nothing else to do. According to research around sixty percent of men think about sex about half a dozen times a day; twenty-five percent think about it no more than ten times a week; for ten percent it's that many times a month; and around five percent of men think about sex no more than once a month.

2. Other women must be much more "up for it" than my partner

Probably not. As men progress in a steady relationship their sex drives remain pretty much on the same level. Women's, however, will often decline progressively as the relationship goes on, and a desire for physical affection rather than sex takes over.

3. It's not very big

It never is if you look down at it – for some reason the rule that makes your feet look bigger doesn't apply to your penis. Five studies taken over the last eight years put the average erect length at 12.9cm (5.08 inches), so don't stress about anything you might have seen in a porno film. Those blokes were never chosen for their acting abilities.

4. I can't keep going forever

Whatever you may have seen on screen or read about or heard about from friends, as regards marathon all-night sessions, the average sex act lasts between five and fourteen minutes.

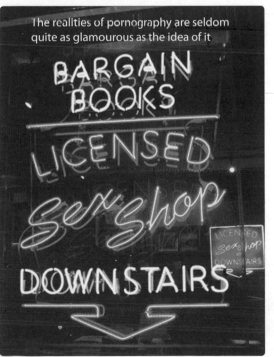

The realities of pornography are seldom quite as glamourous as the idea of it

How it all works: Viagra

Although it has passed into language as your erection's magic bullet, or "Vitamin V", Viagra is actually just a trade name for one of the many brands of sildenafil citrate tablets on the market. Albeit the first and biggest selling of them (92 percent of all sales). Developed in the UK by the pharmaceutical giant Pfizer as a drug to treat high blood pressure or angina, the erection-boosting aspect of it was discovered almost as a side effect. Patented in 1996 and given official approval as an erectile aid in 1998, it went on sale in the US that year and did more than $1 billion's worth of business in the first twelve months.

It works by assisting the tissues within the corpus cavernosum of the penis to relax sufficiently to allow the arteries to smoothly and easily fill up with blood. To do this, a hormone called cyclic guanosine monophosphate (cGMP) has to be present in relatively large quantities, and sildenafil citrate blocks production of the enzyme cGMP-specific phosphodiesterase type 5, which, as the name suggests, specifically inhibits the production of cGMP. It takes about forty minutes to take effect, and a 50mg dose is usually good for about four hours.

It should be remembered that this medication is not an aphrodisiac; it will only assist with the physical aspect of your erection once psychological arousal has been achieved. Thus the usual erotic stimulation will be required and the notion of a four-hour unprompted boner is best left to the stand-up comedians. Side effects, meanwhile, include headaches, reduced blood pressure, hot flushes, nausea, nasal congestion and blurred vision.

It will come as no surprise that almost as soon as they hit the pharmacies an alternative market for erectile dysfunction drugs emerged, one that was well under the official target age group and rarely suffering from any problems in that department. Bought without prescription, usually online, it is used to either enhance sexual experience or, as is increasingly the case, in conjunction with other drugs to combat their negative erectile effects – there is a mix of ecstasy and sildenafil citrate currently in vogue, known as "Sextasy".

What may come as a shock though is that there have been, in the US, between five hundred and a thousand deaths per year related to the recreational use of ED medication. Mostly among young healthy men, and mostly, when used in tandem with other drugs, for cardiovascular reasons. This is because the combinations of drugs can put enormous strains on the heart, and in the case of amyl nitrate dangerously reduce blood pressure.

5. I'm not very adventurous

Neither are most other men it seems: in a worldwide survey conducted by Durex, 29 percent favoured their partner on top; 28 percent doggy style; and 20 percent good old missionary. Not exactly swinging from the chandeliers, are they?

6. It takes too long before I can do it again

Thanks to the wonders of an editing room, porn stars can hop from bed to bed to bed to bed with barely a pause for breath. In the real world the more you orgasm the longer you're going to have to wait to achieve the next erection. After three or four times it might not happen at all, simply because your brain will have had enough propagating the species for one day and will switch that circuitry off.

A healthy sex life

Remarkably, although awareness of and education about the dangers of careless sex seem to have been rising sharply during the last 25 years – post-AIDS – the incidences of sexually transmitted diseases (STD) in the UK have been escalating. During the

Buy me and stop one

The most popular methods of contraception in the UK and US are:

Method	Involves	Reliability	Pros	Cons
Vasectomy	Vas deferens cut to prevent sperm reaching the semen; local anaesthetic	Around 100 percent*	Never having to worry about contraception again	No protection against STDs; not always successfully reversible
Female sterilization	Fallopian tubes cut or blocked, preventing eggs reaching the womb; general anaesthetic	Around 100 percent	A one-off op; you'll never have to worry about contraception again	More serious procedure than a vasectomy; no protection against STDs; very difficult to reverse
The Pill	Combination of two female-type hormones, oestrogen and progestogen, that prevent ovulation	Around 100 percent	Relatively convenient, allowing for a spontaneous sex life	Must be taken every day; no protection against STDs; side effects include weight gain and cardiovascular problems; not recommended for smokers
Condom	Latex sheath covering the penis	90–98 percent	Protects against STDs; always available	Unreliable; putting on reduces spontaneity; some find it reduces sensation
Contraceptive injection (for women)	Injection of female-type hormones, similar to the Pill	Around 100 percent	Each injection protects for up to three months; some types protect against cancer of the womb	Remembering to get re-injected; no protection against STDs; some weight gain; takes a while to leave the system after coming off it
The Coil (Intra-uterine device)	Fitted into a woman's womb to block sperm entry, making womb less likely to accept an egg	97–98 percent	No surgery required; each insertion lasts between five and eight years	Risk of infection; possibility of expulsion; no protection against STDs
Diaphragm with spermicide	Rubber shield, smeared with spermicide cream, inserted into vagina prior to sex	90–96 percent	Can be inserted hours before sex to preserve spontaneity	Relatively unreliable; no protection against STDs; spermicide may cause allergic reaction in either partner

* No method of contraception – other than not having sex – can be described as one hundred percent reliable, because none of them are.

The A–Z of STDs

Condition	Symptoms	Transmission	Treatment	Observation
Chlamydia – infection of the urethra	Painful urination; itching at penis opening; milky discharge	Vaginal, oral or anal sex; very rarely in fingers	Antibiotics – it is a bacterial infection	Symptoms appear a week after exposure; seventy percent of women infected have no symptoms
Crabs – aka pubic lice	Itching in pubic hair and around genitals	Genital contact; an infected person's bed; can be passed on during non-penetrative or protected sex	Specially medicated shampoo	Crabs are not crabs, but tiny insects hatched from eggs laid at the base of pubic hair shafts
Genital herpes – the HSV-2 strain of the herpes virus	Itching in genital or anal area; small circular blisters that burst into painful sores	Contact with a carrier's infected areas – can be passed on during non-penetrative or protected sex	Antiviral medication, although will usually clear itself up within a week	Never fully clears up and symptoms may re-emerge at any time
Gonorrhoea – aka the clap	Thick, yellowish discharge from penis; burning pain during urination; inflammation of the anus	Vaginal, oral or anal sex	Antibiotics – it's bacterial – and if caught early can be cleared up with a single dose	If untreated can lead to infection of the urethra, testicles and prostate; can cause infertility
Genital warts – a symptom of HPV (human papilloma virus)	Small white bumps on the end of the penis; larger uneven lumps in the genital area	Contact with infected skin – can be passed on during non-penetrative or protected sex; infected genital fluid	Application of prescription creams or liquids; in extreme cases laser treatment or minor surgery	Genital warts can spread to the anus, even if there has been no anal sex

last twelve years, cases of chlamydia have increased by 300 percent, gonorrhoea by 200 percent, HIV by 300 percent and syphilis by 2000 percent, although, numerically, the latter is still a small figure compared with the others. In over two percent of UK men a year – almost 400,000 in total – are treated for an STD. This is a rise of 68 percent in the last decade.

Who's Chlamydia?

These increases are massively skewed towards the under-25 age group, who in spite of enjoying a much more comprehensive level of sex education than previous generations, have the highest rates of STDs and teenage pregnancy in the EU. It's believed that teens having sex at younger ages, and a

Condition	Symptoms	Transmission	Treatment	Observation
Hepatitis B	Flu-like symptoms; yellowing skin and whites of eyes; weight loss	Unprotected sex; it's spread through bodily fluids	Usually clears up by itself; antiviral medication if it persists	Eighty times more infectious than HIV; if untreated the chronic condition can cause liver damage
Hepatitis C	Flu-like symptoms; yellowing skin and whites of eyes; weight loss	Unprotected sex that involves bleeding, it's spread via blood	A combination of antiviral drugs; regular check-ups in case it comes back	Sufferers should avoid alcohol because of the strain it puts on the liver
HIV – Human Immuno-deficiency Virus	Continuing and escalating propensity for illness	Blood and sexual fluids of an infected person	Antiretroviral medicines slow the transition from HIV to AIDS, but there is no cure	You are very unlikely to become infected with HIV through saliva
Syphilis	Stage One: ulcers on the penis. Stage Two: flu-like symptoms; itching all over; hair loss; white patches on tongue. Stage Three (tertiary): affects the heart and nervous system; can cause mental illness	Vaginal, oral or anal sex with an infected person	A course of penicillin injections	Incidences of syphilis were falling in the UK, but have recently started to rise again; in the US they have been escalating for decades

widespread notion that HIV belongs to a previous generation are among the main causes. Youthful drinking and drug taking is also seen as a huge contributory factor to this age group's sexual recklessness, as around 35 percent of teenagers admitted to being drunk or stoned when they first had sex.

Interestingly, among men under the age of 25, while the last fifteen years' AIDS and HIV education has hit home, recent research has found that this seems to be at the expense of other STDs. A worryingly large percentage of that age group doesn't even seem to know about them, let alone take precautions.

F

Fact: There are an estimated 62.4 million new cases of gonorrhoea in the world every year, around 8000 of them being in the UK.

Sex and drugs and middle age

In the UK and US men and women are staying single for longer, and continuing their twenty-something approach to a social life into their thirties and beyond. It's led to a rise in what's known as "risky behaviour" – binge drinking, drug taking, casual sex – among the almost middle aged that is believed to be fuelling the present increase in STDs among older men.

According to recent research, women who ten years previously would have brought proceedings to a swift halt if he didn't have any protection, are now likely to be at least as drunk and just as liable to instigate reckless sex. It has, according to the World Health Organization, removed one of the most effective preclusions to unprotected sex – women old enough to know better.

Also, this extension to staying single means each gender now, on average, will have considerably more sexual partners than previous generations, which is directly contributing to the rise and spread of STDs among older people.

No pain no gain

Another important factor in the recent rise of STDs is how easy and relatively painless it is for the lower-level infections to be cleared up with today's antibiotics and antiviral medication. As treatment for men no longer involves a needle and tiny scoop down the urethra, many people are showing such infections less respect. Casual sex is often taken for granted as part of an active social life, with "a dose" being seen as little more than an occupational hazard, thus the need for precautions is seen as less urgent.

While modern medicinal remedies may be reliable, the big danger that comes with taking frequent courses of antibiotics is the damage that can be done to the bacteria that keep your immune system functioning. Unless care is taken to restore a healthy balance within the gut it could leave your body vulnerable to all manner of other infections.

The best of the web

body.aol.com/condition-center/mens-sexual-health
Covers all aspects of men's sexual health, and offers access to collected articles on the subject.

4-men.org
The more intelligent end of the lad mag approach, that offers plenty of advice for young single men without being totally selfish.

Netdoctor.co.uk/sex_relationships
Comprehensive site for men and women, discussing sex and relationships from the emotional point of view as well as the physical.

Brook.org.uk
The website for the Brook Advisory Centres, a charity that has been providing advice and assistance on contraception and sexual health since the 1960s.

realsextips.com
Interesting, varied and generous performance pointers, taking into account the emotional as well as the purely physical.

Ten top tips for a better sex life

▶ Give up smoking It will have a detrimental effect on both your erection and your sperm count.

▶ Don't worry about not getting an erection Unless it starts to happen more than fifty percent of the time it's not a serious problem.

▶ Viagra isn't an aphrodisiac It won't help you function if the stimulation isn't there to start off with.

▶ Losing weight will improve everything as it will take strain off your heart, improve your breathing and allow your testicles to keep cooler.

▶ Don't feel you have to be wildly inventive all the time Most other people's sex lives are far less interesting than you might imagine.

▶ Drink water towards the end of an evening Brewer's droop is not an urban myth, and you will feel better in the morning.

▶ Take your partner with you if you ever have to visit a healthcare professional to discuss a sexual matter It concerns both of you, so you should both be there to talk about it.

▶ Beware of taking Viagra in tandem with other recreational drugs Such cocktails led to over five hundred deaths in the US last year.

▶ Don't ever admit your morning erection has nothing to do with your partner's inherent, unturnoffable sex appeal.

▶ Relax You're supposed to be enjoying it.

There's never a good time for erectile dysfunction, but it needn't be the end of your evening

In the gym (8)

The way humanity's energy equation evolved was pretty much like this: calories taken in equated to calories expended. Then, even after we no longer needed to expend these calories catching or digging up the food that supplied them, we still walked places or rode horses and the only labour-saving devices were called "servants", which weren't available to everybody. In today's developed world, however, our day-to-day existence seems to see us expending as little energy as possible, and thus our fuel in/fuel burned ratio has become alarmingly overbalanced, and redressing this imbalance involves going out of our way to keep fit.

Why keep fit?

The obvious answer to this question is staring you in the face practically every time you leave your house: virtually everywhere you look there is vivid evidence of the West's growing obesity crisis. And if you can't see fully fledged examples, then there's the even more commonplace casual overweightness that is so often the overture to obesity. Regular exercise is the key to preventing weight gain – together with eating healthily, see Chapter 1 – and will not only keep your weight down, but also reduce your risk of heart disease, high blood pressure and type 2 diabetes.

More than that, it will boost your entire metabolism, meaning everything in your body will start to function more efficiently, causing your all-round health to improve.

This is because exercise is part of what we are supposed to do as human beings, so by making sure you're getting enough you are simply functioning correctly. However, given that so many of us continually operate somewhere below par, just getting up to normal levels of fitness can make a huge

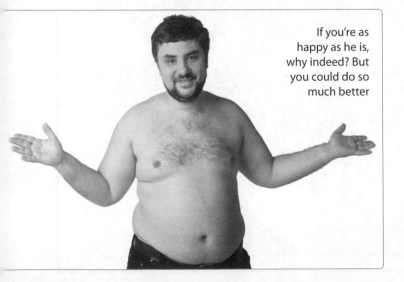

If you're as happy as he is, why indeed? But you could do so much better

How it all works: fitness

When people talk about measuring how fit a person is they are talking in terms of his cardiovascular (heart and lungs) efficiency, which will be gauged by his VO₂ max. This measurement is the maximum volume of oxygen he can make use of to power his muscles in one minute, and it is measured in millilitres of oxygen per kilo of body weight. The higher the figure, the higher your performance is likely to be, as oxygen is the key to effectively converting the carbohydrates you have consumed into the energy needed to power your muscles.

Energy is produced from carbohydrate or fat becoming fuel for the working muscles, but before these nutrients can be delivered to and utilized by the muscles they have to be converted into a substance called adenosine triphosphate (ATP). This process is the "burning" stage and requires oxygen for it to happen. As you exercise – or do anything, for that matter – the oxygen from the air you inhale is delivered to the bloodstream via the lungs, meaning the oxygen-rich blood cells can be transported to the muscles that need it. Once arrived, it metabolizes with the carbohydrate, which has now been broken down into glycogen and glucose to produce the ATP which actually makes the muscles work. A by-product of this intra-muscular process is carbon dioxide, which is removed from the muscles by blood flowing in the other direction. It is taken to the lungs where it is discharged into the atmosphere as you breathe out.

As exercise intensifies, the demand for oxygen to metabolize increasing amounts of fat or carbs will increase proportionately, which is why you gasp for air when you raise the effort you are putting in. This means VO₂ levels have to increase, and as they do your cardiovascular fitness improves – the lungs provide more oxygen and a stronger heart delivers it to the muscles quicker. You can raise your VO₂ max with aerobic training that increases in intensity and endurance over a period of time, during which your stamina levels will rise appreciatively. However, there will be a limit to which you can take it, and if after about three months you are no longer noticing any improvement you have probably reached it.

5. Where it takes on fat to be delivered to the muscles along with the oxygen

1. Oxygen is breathed in through the windpipe into the lungs

2. Blood is pumped from the heart to the lungs

4. It is pumped up to the liver

3. It becomes oxygenated in the lung tissues

159

Fact: Overall, sixty percent of American men do no exercise activity at all, which compares with fifty percent in the UK; this is against forty percent (US) and 29 percent (UK) of women. The figures also show, in each country, men under thirty are twice as likely to exercise as those over fifty.

difference. An exercise routine will also help you sleep as you will be physically tired and have less nervous energy keeping you awake.

There's also a huge psychological aspect to keeping fit. The increased blood flow will boost the oxygen levels in your brain, making thinking clearer – it's not by accident that you'll find yourself able to think things out on a good hard run. Exercise releases endorphins, the brain's feel-good neurotransmitters, which can promote an "exercise high". Equally, the act of physical movement or having to think about an activity, such as tennis or basketball, can dominate the brain to the degree that you forget the tensions and problems of the day. And when you've finished working out, those same tensions won't seem so immediate or pressing. All this will conspire to reduce your stress levels – indeed, research has shown that regular exercise can relieve the symptoms of mild depression and persistent anxiety.

But I haven't got the time

The real problem with keeping fit in today's society is that people have so many excuses not to bother. By far the most popular single barrier to keeping fit is time, or the lack of it, and this tends to be cited as much as a reason for not keeping up with a fitness plan as it does for not getting started on one in the first place. The thing to do is to sort out something that fits in with your life rather than causes you to make huge amounts of changes. That way, provided you accept that there is going to be some element of disruption, you are far more likely to logistically be able to do your exercise, and also much less likely to resent the time it's taking from all the exciting things you could be doing instead.

There are so many options when it comes to keeping fit, and such a vast array of practical and affordable home gym equipment available, it's virtually impossible not to be able to find something that can fit in with your life. Running can be done at any time, almost anywhere. Most gyms and swimming pools have extended opening hours; many keep fit classes, martial arts clubs and five-a-side football squads hold lunchtime sessions; or you could always buy a bike to get around on and in the process

Regular exercise will:

Raise your overall energy levels.

Stimulate your brain and increase its activity.

Contribute to lowering your stress levels.

Reduce everyday aches and pains.

Help you sleep better.

Keep your heart and lungs healthy.

Get rid of excess calories that would end up being stored as fat.

Boost your overall health, meaning fewer niggly coughs and colds.

Improve your sex life as you will be more energized in general.

Increase your confidence, as you will feel better about yourself.

Activity	Pros	Cons	Expense
Cycling	Excellent cardiovascular exercise; the quickest way to get around our cities; cuts down on fares; you can cycle practically anywhere at any time.	Will not develop upper body or arms; inconsiderate fellow road users; exhaust fumes; a bike is stolen every seventy seconds in the UK	Once you've bought the bike it can actually save you money
Running	Excellent cardiovascular exercise; you can do it anywhere and at any time; it can be used to get you from A to B	Wear and tear on the joints can cause problems later in life; if you run to work, you'll need to take a shower	A good pair of shoes will set you back about £80 ($150); after that all you need is shorts and a shirt
Rowing	Excellent cardiovascular exercise; good for all-round conditioning; being on the water can be very relaxing	You'll need a large body of water and a boat	Hiring a boat or joining a rowing club needn't be too expensive
Karate	Good for cardiovascular exercise, strength and flexibility; boosts confidence; encourages mental discipline; has a spiritual side	You'll need to join a club; difficult to start off with; requires a strong dedication over a long period of time	Club fees are seldom overly expensive; a gi (suit) will cost about £40 ($25)
Basketball	Good cardiovascular exercise and improves coordination; sociable – at the gym or a pick-up game; relatively easy to find somewhere to play	You can't play by yourself; the injury rate among leisure-time basketball players is high	A ball and a decent pair of high tops. Other than that you can wear your regular gym kit
Walking	Mild cardiovascular exercise – excellent for seniors or those starting exercising; you can do it anywhere, at any time; will get you from A to B without needing a shower	It might not be intense enough for everybody to use it as their main form of exercise	It will save you money with no initial outlay needed
Football (soccer)	Reasonable cardiovascular exercise and improves coordination; sociable; easy to find somewhere to play; practically everybody in the world can play it	Because it's unlikely you'll play more than once or twice a week, it should only be part of a fitness plan; the injury rate among Sunday footballers is high	A ball and suitable footwear
Tennis	Excellent cardiovascular exercise and improves coordination and reactions	You can't play by yourself; there are relatively few facilities (compared with football and basketball); many public courts shut for the winter	A racquet, balls and appropriate shoes if you use public courts; joining a club could be costly and you will need all the gear

A

Expert advice: "If you're going to do one thing towards getting fit then it should be breathing. Sit down and take three minutes a day to get diaphragmatic breathing back into the body. Most people, through stress, breathe through their chests and not very deeply, but breathing exercises help in that they aid your posture, energy levels … everything. Once you can get them to work it'll make a difference in so many other areas and provide the best basis for getting fit."
Gideon Remfry

end up saving yourself some time.

In the beginning, look to spending about three hours a week on your keep fit schedule – time that pretty much anybody can spare. Split that up into chunks of no more than one hour and no less that thirty minutes, then allocate a convenient time of day, such as early morning or lunchtime, and look for an activity and location that will fit in with what you do. Importantly, though, once you have arrived at what you are going to do

make sure you genuinely incorporate it into your schedule so you look at it as being as much an intrinsic part of your routine as, say, taking a shower in the morning.

I've tried a gym, but it didn't work out

This has become increasingly commonplace as a reason people don't keep up with a fitness regime, and it can be as much a fault of the gym itself as it can be of the individual. In the first instance, gyms too often fail to keep up the level of instruction members receive when they have just joined, and after half a dozen or so visits newbies will be left to get

T

Tip: Don't be swayed by a gym that seems populated with bodybuilders. An over-muscled physique is not something most people are trying to achieve, thus it isn't relevant to the majority of members. Also, too often that gym's staff will devote their time to these guys as they might be entering competitions from the gym, or they just see them as a good advertisement.

Find the time

According to our fitness expert Gideon Remfry, there is no reason at all why you can't make time to work out.

"Everybody has time to keep fit. If anybody says they don't then that's a time management problem and they should sit down with their weekly diary and discover all those times when they've wasted an hour or half an hour doing something useless or doing nothing at all. They've got to literally plan out their week and pinpoint all the spots when they have down time – and they will be there – then say to themselves, what's the easiest way to do this? Shall I do this at home? Shall I join a gym? How best can I factor keeping fit into my life to make it work? I guarantee there's nobody who hasn't got thirty minutes three times a week."

on with it by themselves. Not only can this be dangerous, but it's demoralizing because members tend to stay doing the same things for too long, as they don't know when or how to advance their routines.

In the case of the individual not getting much out of it, going to a gym and working out with weights or on machines in a crowded, noisy and brightly lit environment simply might not be right for them. This isn't unusual and is perfectly understandable – you might not relish the showing-off factor that will never be too far away at these temples of the body beautiful. Perhaps you feel more confident working out by yourself, or you may simply be better suited to a different way of keeping fit. The problem is that you probably won't find out you aren't the ideal candidate for gym membership until you've actually joined one.

Choose carefully when considering which gym to join (see box on p.173), and read the small print on any contract – make

Calories burned

Per hour by a 77 kilogram (168lb) man; the sports figures err on the side of the casual participant rather than someone fiercely competitive. Ideally, your exercise plan should involve the burning of at least 1500 calories per week, falling to 1200 once you reach the age of sixty.

Activity	Calories burned per hour
Running (ten-minute miles)	710
Skiing (general)	450
Football (US)	560
Football (soccer)	550
Badminton	350
Swimming (freestyle)	600
Squash	850
Walking (moderate-to-brisk pace)	300
Basketball	550
Cycling (on the road)	620
Golf (walking, carrying your clubs)	290
Circuit training	570
Rugby	700
Raquetball	500
Weight training	220
Tennis (singles)	570
Rollerblading	500
Rowing	600
Martial arts (judo, karate, kickboxing)	710
Boxing	850

F

sure you can stop your payments if you opt out, because there have been many horror stories of people locked into twelve-month deals when they thought they could get out after three.

I can't afford it

Keeping fit can cost as much or as little as you want it to. At the affordable end of the scale there is walking – to work, to college, to the shops, to the pub, and so on – anywhere you'd normally drive or get the bus. Walking at a medium-to-brisk pace can burn between 280 and 320 calories per hour, and that figure rises considerably if there are hills involved. It won't cost you anything and will even save you money if it's a journey you'd usually make on the bus. Running or cycling involves minimal initial outlay – about £250 ($450) should get you started for either – and won't cost anything more after that. All you need to go swimming is a pair of trunks and the cost of admission to the local baths, at which you should be able to find details of municipally run gyms and keep fit classes, which shouldn't cost you an arm and a leg. Any activity that will require a

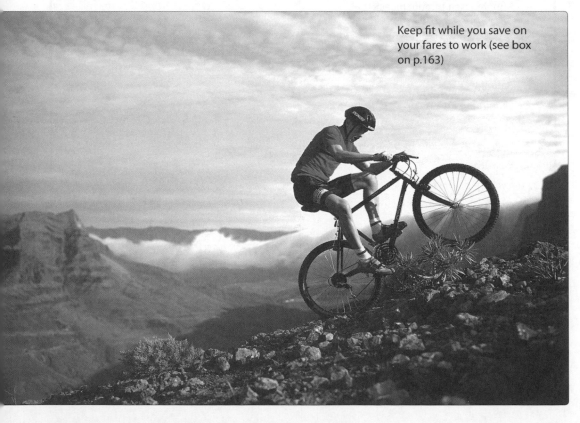

Keep fit while you save on your fares to work (see box on p.163)

B

Best investment: heart-rate monitor, between £30 ($60) and £300 ($590) A vital piece of kit to enable you to train smart as well as hard, these send a signal from a band around your chest to a read-out on your wrist. They allow you to monitor your cardio improvement, to check when you have warmed up, or to regulate your intensity levels. Most can be set to warn you if you stray outside prescribed limits, and incorporate stopwatches and lap-timers. Top of the range models store your previous performances and with some you can download data into your computer.

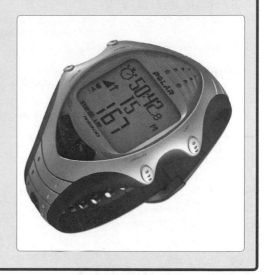

huge investment in kit ought to have facilities for you to borrow or hire equipment before you decide to commit to the activity – if you are not offered this helping hand, look for a more amenable club or fitness centre.

I don't like team sports

Then don't do them! Team sports are brilliant for those who want to attach a social element to their keeping fit, but they are definitely not for everybody. There is so much choice on offer (see p.163), so don't feel you have to join just the local football team or cricket club.

It wasn't making any difference

Be patient; anything as beneficial as getting fit is worth waiting a little while for. Don't expect to see differences immediately as it will take three or four weeks for your body to start noticeably changing shape. But, if you are following your plan correctly, your fitness levels will have been improving from the very first session. Simply stick at it and, as well as looking better, you'll find you can

perform whatever exercise you have taken on a little better and easier each time. Then before too long it will be time to pick up the pace or increase those weights.

It hurt

Although the phrase "No pain, no gain" is usually a justification for somebody doing something dangerously wrong, there will always be a certain amount of physical discomfort following a good session of physical exercise. When you start a programme, the chances are you will be exercising muscles and aspects of muscles you haven't used much in the past, so there will be a degree of soreness afterwards as they will have suffered microscopic internal tearing. However, this will ease up as you use them more and more, and to minimize

T

Tip: Be flexible when you start your fitness routine, as it will take time for you to work out what works best for you.

Aerobic exercise

This is exercise that raises the amount of oxygen the body can process to power the muscles. Such exercises are best for burning fat, lowering blood cholesterol and increasing endurance – cycling, distance running or swimming are all aerobic.

Anaerobic exercise

Workouts that build strength and muscle mass to increase power, these would be used to train for events that require explosive power, brute strength or do not last more than a couple of minutes – sprinting, weightlifting or throwing events benefit from anaerobic training.

post-workout discomfort, or risk of muscle damage while exercising, make sure you follow the warming up and cooling down routines as described on pp.177–178. Don't let a bit of stiffness put you off.

The elements of a fitness programme

For an all-round healthy and fully beneficial exercise programme to work it needs to boost your cardiovascular levels, increase the strength and size of your muscles andgimprove the flexibility of your joints and tendons. For this it needs to incorporate three elements: aerobic exercise, strength training and stretching. Some activities will provide all of this as an intrinsic part of the training, or organized clubs will make sure all are covered in each class's schedule. But under some circumstances you may need to incorporate some extra routines, for yourself, at the beginning or end of an activity.

Aerobic exercise

This is the continuous, heart-pumping, fat-burning variety of exercise that involves working the large muscles in the legs, arms

It's never too early to start

One of the biigest problems with men's approach to keeping fit is we don't get into the habit soon enough, or if we did we stopped right after we left school. Gideon Remfry explains:

"Guys over thirty are the most likely to start worrying about general fitness because that's when things start to really change for them and they're taking on a different body shape. Men of thirty-five will suddenly realize they're about forty pounds heavier than they were when they were twenty-five and they're taking trousers with waists that are suddenly four inches bigger. While it's a good thing they're doing something about it at that point, it would have been so much easier and better for them if they'd started ten years earlier or kept up their fitness levels from the time they left school.

"The trouble is that so many men don't really consider fitness for fitness sake when they're young, and unless they get involved with a team sport or take up some sort of specific activity then their fitness efforts tend to stop dead as soon as they finish school. It has been getting better during the last few years as there is so much more opportunity to keep fit – so many more home gyms, so many more health clubs, so many more local authority gyms and classes – but it's changing slowly and it's still something men need to positively address."

and trunk, and should be the basis for every exercise routine you take on. Regular cardiovascular exercise will strengthen your heart, increase your lung capacity and lower your blood pressure. All of this goes a long way to preventing heart disease, while it is also the best form of exercise for keeping your weight down (see box on p.155). Beyond that, the immediate effects of a good aerobic workout are to help you release stress after a hard day; lift your mood, as it can release endorphins in the brain; and improve your cognitive powers thanks to increased oxygen flowing through the brain. In the long term, an aerobic exercise schedule improves bone strength and boosts the immune system; also the increased overall stamina boosts your sex drive and makes life in general seem a bit easier. Plus you will be less likely to suffer from osteoporosis or chronic muscle pain in later life as you will be strengthening your bones and promoting the growth of capillaries within your muscles.

F

Fact: any exercise is better than nothing, so if when you start off short periods suit you better, do them instead of doing a scheduled hour. But do this with a view to increasing the lengths of these periods as you get fitter.

Your resting heart-rate (in beats per minute)	Your level of fitness
80–100	Grossly unfit
70–80	UK average, but still unfit
50–70	Fit
30–50	Extremely fit

Running, cycling, walking, swimming, rowing and elliptical training are all good aerobic exercises, as is dancing or anything that involves constant movement, like squash or basketball.

Strength training

This doesn't necessarily mean pumping iron, but is a catch-all term for any exercise routines that are dedicated to increasing a muscle's size, strength and staying power. It could mean stomach crunches or push-ups, as well as bench presses or deep squats. Strength training will cause the most obvious alterations to your body shape and tone, which can do wonders for your self-esteem. Also it will help you enormously with other exercise routines you are doing, as you will last longer and be able to perform better.

Health-wise, strength training helps combat muscle loss which, for an average man, will be between six and eight pounds

Weightlifting rules

Make sure you are thoroughly warmed up before you start.

Have somebody with you if you are attempting huge weights.

Rest between each set.

Be careful not to dehydrate.

Keep the correct posture – if you are forced out of it the weight is too heavy.

Stretch comprehensively after a weights session.

Type of diet	Calorific requirement	Composition of intake
Standard healthy diet	2800 calories per day	50% carbs, 20% protein, 30% fat
Weight loss diet	2500 calories per day	40% carbs, 35% protein, 25% fat
Endurance training diet	3000 calories per day	60-65% carbs, 15% protein, 20-25% fat
Strength training diet	3500 calories per day	60% carbs 25% protein, 15% fat

every decade after his twenties. It will also increase bone density as everything gets stronger to cope with the additional load bearing, which will help to relieve the joints and go a long way to preventing arthritis or will reduce the pain arthritis causes. Putting on a bit of muscle will help keep your body fat down, too, as maintaining a pound of muscle requires more energy that maintaining a pound of fat. Thus, your metabolism increases – you'll be working out even when you're sitting still. Most importantly, though, strength training as applied to your body's core, or torso, is one of the best remedies there is for the lower back pain that seems to afflict so many men past the age of thirty.

If your regular fitness routine doesn't incorporate all-round strength training you should include at least one session a week of something that does. Swimming, weight training, circuit training, martial arts and boxing are all good strength training activities.

Flexibility

Unless you are doing yoga, Tai Chi or a martial art, it's unlikely stretching, or any sort of flexibility training, will be incorporated into your routine, thus it's important you do some. As a long-term prospect, stretching improves overall flexibility and mobility, and allows improved blood flow through the joints, all of which is a vital safeguard against

Is a personal trainer worth the money?

Yes, according to Gideon Remfry. And not just simply because he is one.

"Men seeking to get fit – especially if they've not done anything since they left school – should go and get a good, well-qualified, really reputable personal trainer. That way they'll get a whole lot more out of their training because they will get it right straight away. Even if they don't stick with him or her forever, they'll stand less chance of getting injured, will stay better motivated and because the trainer will be able to address all sorts of areas of the workout they otherwise wouldn't have known existed, it will have much more focus and do them much more good.

"Also, they will get access to the newest technology and the newest training techniques, because a good personal trainer will keep up with what's going on in the word of fitness and see how it can be applied to their clients. Then go and see a nutritionist, to get advice on what you should be eating to complement your programme and what supplements you should be taking.

"Of course, there are some pretty terrible trainers out there who will do you more harm than good. It's best to go on personal recommendation and for a limited period of time at first."

If you are going to take one on, the best way is through personal recommendation. Then make sure they are going to include nutrition advice with your traininng and they have a knowledge of basic physiotherapy. Ask for a trial before committing long term.

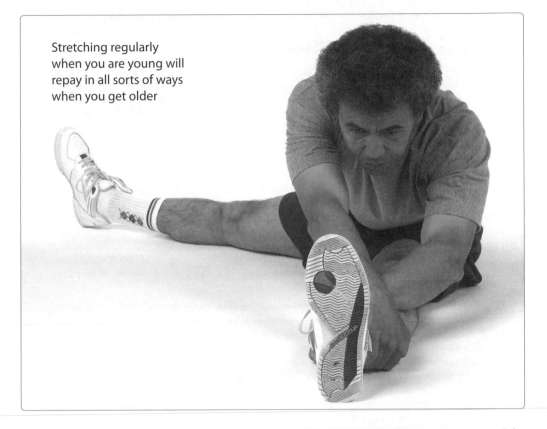

Stretching regularly when you are young will repay in all sorts of ways when you get older

the aches and pains brought on by ageing. It will also improve your balance as you get older, because a supple body's movements will be more fluid and more easily able to correct anything that gets out of line.

In the short term, stretching as part of your warming-up routine will reduce the risk of you injuring yourself, as your joints will be looser when you subject them to the stresses of exercise. If you stretch immediately after you've finished, as part of your cooling down

routine, it will leave you better prepared for your next session.

Choosing a fitness regime

When it comes to deciding what you want to do to keep fit you will be pretty much spoilt for choice, but that doesn't mean you should take your decision lightly. To arrive at your ideal activity, ask yourself the following questions.

What do you want from it?

If you are looking to lose weight you'll need to take up a specifically cardiovascular activity, such as an aerobics class, or look

F

Fact: The reason you feel like stretching when you wake up in the morning is because your tendons and ligaments will have tightened up during the inactivity of sleep.

How it all works: muscles

The muscles in your body fall into three categories: the **cardiac muscle**, which is the heart and the only one which expands and contracts constantly; **smooth muscles**, which perform unconscious internal functions like moving food along the digestive tract; and **skeletal muscles** which cover the entire skeleton, make up around half of the body's weight and are responsible for movement.

Skeletal muscles are made up of long, strong, parallel fibres that connect two bones across a joint and are contracted powerfully to move the body and its parts. This movement begins with a thought, then, once the brain has decided what it wants moved and how, it sends electrical signals along the nervous system to the relevant muscle. This prompts the filaments within the muscle's fibres to cause it to contract, moving one of the bones it is attached to. It's a process that can take place thousands of times in the space of a minute, with thousands of signals being sent to different muscles. After the movement has been successfully completed, the electrical signals are switched off and the muscle relaxes. Muscles can only be contracted and therefore will only produce a movement in one direction, but they are all paired with another muscle on the other side of the bone, which will move the body part in the opposite direction – as one contracts the other relaxes. The stronger and more powerful a muscle is, the faster and firmer the contractions will be, thus the movement is more powerful.

Science is unsure as to why muscles grow bigger and stronger (hypertrophy) as the result of progressive resistance training, but the two most popular theories each involve the body's capacity for regeneration. The first is that as the muscles are subjected to regular overuse in your workout they are internally damaged with hundreds of microtears to the internal fibres. Then, as your schedule progresses, the brain anticipates this abuse and overcompensates the repair process, increasing the muscle's bulk and strength. The other theory is from Russia and maintains that working the muscles hard speeds up and makes more efficient the internal tissue renewal cycle – muscles completely renew themselves every twenty to thirty days. This means an increased demand on the nutrient reserves used to carry out this process – they swell in volume and, as they are situated in the muscle, it grows in size.

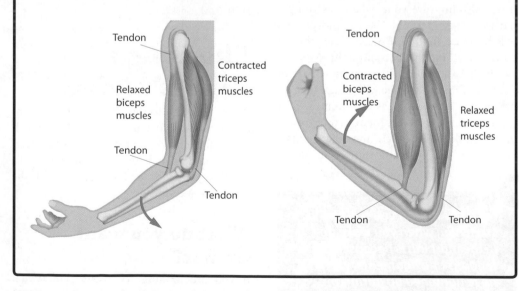

B

Best investment: running shoes, £70 ($130)
Owning a good pair of running shoes means you will never be too far away from an invigorating cardiovascular workout, and even if you have no intention of taking up running seriously, they will be worth what you paid for them. While it may be tempting to go for the occasional run, or go jogging to warm up for something else, in your tennis shoes or high tops, don't – inappropriate footwear is one of the most common causes of running injuries. If you are considering running as your main keep fit activity, then it is impossible to over-stress the importance of good, well-fitting shoes.

There are no "best" shoes, only the best for you, so don't be influenced by advertisements or other people.

Buy them at a specialist running shop where they will watch you run and assess what type of shoes you need.

Shop for them as late in the day as you can, because your feet could expand up to half a size during the day.

They should feel comfortable and well-supporting immediately – if you think you are going to have to break them in they're too small.

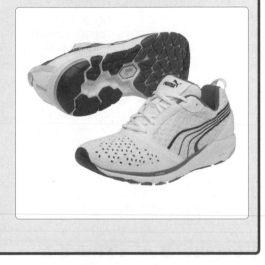

for a sport with a high calorie-burning aspect to it (see box on p.165). Your local authorities or Google are sure to help you locate commercial fitness classes in your area. If you simply want to improve your general levels of fitness and maybe increase your body strength a bit, a mixture of aerobic exercise and strength training will be ideal, and the best place to find that is in a well-supervised gym. Once again, start with your local municipal leisure services, then try the Internet.

To tone up your body, weight training will represent the best value. To achieve this you could join a gym, but it can be done at home with minimum inconvenience and expense if you invest in a set of basic weights (see box on p.178). Or, if you want to take part in a competitive sport, think about what you actually like, what you used to be good at and what you think you might be able to handle at your time of life. Then, do some research to see what is available in your area.

What sort of person are you?

Some people get on much better at a gym than others, and this is perfectly understandable – if you're a bit shy about any visible lack of fitness, a neon-lit room full of adrenalized, Lycra-clad beautiful people won't be your idea of a good night out. And that's even without negotiating communal changing rooms and showers. An activity less open to scrutiny such as rowing or walking might suit you better.

> # RICE
>
> This acronym provides pretty much a universal cure for all minor sporting injuries.
>
> **Rest** Don't try to run or work off an injury; rest up until you no longer feel pain.
>
> **Ice** Icing an injury reduces swelling, numbs pain and speeds up the internal healing process.
>
> **Compression** A tight bandage will support an injured limb and help bring down swelling.
>
> **Elevation** Raising the injured area – preferably above the level of the heart – will reduce swelling.

Team sports, even pick-up games, are good if you're looking for the social side of keeping fit, as the camaraderie following a fierce game of football or basketball can be the perfect end to a session. If you see yourself as more of a solo player, martial arts will give you a club atmosphere but allow you to compete on your own, while tennis or cycling or skating are activities you could do with your partner if you're deciding to get fit together. If you're a more solitary type, then running is an ideal pursuit – it allows you to take off by yourself for hours on end at more or less any time you like.

How much of a routine can you cope with?

Team sports, clubs or regular sessions at a gym or leisure centre will demand you conform to their set times and that may not suit you. If you can't guarantee you will be able to attend most sessions or games, at least during the first three months, you should look for something with a more flexible schedule. This is because if you start missing classes or not turning up for matches so soon, you will not form the exercise habit and probably drift away from it, or you will so irritate your team mates that they will drift away from you.

Getting started

Once you've decided what you want to do and where you're going to do it, actually getting started is going to be quite a major event. It needn't be a traumatic one, though.

Are you well enough?

Unless you are over sixty, asthmatic, arthritic, suffer from uncontrollable high blood pressure, on medication, have a family history of heart disease or are under your doctor's care for an existing medical condition, you shouldn't need to clear it with your doctor before you start your programme. As long as you start slowly you won't do yourself any harm. Push yourself just beyond your limits each time, increasing the amount of

A
Expert advice: "If you're doing resistance training, to recover as efficiently as possible you should drink a really good protein shake drink within ten minutes of stopping your workout. Natural Super Red and Super Green are the best and can be found in any fitness or nutrition store."
Gideon Remfry

F
Fact: Of the UK adult population 39 percent have not set foot in a gym since they left school.

Choosing a gym

If you've decided to join a gym, follow the guidelines below before you sign on the dotted line:

• **Check the opening hours** and make sure they are going to be convenient for you.

• **Check out the journey time from home or work** – the more awkward it is the less likely you are to keep going.

• **Make a couple of visits** at different times of the day/week to get an overall feel of the place. It's best to do so without an appointment, and be wary if they object to you looking around more than once.

• **Does it have all the equipment you think you will need?** A good gym should have a wide selection of resistance machines, free weights and cardio equipment, including treadmills, bikes, elliptical trainers, rowing machines and stair climbers.

• **Is it crowded?** You want the place to be buzzing and not deserted, but it is not a good sign if people have to wait for machines at certain times.

• **Is it clean?** Not only should the changing rooms and the showers be hygienic, but if there is a low standard of general cleanliness and tidiness it could be dangerous.

• **Are there sufficient changing facilities?** Just as the gym itself may get crowded, it will be equally frustrating if you are bumping into people in the changing rooms or have to wait for a locker or a shower.

• **What are the staff like?** Are there enough of them? Are they sufficiently attentive and knowledgeable? Do they look fit themselves?

• **Will they let you try out before you sign a contract?** There is no reason why they shouldn't.

---

time and effort you are putting in as those limits get higher. If you can't manage the half-hour sessions straight away, then that's no problem – schedule fifteen- or even ten-minute sessions to start off with and work up from there. Crucially, remember to warm up properly before you start.

Got the right gear?

Make sure your kit fits before you arrive at the session. This is especially important when it comes to shoes, but the rest of what you're wearing needs to be comfortable, too. It shouldn't chafe anywhere, must allow full movement for your activity, yet not flap about to an irritating or dangerous degree.

(M)

Mythbuster: you can "spot reduce" to shed fat from parts of your body by exercising that specific area

Burning fat is an overall body experience, and it cannot be targeted. Although it may appear that doing hundreds of sit-ups and stomach crunches is blitzing your belly fat, what you are doing is toning your stomach muscles so that it all tightens up – any fat-shedding that is going on is happening everywhere. If you were able to spot reduce then people who ate too much would all have thin faces.

F

Fact: Gym membership spikes in January, with an increase of around fifty percent in new recruits, but almost one third of those will have thrown in the towel by the end of March. However, statistics also show that if you are still there in April you are unlikely to quit. Ever.

Clothing should be made of a specialist performance fabric that will wick the moisture away from your skin to be evaporated on the garment's surface, unlike anything as old school as cotton which will collect sweat, weigh you down, rub and disrupt your body's temperature regulation.

Stay on track

Don't expect to see too many huge changes in your physique too soon. This can be a major demotivator, so set yourself achievable short-term goals – shed two pounds each week … run for ten minutes … cycle all the way to work – and reward yourself in some way when you reach them. Stay focused on your programme as a long haul project, regularly marking your achievements along the way.

Be prepared to adjust your diet, whether you are working out to lose weight or not. Losing weight through a combination of diet and exercise will involve cutting out the fat and cutting down on the carbohydrates, forcing your body to burn fat to power your muscles. If you have no weight to lose but want to improve your fitness levels, you will need to increase the amount of complex carbohydrate you eat in order to provide that extra energy.

What to do first

When starting an exercise regime there will be three aspects to it: what you eat, what you do and, importantly, what you don't do. Gideon Remfry breaks it down:

"As regards working out, nutrition has to be supplementational to exercise as you have to eat properly if you want to exercise. It's vital that you take on the fuel to get you through it and the nutrients you need to make sure your system functions properly under the stress of working out and to make your muscles grow. Think of it as putting the wrong or bad fuel in your car – it wouldn't go very far, especially if you wanted to put your foot down, and something's going to break down.

"Then there has to be a really good rest cycle in between workout sessions, because you have to make sure you are fully recovered before the next time you train. The rest cycle is probably the most missed component among men trying to get fit, because they've set themselves slightly overambitious targets or are trying to get fit or lose weight within a certain time frame. This isn't necessarily about being sedentary either, but if you're going to hammer it in the gym then you have to alternate it with light exercise, and this goes for resting in between sets as well as getting rest days in between sessions. The rest period is the only time when your body is going to get the chance to regenerate.

"Overtraining is a common problem, especially among younger men who think they are invincible and the more they work out the more benefit they will get from it. But the reality is they are far more likely to do themselves damage. Every time you do some sort of resistance training what you're doing is something the muscles aren't used to, so they are having to overcompensate. To do that, they will break down and rebuild and regenerate bigger and stronger to cope with the load you're throwing at them and they can only do that while you're resting."

What to do next

Gideon continues his advice for those starting off on a fitness programme:

"When you start an exercise programme give yourself six months, then take a look at yourself and evaluate where you've got to. You have to do it consistently, and do it for a small amount of time but over a long period and then you'll start to see results. The problems come when the very goal-dependent go into a programme with a definite idea of what they should be doing and what they want to achieve, and they hammer it for two weeks and end up in a lot of pain. They often get into so much pain that they don't go back to it at all, or don't go back for a few weeks and then they're back to square one. Or, at the other extreme, they don't go often enough or do enough when they do, so there's not nearly enough result coming out at the end of it and they get dispirited with the whole idea. You have to strike that happy medium.

"That said, goals are very important on two distinct levels. Anybody will stay motivated much better if they have a target to aim for – lose a stone or get rid of that gut – rather than just starting to do exercises and seeing where it takes you. Then there is a deeper level, at which goals help you keep real records of what your progress is, and that will keep you improving as well as keeping you motivated.

"During that initial period don't pay too much attention to the scales. What will happen is when you start to lose fat and increase lean muscle tissue, you'll also be increasing your bone density and blood volume, and your weight will go up. However, there will be very little change in your body shape initially, and although you will have got slightly smaller your weight will have gone up. You have to look at it long term and ignore the scales in the beginning."

Drink water before, during and after your workout, and once you have finished, don't forget to cool down (see p.178).

What's the worst that could happen?

If you are careful and follow the correct procedures before, during and after you work out, you should be reasonably injury-free. You are bound to pick up something, though. These are the most likely occurrences:

Ankle sprain

A sharp pain in the joint, caused by the tearing or stretching of the ligaments due to suddenly twisting the ankle into an unnatural position. Treat with RICE (see box p.172) and stay off that foot as much as possible for at least two weeks.

Cramp

A contracted muscle that goes into spasm as the result of fatigue, dehydration or salt deficiency. Gentle stretching and deep massage along the muscle fibres will relieve the stiffness; make sure you rehydrate.

Delayed Onset Muscle Soreness

Your muscles start aching at least 24 hours after you've finished exercising because of the microscopic tears in the fibres caused

F

Fact: Failure to warm up is the biggest cause of injuries among amateur sportsmen and casual keep-fitters. This is because the body will be too tight when it is called into vigorous action and something – usually a muscle or a ligament – has to give.

Strains & sprains

A strain is a stretch or a tear in the muscle itself or the tendons that directly connect it to the body.

A sprain is a stretch or a tear in the connective tissue (ligaments) that joins one bone to another inside the joint. These usually take longer to heal because there is a less-efficient blood supply to these ligaments.

by the unusual strain you have been putting them under. This will be particularly acute for people who are just starting an exercise routine, and old hands will feel it when they try something new. Treat with RICE, gentle stretching and massage.

Groin strain

Tearing or straining of the large muscle that runs down the inside of the thigh, due to overstretching or sideways stretching of the leg, which results in swelling and soreness. Stop your activity immediately and treat with RICE. Don't attempt to work it off as you could do yourself much more damage.

Hamstring damage

Sharp pain down the back of the thigh as muscle fibres have been torn – how great the pain is will depend on the severity of the tears. The muscle will have either been moved too violently while not sufficiently warmed up or it's been put under too much strain. Stop what you are doing, apply RICE and try to stay off that leg for a few days; don't attempt to exercise again until you can stretch your leg out gently with no pain. Wear a support around that thigh – a bandage or compression shorts – for your first couple of comeback sessions.

Knee ligament damage

Pain and swelling from inside the knee; may be the result of an unnatural sideways or backwards movement that has ruptured or stretched the ligaments holding the joint together. Stop what you're doing immediately and apply RICE. Stay off that leg as much as possible for the next two weeks, icing frequently for the first few days, and if there is no improvement seek medical advice as you may need surgery.

Lower back pain

Pain in the small of your back or at the top of your buttocks is usually symptomatic of something else, such as tight hamstrings or weak abdominal muscles, or, if a distance runner, a bad posture. Massage the painful area and treat with RICE, then address what might be causing the problem. A good trunk-

Just say no

Anabolic steroids – factory-made substances that approximate the male sex hormone and stimulate muscle growth – are only legally available on prescription, yet their use is more widespread now than it has ever been. High-school kids, weekend sportsmen and regular gym-goers are increasingly taking on some chemical help to improve their performance or achieve that ripped body. Even aside from instant disqualification from sports, the stigma of being branded a cheat and possible criminal prosecution, steroids are bad news. The most serious side effects are liver tumours, jaundice, hepatitis and a hugely increased risk of prostate cancer, and steroid abuse will also cause fluid retention, acne and extreme and often violent mood swings known as "'roid rage". Add to that the prospect of infertility, shrinking of the testicles, high blood pressure and an increase in LDL cholesterol and is that couple of extra inches around your biceps really worth that much?

stretching and loosening session before exercise can help prevent lower back pain.

Side stitches

This stabbing pain just underneath the ribcage is caused by the jolting of your internal organs, straining the ligament that holds the liver in place. Deeper breathing can prevent it, and as a remedy push your fingers up under your ribs to lift your liver, or stretch that side out with the corresponding arm over your head.

Before and after your workout

If you take the correct steps before and after you work out, not only will you be much less likely to injure yourself, but your body will perform better, thus you will get more out of your routine.

Warming up

This does exactly what it says it does by bringing up your body to the ideal operating temperature for exercise, plus it loosens the muscles and will provide a zone for you to get ready mentally for the tasks ahead. It is absolutely vital to warm up before you start exerting yourself; if you pitch yourself straight in, then your cardiovascular system won't be able to deliver the oxygen required and you'll struggle. Also, a cold, tight muscle is much more susceptible to tearing than a warm, loose muscle – not warming up properly is the number one cause of injuries among amateur sportsmen and gym users. Your warm-up routine should consist of three parts, carried out in this order:

1. Pulse warmers

Light jogging or jumping or skipping, slowly gaining in intensity, to raise the cardiovascular levels. This allows increasing amounts of oxygen to be transported by a faster blood flow, which in turn expands the blood vessels in the active muscles, meaning the tissue becomes looser. It will also raise the body's internal temperature ready for action.

2. Dynamic stretching

A series of slow, controlled movements that loosen joints and increase mobility by gently stretching out the muscles, tendons and ligaments. It will cut down the risk of sprains or strains and mean your joints will be better prepared to move efficiently. Dynamic stretching includes rotating the hips, knees and trunk – in both directions; flexing the

---

Keep it safe

- Make sure you are in good physical condition and don't work out or play sport if you are ill or injured.

- Wear the correct clothing, and protective gear if required.

- Stay hydrated.

- Don't take part in any exercise if you have had less than five hours' sleep the night before.

- Always warm up before starting.

- Understand and abide by the rules or guidelines for whatever you are doing.

- Rest between sets or matches and allow recovery days in your schedule.

- Listen to your body – if you are in pain it's telling you to stop because something is wrong.

B

Best investment: weight set, £100 ($190) Keeping a set of weights at home removes any last vestiges of excuses for not working out, as you'll be able to put in half an hour or so any time you like. Although what you're likely to buy and keep at home is unlikely ever to be enough to turn you into Mr Universe, it will be plenty for you to get good toning or for a mildly cardiovascular workout. Also, the companies that make weights for home use have finally got wise to the idea of them being in your house and have designed some very nice-looking pieces of kit.

Go for a set with a bar as well as dumbbells so you can do squats and presses too. Look for quick change collars, rather than anything involving keys: you will appreciate the trouble saved in between exercises.

Buy a set with as many different weights as possible to allow maximum flexibility. And invest in a weight training instructional book; don't just hurl yourself into it.

ankles; loosely swinging straight arms; and turning the head from side to side.

3. Skills rehearsal

As the final part of your warm-up, practise the movements you will be using during your activity. This will reactivate the neuron path from brain to muscle, or "muscle memory"; and put you in the right frame of mind.

Cooling down

This end-piece to a session is often shamefully neglected and has two major effects: it will go a long way to preventing stiffness later in the day; and will prepare you for your next workout or event. It falls into two parts:

1. Tapering off

This is like warming up backwards, as it allows the system to gradually return to normal – cardiovascular levels drop, adrenalin production stops, etc – and is important to remove any surplus lactate from your muscles. Lactate is produced in the muscles as a waste product of carbohydrate metabolization, and normally your high pulse rate while exercising will pump it away. If you stop dead, however, any excess stays there to produce soreness.

2. Static stretching

This involves putting gentle pressure on muscles to, quite literally, stretch them out, and over time it will permanently extend and loosen the fibres. The idea behind this is to make future workouts easier, rather than to affect your recovery from the session it follows, but it's carried out now because it is much easier and safer to stretch a warm muscle. Static stretching involves stretching the major muscles just past their point of comfort and holding it for twenty or so seconds. Always achieve a static stretch with very gentle pressure rather than a bounce.

The effects of dehydration

Percentage of body weight lost through sweat	Stage	Symptoms	Effect
1–2%	Normal	None	Won't affect performance
2–4%	First stages of dehydration	Thirst and dry mouth	Reduced endurance
5-6%	Reduced aerobic capacity and rising body temperature	Raised heart-rate and shortness of breath	Exercise will become harder and decision-making will suffer
7–9%	Dangerously high body temperature and blood thickening through lack of oxygen	Difficulty breathing and impaired vision	Loss of balance, dizziness and overall weakness, meaning working out is virtually impossible
+10%	Potential heat exhaustion	Confusion and possible hallucinations	Blackouts and collapse as your system is on the verge of shutting down

Hydration, hydration, hydration

When working out, or running, or playing sport the golden rule is to keep your fluid levels topped up, as nothing will affect your performance more or put you in more danger than if you start to dehydrate.

Once you are warmed up and into your routine you will start sweating – this is because while one aspect of your system has raised your body temperature a few degrees, another part of you is producing sweat to try to cool you back down to normal. As you can't stop yourself sweating, you have to constantly replenish the fluid you are losing. If you are perspiring freely you should be drinking water at a rate of about 200ml (6 fl oz) every twenty minutes or so, increasing that amount if the weather is warm. Keep this intake up regardless of whether you think you need it or not, as if you wait until you feel thirsty you are already in the first stages of dehydration. After you have finished, continue drinking water at the same rate for about an hour.

T

Tip: Make your own sports drink with water, fruit juice, sugar or powdered glucose, and salt. A good isotonic mix is 500ml (17 fl oz) with three large spoons of demerera sugar and a pinch of salt. Adjust the sugar for hypertonic or hypotonic, or substitute it for fruit juice or squash stirred into the water.

T

Tip: Getting off the bus or train a stop or two early and walking the remainder of the journey can really add up, in exercise terms, over the course of the week.

Sports drinks

These are a blend of carbohydrate, water and electrolytes, and can prove more effective than plain water – especially if you are in an endurance event – because the carbohydrate content will provide energy and help your body to absorb the water quicker. Sports drinks come in three types: isotonic, where the dilution of the carbs and the electrolytes in the water is about the same as your body, so it is absorbed at the same rate as water; hypotonic, which has less carbs than the above, and therefore won't provide so much energy but will be absorbed quicker; and hypertonic, where there are more carbs than either of the other two. Hypertonic drinks are best for energy replenishment but will be absorbed the slowest and are very good for post-workout recovery.

The best of the web

keepfit.org.uk
Website of the Keep Fit Association, a body supported by Sport England, which offers advice and guidance on all aspects of keeping fit, either at home or as part of a class.

buiding-muscle101.com
An American site dedicated to weightlifting; although its primary purpose seems to be to sell you stuff – videos and supplements, mostly – it has a vast amount of tips, instruction and advice.

runnersworld.com or co.uk
Everything you need if you're going to go running or are already doing so. Packed with fitness and training routines, technique tips, gear guides and injury advice, it also has a lively runners' forum and a comprehensive race calendar.

mensfitnessmagazine.co.uk
The website of the magazine of the same name; includes exercise, nutrition, weight loss and gear-buying advice, and even offers an online personal trainer.

menshealth.com
The website of the magazine that claims to offer "tons of useful stuff", and it isn't lying. Every aspect of fitness for men is dealt with here.

Ten top tips for getting fit

▶ **Build keeping fit into your routine** make it an intrinsic part of your life. Keeping it as some sort of optional extra will only encourage you to miss sessions.

▶ **Set yourself goals** But make sure that, although they will stretch you, they are achievable goals. Then reward yourself when you attain them.

▶ **Be flexible about it** Don't adopt an all-or-nothing approach. If you have to miss a session don't worry, just put a bit extra into the next one.

▶ **Don't overdo it** Overtraining is common among beginners and can sneak up on you without you realising. It can lead to all sorts of injuries, bring on fatigue and eradicate any exercise-related feeling of well-being.

▶ **Don't expect immediate results** You are in this for the long haul and it will take time for you to start to see changes in your body shape or attain a noticeable increase in fitness – be patient!

▶ **It's supposed to be fun** If you're not enjoying whatever activity it is you've started then stop it and do something else. There's masses of choice out there, and if you're not motivated by what you're doing you are unlikely to keep it up.

▶ **Anything is better than nothing** If you can't run then walk, and if you can't walk for thirty minutes walk for fifteen. Everybody has to start

There's no need for your good lady to become a gym widow either

somewhere, so don't get discouraged if you can't work out like a madman from Day One.

▶ **Sneak in some extra exercise** Take the stairs instead of the elevator or get off the bus early and walking the rest of the distance, or dump the power mower in favour of an old-school push model.

▶ **Hang with a fit crowd** Find yourself some like-minded friends, or, better still, encourage the friends you've got to keep fit with you. You'll have more fun, and you're bound to end up motivating each other.

▶ **Eat correctly** You will have the energy to work out and the nutrients to speed recovery. This will probably mean alterations to your diet even if you were a healthy eater to start off with.

On the town

Every man needs a night on the lash every now and again. Even men that make it a point not to would probably benefit – or should that be especially those men? Worryingly though, in recent times "occasionally" has become "regularly" for far too many men, meaning drink- and drug-related issues are affecting an increasing number across the world, particularly in the UK.

Got a problem?

Skim through practically any of those magazine surveys on how much you drink or take drugs and the chances are you'll rack up a score in the "problem" category. Indeed it's not unusual for those multiple choices to make even the most restrained among us feel uncomfortable about our indulgences. But astonishing as this may seem, it's making a valid point. Essentially alcohol, nicotine and most illegal drugs are toxins and those ticked boxes are designed to recognize the notion that any amount greater than None At All will be doing you some sort of harm. Therefore, the idea that you should actually enjoy/look forward to/derive some sort of

benefit from introducing a poison into your system has to be addressed in some sort of way.

However, as apparently unnecessary as drinking, smoking or taking drugs might be – and, let's face it, you'd need a Sid Vicious-level IQ to truly believe anything different – it's naïve and potentially alienating to assume everybody's going to give them up completely. Prohibition didn't work seventy-odd years ago, and in the War on Drugs the authorities are being outfought in every major city across the world.

Indeed, current figures show that, in the UK, one-third of all men drink over the recommended limit of twenty-one units of alcohol a week, twenty percent of us worry

---

Measure for measure

A unit of alcohol is half a pint of regular strength beer, a small (125ml) glass of wine or a single measure of any spirit, and the recommended consumption for men in the UK is 21 units per week (it's 14 for women). These days, however, drinkers need to take extra care if trying to stick to these guidelines. Strong ales or lager can supply more than one unit of alcohol per half pint; many pubs and bars now serve wine in 250ml glasses; wine in general has increased in strength from eleven or twelve percent to fourteen or fifteen percent; and alcopops can contain two or three measures of spirit per bottle.

How it all works: the drunkometer

Every drink you take during a night out has a cumulative effect, slowly disrupting different aspects of your system until it more or less shuts down and you pass out. Everybody's tolerance levels to alcohol will be different and they will go up the more and more regularly you drink. The sequence here is for the casual/social drinker. It assumes one drink every 25 minutes or so, and as it takes the liver almost an hour to process one unit of alcohol, drinking at this rate quickly builds up.

This sequence assumes two units per drink, as most men in a social drinking situation will be drinking pints of beer or large glasses of wine.

First drink — The instant effect you'll feel from downing that first pint is a small amount of alcohol passing directly from your stomach into your bloodstream. As most of it passes into your small intestine, this will be mild and short term. — Alcohol/blood approximately 25mg/100ml

Second drink — Brain activity is starting to decrease as the alcohol affects the frontal cortex, where conscious thought is processed, which means your inhibitions start to disintegrate. You are probably talking too loudly and are unaware of it. — Alcohol/blood approximately 75mg/100ml

UK legal drink/driving limit 80mg/100ml

Third drink — As logical thought centres get further suppressed your confidence soars and you'll know very little fear. The booze will be working on your cerebellum by now, throwing your coordination out – slurred speech, wonky balance, misjudging of distances – but because of your new-found confidence, you'll probably find it quite funny. — Alcohol/blood approximately 120mg/100ml

Fourth drink — As alcohol suppresses the anti-diuretic hormone vasopressin, your kidneys will direct fluid straight to your bladder and you'll be popping to the gents with increasing regularity. Coordination will be very poor, but confidence will be so great you'll be convinced you are actually doing better than normal – it's why so many people will drive very drunk but wouldn't dream of getting behind the wheel when just a bit pissed. — Alcohol/blood approximately 160mg/100ml

Fifth drink — Your lack of inhibitions will be such that your emotions swing to extremes – enthusiasm, aggression, affection, misery… Or you could start to feel maudlin, as the alcohol's depressive qualities suppress the production of glutamine, one of the brain's stimulants. You may well be staggering too. — Alcohol/blood approximately 200mg/100ml

Sixth drink — Your central nervous system will be greatly affected, slowing down communication between brain and muscles, meaning everything you do or say will be sluggish – not that you'll be making a great deal of sense at this point. You should also be feeling hungry as frequent urination has been depleting your system and blood sugar levels will be falling. — Alcohol/blood approximately 240mg/100ml

Seventh drink — Confusion and disorientation sets in as the brain and central nervous system are on the verge of shutting down. Drowsiness and overall tiredness will result as increased glucose from the sugar in the alcohol means massively raised insulin levels have removed nearly all your blood sugar. You may start throwing up as your body finally rebels against the poison you've been feeding it since you left home. — Alcohol/blood approximately 280mg/100ml

Eighth drink — The brain ceases all conscious activity and you pass out. There will be so much alcohol in your bloodstream it may take a couple of days to clear, and you will definitely fail a breathalyser the next morning. — Alcohol/blood approximately 300mg/100ml we drink too much and one in six admits to regularly binge drinking, which is officially defined as more than twelve units in one session. The trick is to keep recreational intakes under control and to know when and how to cut back or stop if it starts getting out of hand – to use it without it using you.

What those limits will be is going to be a matter unique to every individual's metabolism and circumstances, and a broad-brush approach will never be too practical when judging what constitutes a "problem". In real terms, the definition of such is when your actions-under-the-influence start adversely affecting other people like your family, your co-workers, your friends, fellow road users, the police, the health service, society in general. After all, if your habitual substance abuse isn't impacting on anybody except you and yours – that is your health, your bank balance and your liberty – why should anybody else care? Therefore, how can it be a "problem"?

But because it can be a scarily short step from merely behaving like a berk to shouting at traffic, it helps enormously to understand what it is you're doing to yourself. That way you will have the best chance of staying in control.

Fit to drink

Much like anything else, going on the lash will be much easier for your body to cope with if it's in good shape. If you eat healthily, there will be far less rubbish floating around in your system for your liver to have to deal with as it sorts out whatever toxins are contributing to

There is no such thing as "a quick one after work"

your good night out – this will ease the next day's hangover too. A good strong heart, at the centre of a healthy cardiovascular system, will make sure that toxins are processed and despatched as efficiently as possible. And not being overweight will minimize strain on your liver when it puts fat conversion on hold to process the poison you've just brought to it.

It's because professional athletes are so much fitter than us mere mortals they can survive going on benders with few apparent performance problems. Also why so many of them get into trouble with drink or drugs when they finish playing – they carry on at much the same levels, but are no longer fit enough to cope with it.

Provided you look after yourself for the rest of the week, there is no reason why one night off from such responsible behaviour will do you too much harm. Indeed, it will do you good to be able to relax and not worry about what's best for you for an evening. Provided one doesn't turn into two or three, and if you find yourself feeling the effects to an increasing extent you address the issue before it gets out of hand.

Fancy a drink?

The chances are you do. In Britain, like so many other Western countries, alcohol oils the wheels of just about everything. We think nothing of hanging out in the pub, or sealing

F

Fact: In vino veritas – with the drastic lowering of the inhibitions, tactful behaviour or self-preservation disappears, and around the fifth drink are replaced with a dangerous compulsion to tell the truth.

a deal over lunch, or ordering a decent bottle of wine on that potentially awkward first date. If imbibed responsibly it is unlikely to do you too much harm; indeed a moderate alcohol intake definitely can be good for you. After all, our love affair with beer dates back six thousand years, when the Ancient Egyptians and Mesopotamians began brewing, and the human race is still going strong.

First the good news

Everybody is aware of strong drink's relaxing qualities. Recently though, it's been found to have physical benefits too. And this isn't merely the "glass of red wine a day" mantra. A British survey of 20,000 moderate drinkers – one or two glasses of wine or pints of beer per day – found there was no difference in health between the exclusively beer drinking and exclusively wine drinking halves, and both had made the same improvements over the teetotal sample. In other research, moderate

Dying for a drink

During the last fifteen years the alcohol-related death toll in the UK has doubled with an increasingly steep upward curve – a rise of twenty percent in the first five years of the twenty-first century.

In the UK in 2007 almost 25 people per day died through excessive drinking; 9.09 percent of men admitted to hospital during that year were for alcohol-attributable complaints, which is up one percent on 2006. Eight percent of British men will have a problem with alcohol at some time in their lives. In the US, that figure is eleven percent.

How it all works: the liver

The largest, heaviest organ in the body, the liver is also the most complex – after the brain, obviously – and carries out over 1000 functions, around half of which are vital to keeping us alive.

The three main duties are the storing of fat extracted from food and its controlled release into the bloodstream as cholesterol; the chemical processing of nutrients that have been taken from food and metabolizing them into a usable form for delivery around the system; and the filtering out and breaking down of toxins that have found their way into the bloodstream, such as alcohol. It also manufactures the bile used to break down fats in the small intestine, produces and regulates the proteins needed for blood clotting, converts excess glucose into glycogen and stores it ready to provide energy bursts and creates the factors that form the basis of the immune system.

It manages all of this by processing oxygenated blood that is delivered from the heart, via the hepatic artery, and nutrient-rich blood arriving from the intestines through the hepatic portal system. This is a network of capillaries and blood vessels that feed into the hepatic portal vein at the base of the liver. All the body's blood passes through the liver, and at any point it will contain around thirteen percent of it.

Once inside the intricate lattice of veins inside the liver, blood passes through thousands of tiny lobules, themselves made up of billions of cells called hepatocytes, that are miniature chemical processing plants. They extract food's nutrients and fats, modify them into usable form and store them to be despatched to tissue and organs around the body. They will also distribute the oxygen delivered from the heart. Once everything has been removed, the blood is pumped back to the heart via the largest vein in the body, the inferior vena cava.

4. Once in the liver the toxins are filtered out before the blood flows back to the heart

1. Alcohol is taken into the stomach and the intestines

3. It is delivered to the portal vein, which feeds it into the liver

2. It is then absorbed through the walls into a series of blood vessels and capillaries

The lobules in the liver will also cleanse the blood, removing bacteria and damaged blood cells and filtering out toxins. These it processes into a form that can be passed back into the intestine to leave the body in faeces or urine. It's this that is related to alcoholic liver disease, as removing the high concentration of toxins in alcohol occupies far too many of the liver's resources and capabilities.

A

Expert advice: "If you keep yourself fit and look after yourself you'll stand a better chance of getting away with going on the lash. If you have got a high basic level of fitness and your everyday nutritional level is good, then you're going to bounce back much quicker. Your metabolism will go much faster, therefore, you're going to get the toxins through your system much faster, and if your nutritional level is high and you've got a good level of antioxidants in there, then that's going to cure a lot of the lingering problems you get from going on the lash. You're going to get away with more, big time, and while that shouldn't be the biggest plus point of getting fit, it's certainly one of them."
Gideon Remfry

drinkers have consistently scored higher on the "how healthy do you feel" charts.

Science has yet to fully explain why modest amounts of alcohol – a poison, after all – seem to promote several different types of good health. For a long time the idea

of Mediterranean men living longer and healthier was attributed to the diet and air quality as much as the regulation red wine, but more modern findings are isolating the drink as being equally beneficial. Again, this is down to large study groups rather than scientific research. Moderate drinking has cardiovascular benefits, as it seems to raise HDL (good) cholesterol and lower LDL (bad) cholesterol, while test subjects have also experienced fewer incidents of high blood pressure compared to that of teetotallers. The antioxidants in red wine are believed to help protect against cancer, while it is the richest known source of reserpine, a substance that activates protein metabolization and in doing so could increase longevity.

There's also good reason to drink before, during and after a meal. When the Italians first coined the word aperitivo toward the end of the eighteenth century to describe an alcoholic drink taken before a meal (it means "opener") they were formalizing a tradition that dated back to the Ancient Egyptians. It was they who discovered that such a drink before a meal stimulated gastric juice production to increase the anticipation and digestion of food. The right wine with a meal can heighten the perception of different tastes on the tongue, particularly sweetness or spices, and will take the edge off the sharpness of overly acidic dishes. Then whoever invented the *digestif* after the meal knew what they were doing too, as small quantities of alcohol can help break food

Get something in your stomach

Have that post-piss-up fry-up before you go out drinking, rather than mopping up remaining alcohol after the event – there won't be much left in your system by now anyway, hence the hangover. Fatty foods serve to line the stomach more effectively, thus slowing down the absorption of alcohol into the bloodstream. This will mean you'll get drunk slower and your system has more time to process the toxic, hangover-inducing by-products, meaning you won't feel so bad in the morning. It is a custom in southern European countries to swallow a spoonful of olive oil before a night on the drink, for precisely this purpose.

Getting drunker younger

More and more people in their twenties and thirties are being treated for alcohol-related liver disease, a condition which was previously almost exclusive to the middle-aged and elderly. The toll among women is rising faster than among men, but that's no reason to feel at all smug as, according to the World Health Organization, the UK's level of drink-related disease is twice the worldwide average.

down in the stomach to aid digestion long after the plates have been cleared away.

Too much of a good thing

The key word in all of the above is "moderation" because it's when responsible or occasional drinking becomes heavy and/or regular that alcohol's true toxic nature reveals itself. Quite apart from potentially destroying any relationship or home life you may have, removing your means to earn a living and easing you over on to the wrong side of the law at some point, there's also the physical cost.

Alcohol abuse will seriously damage your liver. Everybody knows that. But how it can creep up on you and quickly become very serious indeed is less widely acknowledged. One of the liver's vital functions is filtering toxins out of the system, those internally produced and introduced from outside – like

F

Fact: If alcohol, as a drug, was up for consideration for legality in 2008, it is so dangerous in terms of the damage it causes to people and society, it would never get passed.

World-class drinking

Alcohol consumption around the world is rising, although in France and the US it is falling. Currently, the per capita average of alcohol drunk in developed, non-Muslim countries across the world is just over five litres per annum. These are some of the top thirty drinking nations:

Germany 19.2 (highest in the world)
Luxembourg 15.5 (second)
Ireland 14.4 (third)
France 14.2 (fourth)
UK 11.2 (ninth)
Australia 9.8 (fourteenth)
Russia 9.29 (eighteenth)
US 8.3 (twentieth)
Canada 7.8 (twenty-third)
Japan 7.6 (twenty-fifth)

Source: World Health Organization

After two drinks you'll be talking too loudly. After two more, women will no longer be listening

alcohol. Thus, when large amounts are taken on board, it neglects other operations to cope with this poisonous overload, and the first to be affected is the regulation of fat in the bloodstream. Fat will be held back for processing later, but if large amounts of alcohol are regularly coming in, the fatty deposits build up to dangerous levels, causing fatty liver disease. It swells the liver, causes discomfort in the upper abdomen and is a reliable first physical sign that you are drinking more than your system can handle. This will be experienced by every heavy drinker, but will clear up as soon as you cut down to more sensible levels.

The next stage is alcoholic hepatitis, which comes about after the liver is so overworked and clogged up over a period of time it can no longer process all the toxic elements being shipped in. Cell damage and tissue inflammation will result. Around one-third of heavy drinkers will suffer from this

M

Mythbuster: you can sober up the next day by sweating out alcohol

Exercising wearing a bin bag or sitting in a sauna won't remove any alcohol lingering in your bloodstream, but it will make you feel a great deal worse as you will be further dehydrating yourself.

189

condition of which the symptoms include abdominal pain, nausea, headaches, jaundice and fever. Again, it is not permanent, and will reverse itself if you stop drinking completely for an extended period – six months – but if ignored it can easily lead on to cirrhosis.

Alcoholic cirrhosis comes about after years of heavy drinking, and is the result of persistent damage that has resulted in scar tissue building up inside the liver, meaning it has become progressively less efficient. Cirrhosis is a permanent, irreversible condition suffered by between ten and twenty percent of those who have been drinking heavily for ten years or more. Its progress can be halted if you stop drinking, but if you don't your liver will eventually give up the ghost.

Infertility and impotence are another side effect of drinking too much. Alcohol can inhibit testosterone production and interfere with the testicles' sperm-producing cells, while its suppression of the central nervous system will impede the complex set of responses needed to bring about and maintain an erection (see p.144).

Whereas moderate drinkers are around fifty percent less likely to suffer a heart

F

Fact: Globally, 1.8 million deaths per year are directly related to alcohol.

attack than non-drinkers, heavy drinkers are liable to all sorts of cardiovascular problems. Failings in the liver can mean too much fat is getting into the bloodstream, which can raise blood pressure and even cause heart failure. Alcohol's high calorie content can lead to obesity and all of its attendant cardiovascular complaints, including diabetes, which won't be helped by a malfunctioning liver.

And if all of the above wasn't quite enough, persistent alcoholic assaults will attack your stomach lining, causing sharp pains and maybe even ulcers.

From social drinking to antisocial behaviour

If drinking too much is so bad for us, why do nearly all of us do it on a fairly frequent basis? The simple answer is because we like it. It's part of a situation called "positive reinforcement" in which our brains are hard-wired to make us want more of anything we find particularly agreeable. This is also known as the brain's reward pathways, and they are remarkably easy to escalate, causing us to increase the amount of stimulation involved to achieve more pleasure.

Although alcohol is a depressant it registers pleasure because it depresses the parts of the brain that restrain our behaviour and feelings, to allow a usually enjoyable state of abandonment. (Alcohol is categorized as a sedative-hypnotic type drug, along with

The cost of a drink in Britain

The NHS spends £3.7 billion per annum on alcohol-related conditions, spending that has doubled in the last five years. Drink-related crime and public disorder costs the police and the judiciary in the UK £9.3 billion a year – it is estimated that half of all crimes of violence involve alcohol.

UK employers estimate they lose around £7 billion per year through drink-impaired performance or absenteeism caused by drink – that's between three and five percent of all absences, adding up to eleven million "sickies" being taken each year.

Valium, Librium, Seconal and Rohypnol). As the system becomes used to this state of affairs, however, it builds up a tolerance and requires larger and larger doses to achieve the same effect, and will push us into administering them. Which is where the health problems start.

There's also a psychological "tolerance" aspect to this, whereby behaviour becomes progressively outrageous, as general drunkenness levels increase often without the drinker being aware of it. Standards get recalculated for what is acceptable on a night

T

Tip: Black coffee will not sober you up. All a caffeine fix does is turn a sleepy drunk into a wide-awake drunk, which will probably cause more problems, unless, of course, you're trying to get him off your sofa and out the front door.

Twelve tips to cut down on the drink

1. Start the evening off with a big drink of water
It'll quench your thirst and stop you downing the first in one and going straight on to the second – if that happens your inhibitions will be instantly lowered and you'll be liable to drink more.

2. Drink water alongside your drink
This will help with the hangover and the next point.

3. Drink slower
This one's not rocket science, and if you're gulping down glasses of wine then switch to beer.

4. Miss yourself out of your own round
That way you won't have to make a big deal about refusing a drink.

5. Don't stand at the bar
It's much too easy to buy more drinks or for the bar staff to offer you one.

6. Avoid salty bar snacks
Their whole purpose is to make you drink more.

7. Have a couple of days off a week
Even if you have cut down the amount you drink, a couple of teetotal days will prove you're in control.

8. Be the designated driver
If your friends have any instinct for self-preservation they won't let you drink too much.

9. Don't keep booze in the house
Otherwise you'll drink it at some point.

10. Stop hanging out with people you only ever meet in pubs
The chances are all you really have in common with them is drinking, so it's all you're ever going to do with them.

11. Arrive later if you're meeting in a bar
By turning up at eight instead of seven you'll probably save yourself three drinks.

12. Get a hobby
But not collecting beer mats.

Help is at hand

addaction.org.uk
Britain's largest specialist drug and alcohol treatment agency, offering help and advice to anybody who has a problem or has to deal with somebody who has.

alcoholics-anonymous.org
The international AA site, explaining how the organization works and where to find a meeting.

aa-uk.org.uk
Alcoholics Anonymous in the UK, with the 24-hour helpline 0845 769 7555.

al-anonuk.org.uk and al-anon.alateen.org
The support service for the families and friends of alcoholics, or for those affected by somebody else's drinking – the latter is aimed at young people.

out, an escalation which can have a herd-like mentality as people see what others are getting away with and, drunkenly, follow suit. Then, when enough people are carrying on like that, "normal" becomes redefined.

But while this is about recreational drinking there's another even more insidious side to alcohol abuse that involves being drunk as a desired default setting. This used to be largely the preserve of the less outgoing who needed "dutch courage" to put themselves at ease and found their tipsy-self to be preferable to their usual comparatively flat-self. Nowadays, however, it appears far more widespread, among both men and women.

Twenty-first century men are becoming so stressed maintaining a decent work/life balance that the bottle is an increasingly convenient pressure release valve. Once again, through the reward pathway mechanism, life as viewed through the bottom of a glass can become far too desirable a situation – it's no coincidence that the areas in Britain with the highest levels of alcoholism are the more deprived parts of the country.

Curb your enthusiasm

Provided you're not a fully fledged alcoholic, in which case you should seek professional help (see box above), cutting down your drinking to a reasonable level isn't all that hard. It's mostly a matter of changing habits

Old enough to know better

Binge drinking and persistent overindulgence is far more common among the young. This is largely because, as men grow older so their work/life balance shifts and career, domestic and relationship responsibilities preclude the behaviour of their youth. This is just as well, because although moderate drinking has been shown to help protect against heart disease, with age comes a reduced tolerance to drink and drugs. It's simply because, as the body ages, it becomes progressively less able to break harmful substances down, thus the prospect of liver disease rises as toxins linger longer to do more damage. You'll also feel worse the next morning, as less poison will have been processed while you sleep, and that sleep will be of greatly reduced quality.

Although working harder to keep fit will hold this off, you will start to notice the adverse effects increasing from your mid-forties onwards. Then by the time you hit your sixties, you should even be reducing levels of indulgence that were previously considered "responsible".

and altering the sort of behaviours that for a long time have been drink-related. Not unlike rewriting your eating plan or giving up smoking, the key to cutting down drinking is to address the situations in which drink is a (if not the) vital component.

The biggest hurdle for British men though, is pub culture and the kind of heroic associations that go with drinking far too much. Too often what, logically, ought to be a simple matter of announcing that you're on the Diet Coke, turns into a night of humorous remarks directed at you about your sexuality, gender or whether or not you've got "a dose". Often it can be far less painful just to get sloshed.

However, if you're prepared to put a bit of effort into it you can climb on the wagon without looking like a complete girl.

He'd feel so much worse if he wasn't fit and healthy to start off with (see boxes on p.187 and p.198)

Climbing aboard the wagon

In the beginning, give up by stealth. Tell as few people as possible you're giving up/ cutting down, and make as small a deal as possible of it as this immediately removes pressure. If you make an announcement, it will become a recurring topic of conversation and you'll end up having to think much too much about the drinking you're no longer doing. Also, if you do slip off the wagon it's probably best not too many people know about it. To get out of situations when you know you'll drink make excuses that have nothing to do with not drinking – don't meet friends in a pub before an event, see them at the venue, tell them you've got some stuff to sort out first. Or if the activity itself is in the pub it's probably best to give it the swerve for a while, until you've got out of the habit of drinking so much – that way you'll be much more confident about refusing drinks.

When you do come clean, obviously you're going to endure a bit of abuse, but you should expect your friends to support you. If they don't it's their problem not yours, and you should drop them in the same way as you're dropping the booze.

Anatomy of a hangover

The morning after is never particularly pretty, and the standard legacy of a decent night on the lash can include a dry mouth and eyes, fatigue, irritability, headache, nausea and lack of concentration. And just as that hangover will be so hard to shift, it was painstakingly constructed by a number of different alcohol-related factors.

The most significant is the dehydrating effect caused by the ethanol in the alcohol, which has been causing increased urine production. This will now account for the dry mouth and raging thirst as you strive to re-hydrate yourself. It is also behind the continually throbbing headache because the dehydrated brain has shrunk slightly, to come away from the inside of the skull and stretching the connecting membranes. Any feelings of sickness will be a lingering effect of last night's alcohol acting as an irritant on your stomach lining. Blood sugar will be low because the liver will have been overworked and it is struggling to restore the correct glucose levels. This causes general fatigue, reduced concentration and a fuzziness of thought.

Then something called the "glutamine rebound effect" tops things off with an acute sensitivity to light and sound, restlessness, anxiety and trembling hands. This happens because drinking suppressed the production of glutamine, one of the brain's most effective natural stimulants, so when the alcohol dissipates the body goes into overdrive to replenish it, resulting in over-stimulation of the senses and nervous system.

The bad news is that the only truly

Suddenly, buying tablets from a stranger in a toilet seems like a good idea

The law on drugs

	Drugs	For possession	For dealing
Class A	Ecstasy, LSD, heroin, cocaine, crack, magic mushrooms, amphetamines (if prepared for injection)	Up to seven years in prison or an unlimited fine or both	Up to life in prison or an unlimited fine or both
Class B	Amphetamines, methylphenidate (Ritalin), pholcodine	Up to five years in prison or an unlimited fine or both	Up to fourteen years in prison or an unlimited fine or both
Class C	Cannabis*, tranquillizers, some painkillers, gamma hydroxybutyrate (GHB), Ketamine	Up to two years in prison or an unlimited fine or both	Up to fourteen years in prison or an unlimited fine or both

The specific and separate points covered by the Misuse of Drugs Act 1973 are:

To possess a controlled substance unlawfully (a small amount for "personal use").

To possess a controlled substance with intent to supply (large amounts).

To supply or offer to supply a controlled substance – even if there is no charge made for it.

To allow premises you occupy or manage to be used for the purpose of drug taking or drug supply.

*At the time of writing, the government is debating the reclassification of cannabis from Class C to Class B.

reliable hangover cure is to wait until it goes away (or you could try not getting slaughtered in the first place), so forget spoons full of Marmite, cayenne pepper, burnt toast, raw onions or the hair of the dog. However, you can minimize the next day's misery by drinking plenty of water during the course of the evening, and try a large glass of water or a hypotonic sports drink just before going to bed. The next day, eggs, being rich in cysteine will help get rid of the alcohol-induced toxin acetaldehyde, which lingers in the liver impeding its function. Fruit juice helps too, as the fructose provides a natural energy boost and will speed up the rate at which the body rids itself of toxins. Freshly squeezed juice will also go a long way to replacing lost nutrients.

F

Fact: Cocaine and heroin prices in developed countries have been falling steadily for 25 years, pretty much in inverse proportion to the increase in their usage.

Drug-related

Second to alcohol and tobacco, marijuana is the most popular drug there is, with over eighty percent of the UK's population aged between fifteen and fifty admitting to having sampled it at some point. And the drug arguments continue to rage. Is smoking weed ultimately more harmful than smoking

Coke-crazed Britain

Britain has become the world's cocaine capital. In 2007 6.8 percent of adults admitted to having used it, compared with an EU average of 3.2.

Of people aged between fifteen and fifty, 2.7 percent are regular users, which, for the first time, has overtaken the US where the figure is 2.4 percent.

Cocaine use in Britain has doubled in the last five years making it the second most popular of all illegal drugs.

Since the beginning of this century the price per gram has more than halved, from £70 to £30.

One-quarter of all heart attacks among the under-fifties in the UK last year were cocaine-induced.

Roughly fifty percent of British cocaine users end up with a problem.

Twenty-two percent of all requests for help with drug problems last year were cocaine-related.

cigarettes? Or, if there are far more drink-related deaths than those attributable to cocaine, shouldn't booze be banned? And wouldn't nicotine be banned if its staggeringly addictive capabilities had been discovered today instead of a few hundred years ago?

All this, while making good taproom conversation, is conjecture and the idea that one particular drug is not quite as dangerous as another does not make any of them a good idea. The only difference worth considering between tobacco and alcohol and those drugs listed below is the first two are legal and the others are not. They'll all kill you if you do too much of them and our inherent reward pathway systems form habits in much the same way for all of them. But the two legal ones are much more widespread – hence the higher fatality figures – therefore they are dealt with here in greater detail.

Adulteration alert

Although fags and booze have much higher numerical fatality and hospitalization rates, proportionately the illegals lead the way, largely because they are totally unregulated and nobody really knows what they are taking. Unless you grew the weed yourself, that is. Cocaine and heroin will be cut with all sorts of white powdery stuff from chalk dust to baby milk to rat poison and most of that will end up in your lungs or your veins. No wonder instances of pneumonia and

A

Expert advice: "The most popular illegal drug at the moment is cannabis, 28 percent of young people in the UK use it. A 2006 study of 2790 young people showed an increase in sexually risky behaviour in cannabis users due to increased hedonistic behaviour and them being less likely to take precautions. It would appear that while under the influence they have less appreciation of the consequences of their sexual risks, it seems for many they just don't care or the pleasure in the moment trumps the risks. They need a clear wake up call so that they cannot remain in effective denial."
Dr Sandra Scott

pleurisy are so high among otherwise healthy cocaine users, and hepatitis isn't uncommon among intravenous drug users. Bad ecstasy is all too common, and the make-up of each batch of pills will be something of a lottery as far as the buyer's concerned, while the Hells Angels control much of the speed trade and they're hardly poster boys for hygienic working practice. Plus the environment in which so many illegal recreational drugs change hands or are taken – nightclub toilets for instance – is never likely to promote good health.

However, if you still think there's something cool about drug abuse, it's probably best you're aware of exactly what the most popular of them are capable of.

Why does anybody do it?

Every developed country has a drug problem. In some it's more acute than in others, but every country that can afford one has got one. For example, according to the WHO, in the UK 82 percent of people aged between fifteen and thirty have smoked marijuana at some point; in Australia, overall drug usage has levelled off, but methamphetamines are on the rise. The US has five percent of the world's population, yet consumes fifty percent of the world's illegal drugs. On an average day one-third of German adults will binge drink. Yet, remarkably, everybody knows it's not doing them any good.

How habits can form

Habitual use, or addiction, goes beyond the reward-based psychology of the casual user and is more about the coming down after whatever high has just been experienced and how to avoid it. After a drug's active ingredient has got into your bloodstream via the lungs, the stomach or intravenous injection, it rapidly invades the nervous system to affect parts of the brain and the cardiovascular system. It'll produce a high that will soon start to wear off,

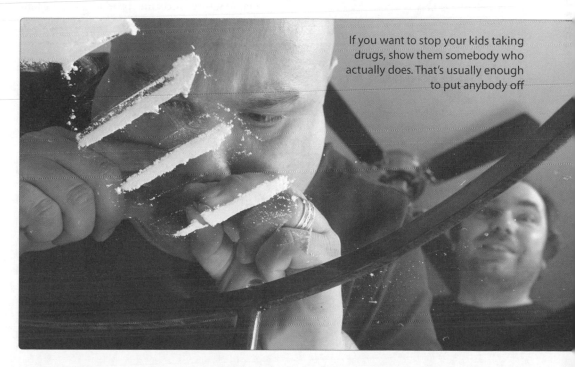

If you want to stop your kids taking drugs, show them somebody who actually does. That's usually enough to put anybody off

Rubbish at football, great at skinning up

Marijuana use among 15–34-year-olds during 2007:

UK 22.3 percent are regular weed smokers
US 22 percent
Spain 20 percent
Czech Republic 19.3 percent
France 16.7 percent
Italy 16.5 percent
Australia 9.1 percent
Canada 7.4 percent
Japan 6 percent

initiating a comedown that the brain will seek to avoid. This is when cravings to get high again start up, and they will be of different strengths and persuasiveness depending on the drug and the individual. Although this is actually the body returning to normal, compared with the high it's no longer what the brain believes is best.

Crack cocaine is particularly effective in this way, producing an intense high followed by a brutal comedown, meaning the user immediately wants to get high again. And, scarily, up there on much the same level of addictiveness is nicotine.

Aided by other chemicals used in cigarette manufacture, nicotine produces an instant

A nutritionist writes:

"The problems brought on by drink and drug abuse are twofold. The first is that it makes it much more likely you won't take on the nutrients you need, because you are unlikely to eat healthily under those circumstances due to time, convenience, money or just because you feel unwell. Then as you recover from the hangover or aftereffects, so you are unlikely to be receiving your requirement for vitamins and minerals from your diet. Food that you are eating is more likely to be high in fat, salt and sugar and nutritionally inferior. If you are going over the top on a regular basis, you are going to be missing out, nutritionally, especially on nutrients like vitamin C, potassium, folate, beta-carotene and vitamin E that are supplied from fruit and veg and whole grains.

"The second problem arises from the fact that more of the body's reserves of vitamins and minerals are needed to protect the body from cell damage caused by the abuse – drink and drugs weaken the immune system, deplete levels of vitamins and minerals in the blood and body tissues and these are not likely to be replaced by eating healthily.

"You have to pay particular attention to what you are eating under those circumstances, otherwise you'll be adding a lot more damage to what you are already doing to yourself."

Dr Sarah Schenker

Drugs: the choice is yours

The drug	The facts	The high	The comedown
Marijuana	The dried leaves of the hemp plant; smoked	A sedative that produces a dreamy state, heightening perception of sounds and visuals	Lack of coordination and inability to judge distances (driving stoned is riskier than driving drunk); hunger pangs; lowers sperm count; long-term demotivator
Cocaine	Powdered, chemically obtained extract of the leaves of the coca plant; once used as an anaesthetic; snorted, smoked or injected	A rush of energy; intense feeling of well-being; massively increased self-confidence	Risk of stroke or heart attack; numbs tissue in between nostrils to the degree it may fall out; crashing comedown; insomnia; aggressive, behaviour; long-term use causes paranoia, anxiety and depression
Crack cocaine	Cocaine purified and reduced down to solid pellets; smoked	More instant, more intense rush than cocaine	High lasts less time; comedown crashes harder; immediate craving for more; long-term use can cause paranoia and suicidal depression
Speed	Amphetamines, a chemically manufactured central nervous system stimulant; swallowed as powder or tablets	Speeds up cardiovascular system to boost energy and keep you awake; rush of euphoria	Can lead to depression and irritability when not speeding; prolonged use can cause insomnia and malnutrition as it suppresses the appetite
Heroin	Chemically refined from the opium poppy; smoked or injected	A dreamy, woozy state of euphoria	Quickly addictive; painful, comedowns; risk of HIV and hepatitis from injecting; prolonged use damages liver and kidneys
LSD	Chemically manufactured lysergic acid diethylamide; swallowed as tablets or liquid	Mind-altering "trip" that distorts perceptions of sound, shapes, colour, time, movement, space, relativity...	A bad trip can be a terrifying experience; long-term use can cause paranoia, depression and schizophrenia
Ecstasy	Chemically manufactured methylenedioxymeth-amphetamine (MDMA); swallowed as tablets or liquid	The "love drug", combining speed's energy boost with a dreamy, huggy euphoria	Raises the body's internal temperature dangerously high; risk of heat stroke; serious dehydration; the amphetamine content can cause insomnia and malnutrition

food, gambling, adrenaline rushes or self-mutilation are not uncommon. But while these cases are on the rise, science is far from in agreement about the root cause of addictions and why some people become addicts when others don't. Because the environment, the substance concerned and the individual will never interact in the same way in more than one case, pinning down specifics has proved difficult. Opinions are split between it being a disease and a personality trait, with the former being favoured by the international medical community.

elevated heart rate and a rush of euphoria, which stops as soon as you finish that cigarette, meaning you'll be starting to come down and will want another one almost straight away. Heavy smoking elevates the notion of what "normal" is, hence during the time without a cigarette – which is what you should naturally be like – you feel awful.

Addictive personalities

Addiction doesn't necessarily have to mean drugs or drink. In the modern world addictions to such things as pornography,

This is more a matter of default rather than positive research though, as the theory of the "addictive personality" becomes difficult to sustain in the light of some aspects of addicts' characters being shared, but equally as many not; and plenty of people exhibiting all the characteristics of an addict without becoming one. The most notable conclusion to be reached by extensive research into personality was that alcoholic

Help is at hand

na.org
The international Narcotics Anonymous site, explaining how the organization works and where to find a meeting.

ukna.org
Narcotics Anonymous' UK-specific site; the helpline number is 0845 373 3366.

ncid.us
The National Institute on Chemical Dependency is an American Christian, non-profit agency offering advice, counselling and treatment centres for addicts and those affected by addiction.

familiesanonymous.org
An international organization offering support and information for those affected by the drug or alcohol addiction of others.

men were slightly more likely to have an alcoholic father, but at the same time huge numbers of sons of alcoholics didn't develop a drink problem.

There may be trouble ahead

Quite apart from the internal harm that can result from somebody's habitual overindulging, there is a great deal of collateral damage to be done, as, once under the influence, the likelihood of risky behaviour soars.

Over a quarter of all unplanned pregnancies in the UK in 2007 were conceived when both partners were drunk or stoned and around thirty percent of STDs were contracted under similar circumstances. But while these have been longstanding statistics, other concerns are rapidly increasing. Last year, around seventy percent of all hospital admissions on weekends were drink/drug-related; and the rise of binge-drinking, often combined with drug taking, exacerbated by extended opening hours, has made city streets at night a far less safe place to be. In the UK, 46 percent of all crimes of violence were alcohol-related, while in 58 percent of all assaults by a stranger, the victim claimed the perpetrator had been drinking.

Perhaps the most worrying figure though is that 44 percent of the victims of violent crime were drunk themselves, a statistic that rose to 65 percent when it was narrowed down to assault by a stranger. So regardless of how mild-mannered and happy a drunk you might be, you stand a much greater chance of getting involved in a fight if you've had a few drinks.

Be extra careful out there.

No smoke without harm

Although still more socially acceptable (just) than swigging from a tin of super-strength lager or shooting up, tobacco smoking is the world's number one dangerous addiction. Currently just over one-third of all adult men in the entire world are hooked on cigarettes. Smoking kills one in ten adults globally – that's one every six seconds – and WHO figures indicate this will rise to one in six by 2030. In the UK, tobacco smoking is recognized as the number one cause of preventable illness, and in 2006 was responsible for 114,000 deaths.

Smoking is directly responsible for

Smoking will:

Lower your sperm count and decrease the frequency and rigidity of your erections.

Vastly increase the likelihood of heart disease, a stroke and high blood pressure.

Cause irreparable damage to your lungs.

Reduce the elasticity of your skin, leading to a prematurely aged appearance.

Increase the amount of LDL cholesterol in your bloodstream.

Make you feel the cold more because it destroys nerve endings just below the skin.

Introduce such toxins as arsenic, cyanide and formaldehyde into your body.

Leave you with much less cash then you might have otherwise.

As well as causing lung cancer, it can lead to cancer of the mouth, throat, kidneys and pancreas.

F

Fact: Less than ten percent of men who contract lung cancer survive the disease.

around 40,000 lung cancer deaths a year in the UK, but it is far more varied a killer than that as the carcinogens in cigarette smoke also cause cancer of the stomach, throat, mouth, kidneys and pancreas. Smokers have a 75 percent higher chance of cardiovascular problems than non-smokers and smoking causes 30,000 deaths by heart attack or stroke each year. Smoking does this by thickening the blood and reducing the amount of oxygen being carried, meaning the heart has to work much harder and the risk of clotting goes up. Also, it will increase the level of LDL cholesterol, which can affect the blood supply to extremities and damage blood

Be a quitter

It won't be easy to give up cigarettes, but it is far from impossible and will be much more manageable if you take these guidelines on board.

Stop dead
Don't try to phase it out. You'll just be putting off the day you actually stop – if you can cut out cigarettes during the day, you can do so in the evening too.

Stay out of pubs
Drinking and smoking for you will go together like, well, beer and snout, and your resolve will be so much less when you've had a couple of drinks.

Change your habits
Vary your routines to avoid the situations in which you always used to spark up.

Change your friends for the time being at least
Don't hang out with people who smoke as it will be very hard for you a) to ignore how relaxed they appear; b) to think about anything other than smoking; c) not to secondary smoke and thus restart your addiction; and d) refuse cigarettes offered.

Don't tell people you've given up
That way your not smoking won't come up in the conversation every time you meet them.

Give up when you are relaxed
Not in the run-up to exams or moving house or getting married, or just after a parent has passed away, or at any other high-stress time.

Sort your fridge out
You will start eating/snacking more, so make sure you've got plenty of healthy, non-fattening snacks readily to hand.

Keep fit
You will put on weight when you stop – it's natural because nicotine is an appetite suppressant – so take up running or going to the gym. It will reduce any increase and give you something else to think about.

Drink plenty of water
It will help get the residual toxins out of your system.

Treat yourself
Save the money you would normally spend on cigarettes to pay for a big treat (you'll be amazed how quickly it adds up) after a couple of smoke-free months.

vessels in the brain through a condition known as ischaemia.

Then quite apart from the smoke itself damaging your lungs, it creates a condition where they are less likely to look after themselves even when you're not smoking. The persistent introduction of hot smoke to your airways destroys a percentage of the tiny hairs that act as filters to keep out particulates we might breathe in during the day. With them no longer functioning as they should, it is much easier for pollutants to get in and cause serious lung damage including pneumonia, shortness of breath and a susceptibility to infections.

Then there's what smoking will do for your looks as it activates an enzyme that destroys the protein collagen. As this is what

F *Fact: In a 2006 survey 68 percent of British smokers said they wanted to give up, nine out of ten who did cited health as the primary reason, with children in the household being a popular second choice.*

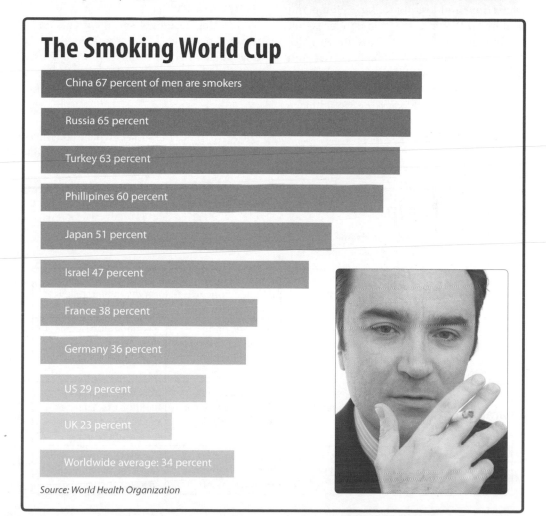

The Smoking World Cup

China 67 percent of men are smokers

Russia 65 percent

Turkey 63 percent

Phillipines 60 percent

Japan 51 percent

Israel 47 percent

France 38 percent

Germany 36 percent

US 29 percent

UK 23 percent

Worldwide average: 34 percent

Source: World Health Organization

Help is at hand

Gosmokefree.nhs.uk
The health service's stopping smoking site, offering help, tips, advice and where to find local groups and clinics.

quit.org.uk
A charity set up to help people stop smoking, offering text message support, events and awards and a telephone hotline 0800 00 22 00.

Bhf.org.uk/smoking
The British Heart Foundation, offering detailed reasons why you should quit, plus support groups and a hotline 0800 169 1900.

gives your skin its elasticity and allows it to stretch and contract as your face changes expression, and keeps it looking plump and healthy, without it the skin stretches but doesn't snap back. This leads to wrinkles and folds, and skin will appear flat and parchment-like, with no natural glow. Knowing all of this, it's hard to imagine why anybody ever thought smoking would make you seem cool.

Give up with ...

Acupuncture

By inserting needles at specific points under the skin, blockages in a person's *chi* (life force flow) are cleared. It is most commonly used to treat chronic pain, but has a high success rate in helping people overcome addictions.

Hypnotherapy

Once in a trance the subject will be convinced that smoking is not a good idea and one

Natural help

The following herbs and natural remedies won't make you give up, but they will help enormously to get you through the miseries of coming off a particular dependency.

Smoking	Ginger; cleanses your bloodstream	Cubeb berry; repairs damage done to lung tissue	Kola nut; calms the nerves to help relieve anxiety
Drinking	Evening primrose oil; helps restore balance of essential fatty acid	Turmeric or milk thistle seed; repairs and rebuilds the liver	Valerian Root; boosts the nervous system
Cocaine/ amphetamines/ ecstasy	Ginseng; energizes and fights fatigue	Turmeric or milk thistle seed; repairs and rebuilds the liver	Kola nut; calms any feelings of anxiety or paranoia, and provides an energy boost
Heroin	Magnesium; reduces anxiety and keeps you calm	Garlic; removes residual impurities from the blood	Turmeric or milk thistle seed; repairs and rebuilds the liver

that shouldn't be indulged in again. Often this can trigger unpleasant sensations when smoke is inhaled. Reasonably successful, but there is a high proportion of charlatans out there, so choose a hypnotherapist by personal recommendation or via the National Council for Hypnotherapy (hypnotherapists.org.uk).

Nicotine substitution

Patches, gum or inhalers are the most common methods, administered in a course of reducing doses designed to wean you away from tobacco. They are not hugely successful, as they merely deal with the nicotine and not the fact that people actually like the whole business of smoking, and thus they don't stimulate any desire to give up.

Willpower

Whatever method you try – including

F Fact: Doctors in the UK are now allowed to write "smoking" on a death certificate as the cause of death.

When you stub that last one out:

Half an hour later
Reduced heart rate and blood pressure.

Eight hours later
The carbon monoxide in your bloodstream has been metabolized and not replaced, normalizing the levels of oxygen in it.

Twenty-four hours later
Your heart is no longer putting itself under added strain as your blood is thinning – odds on having a coronary have already lengthened.

Forty-eight hours later
Damaged nerve endings are regenerating meaning your skin will start to feel more sensitive.

Three days later
Your sense of smell, and therefore your sense of taste returns.

One week later
Your lung capacity will be noticeably improved.

One month later
Your sperm count has risen massively and your skin looks a lot healthier as the collagen is building up once more.

Six weeks later
You get terrible cravings as the last vestiges of nicotine are leaving your body and it means you've successfully given up.

Three months later
Your circulation and immune system have improved to the degree you will feel much more energized and less susceptible to low-level infections.

Five years later
Your likelihood of heart disease or lung cancer is half what it was when you smoked.

Ten years later
Your system is now more or less the same as somebody who has never smoked.

hypnotherapy – you're going to need a fair amount of will power to get out of the habit of how, where and why you smoke. Or you could do it old school, by willpower and nothing else.

None of it's good

Although you won't inhale cigar or pipe smoke it's still not safe, as your mouth, throat and larynx will be exposed to smoke with some of it still seeping down to your lungs. Then the sheer scale of the task means one fat stogie or decent-sized pipe can produce as much smoke as a whole packet of cigarettes, meaning even the small percentage of it getting in your lungs is going to be considerable.

Also, this last point means there will be a great deal of smoke in the air around you. Secondary smoking can affect you as much as the people you are with as you will still be breathing it in.

The best of the rest of the web

britishlivertrust.org.uk
A charitable organization, whose site offers everything you need to know about looking after your liver, recognizing signs that something is wrong and seeking help if it is.

thamesvalley.police.uk/UNDERZONE
Aimed specifically at young people, by a particular police force, but full of good advice for everybody everywhere when it comes to keeping safe and on the right side of the law.

ezinearticles.com/?Herbal-Remedies-And-Drug-Addiction
A fascinating and useful collection of writings on addictions, how to break them and appropriate herbal remedies.

Ten top tips for overindulging

▶ **Drink water alongside your alcoholic drinks** It will go a long way to cutting down on the dehydration that will make you feel miserable the next day.

▶ **Always have a "designated driver"** Even if you all went to town on the bus. You are much more likely to be a victim of violence if you are drunk, so make sure one of your group has their wits about them at all times.

▶ **Don't build your spliffs with tobacco** If you're going to smoke weed at least avoid the addictive qualities and added chemicals of cigarettes.

▶ **Watch that wineglass** Many UK pubs and bars have quietly got rid of 125ml wineglasses and replaced them with 175ml or 250ml glasses, meaning, if it's the latter, you'll have put away a whole bottle but you've still only had three glasses.

▶ **Have a couple of nights off every week** This will allow your system to recover and prove you've not got an uncontrollable problem.

▶ **Don't do drugs in unsanitary surroundings** Chopping cocaine out on the cistern cover or the seat of a public toilet will never be the healthiest preparation for a substance you're about to hoover up into your lungs.

▶ **Beware drunken women who tell you "don't worry about a condom"** The UK statistics for drink-related unplanned pregnancies and STDs are alarmingly high.

▶ **Don't tell people you're giving up smoking** It will seem like it's all they'll ever talk to you about.

▶ **Vodka will still give you a hangover** This is because it will still dehydrate you.

▶ **Make sure you know what you are taking** This is not always possible with unregulated illegal drugs, but don't trust strangers in clubs.

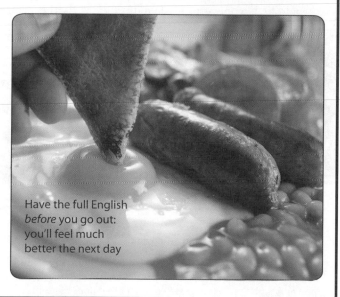

Have the full English *before* you go out: you'll feel much better the next day

In the head 10

What's going on in your head is probably the most important aspect of your overall health, because it keeps you in charge of everything else. However, as modern life increases the pressures on men, this headspace needs some maintenance of its own.

Emotionally speaking

As human beings, emotions are among the most powerful and primal communication tools in our social arsenals – everybody the whole world over understands a smile or any of the other involuntary facial expressions. Emotions are also vital to colour in a world that would be horribly grey if you didn't feel happy when you heard a certain piece of music or sad when your team lost or jealous when your partner flirts with somebody at a party.

As they are unconscious reactions and serve to put the rational brain on high alert, they are the first line of a defence mechanism against awkward or harmful situations. Emotions also provide the glue that holds society together inasmuch as it is the prompting of emotions in ourselves and others that governs how we behave to each other.

F

Fact: The cortex is one of the last areas of the brain to develop, which is why children and adolescents are far more prone to emotional outbursts than adults.

The key to self-awareness

It's through your emotional behaviour that those around you will identify your character – a happy person, a miserable git, a

Brain as big as a planet

The human brain is a masterpiece of electrical and chemical engineering and it is important to realize just how complex it is. The brain is capable of around 100 trillion calculations per second, and although there is one supercomputer that does big sums quicker – Roadrunner, unveiled in 2008 – it cost £61 million ($120 million) and took six years to develop, weighs 22,000 kilograms and requires 21 trucks to move it about. There are so many individual cells in each brain that the connections between them and the signals transmitted are the equivalent of the planet's entire telephone network.

How it all works: the brain

The brain is made up of about 100 billion brain cells known as neurons, which are divided into about fifty different types, each variety dedicated to a different area of activity – balance, pleasure, speech, hearing, memory and so on. These groups of neurons function as individual units and in concert to coordinate thoughts, moods and actions – a relevant analogy is the sections of an orchestra working as entities within themselves and together to create a symphony.

Neurons process and store information, and transmit it by generating tiny electrical impulses to send a chemical along their tendril-like axons and across the gap (the synapse) to a neighbouring cell. The receiving neuron will absorb the information carried on the chemical. Throughout the brain these connections create intricate "road maps" to allow our thoughts to be so varied and precise, and to instruct the body to carry out physical action. These chemicals are known as neurotransmitters and they increase or alter the electrical signals to dictate brain activity and so control our bodies and minds. They apply to different aspects of the brain and among those discussed in this book are dopamine (emotion, movement, pleasure), serotonin (sleep, temperature regulation, appetite) and glutamate (memory and learning).

There are five main areas of the brain that operate different aspects of how we live our lives, and they are split into the categories of the "lower" and "higher" brain. The lowest of the low is the brainstem in which the body's most basic automatic functions are controlled – eating, breathing, the digestive process, heartbeat and so on. This is the first area of the brain to develop in babies. Next up is the limbic system, prompting impulses, instinctive behaviour and involuntary expression of emotion – actions like smiling, frowning, laughing or cussing. This will be the second area to develop, and the next, the cerebellum, is relatively small but contains around half of the brain's neurons. It is responsible for voluntary movement, balance and coordination. It processes information from the senses and translates it for the nervous system to be able to send signals to whatever parts of the body need to be manoeuvred.

All of the above are essentially instinctive, but the last two parts of the brain, the higher brain, are cognitive. They develop as we mature as adults and are the frontal cortex and the prefrontal cortex. The frontal cortex is where high-level thinking goes on, and an astonishing number of electrical impulses zip about between neurons at fantastic speeds to facilitate thoughts or ideas. These ideas can involve future planning, goal setting, or creativity; they can be abstract, or based on what is being received from the senses, or derived from information already taken in – memories; or they can simply set off voluntary movement of the body. The prefrontal cortex is the brain's executive decision maker. It simultaneously absorbs information from all the senses, the memory and our aims for the future, to make the choices we need. It will make judgements between right and wrong or when to take chances; it also governs our behaviour as social beings and exercises restraint as regards emotions or desires. It is the nearest tangible manifestation of a conscience, and is fundamental to what we call intelligence or character.

Frontal cortex

Prefrontal cortex

Limbic system

Cerebellum

Brainstem

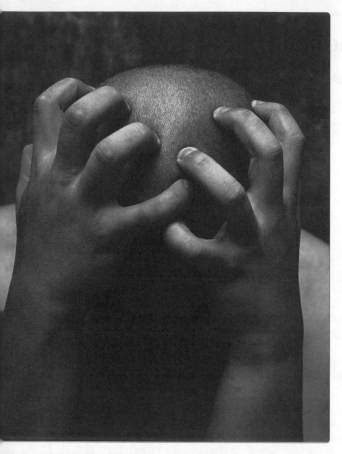

you will be able to better understand what defines acceptable social conduct and how you should behave to achieve it.

This is where it becomes apparent that behaving rationally and emotionally is far from mutually exclusive. Emotions provide an instant, unfiltered assessment of a situation. The rational mind then almost immediately works out how to deal with it and files it in the memory for the next time you come up against something like that. It's actually very easy for the memory to store this information, as emotionally charged situations are always more memorable than bland ones.

Where it can all go wrong, though, is when your conscious mind is not reacting either fast enough or with enough influence, and your emotions are getting the better of you on a regular basis.

Keeping a lid on it

A certain amount of emotional behaviour is a huge advantage. It can sharpen your instincts and reactions, improve awareness of what is happening and introduce a necessary degree of creative – i.e. illogical – thinking. But giving emotions too free a rein can be just as damaging as totally suppressing them. Inappropriate behaviour, such as laughing during a funeral service or looking disgusted at what is put in front

soppy sod, Mr Angry and so on – but, more importantly, it's also how you will define yourself. By being aware of your emotions, you will be provided with irrefutable proof of how you were affected by or behaved in certain situations, which will allow you to define your own personality.

Knowing this, and with your rational mind analysing each incident in its entirety,

Brain vs mind

Your brain is the spongy grey mass of tissue and blood vessels and membranes that supports the neurons and provides the physical environment for electrical activity to occur. Your mind is what is created by that activity as a residual pool of memories, thoughts, emotions, perceptions, imagination and resolve, forming what becomes your intellect, your consciousness and your creativity.

of you at a dinner party, will make sure you have few friends, while not being able to control anger or fear can sput you at serious risk. Violent behaviour is usually a result of a lack of emotional control, and alcohol suppresses the ability to control emotions, hence the high incidences of late-night city-centre bloodshed.

The control of emotions happens in the secondary circuit of the brain's emotional response unit, in the pathway between the amygdala and the cortex, as the former feeds information to the latter to trigger a rational response. Everybody reacts to emotions in different ways because everybody's cortex will have different capabilities; therefore, the

signals it sends out to calm the amygdala will be of varying strengths. In some cases these will not be sufficient to override the

T

Tip: Don't assume that staying late at work, obviously stressing about your job, is going to win you brownie points. It's not unusual for bosses to assume that if you have to stay late it's because you are not working as effectively or as efficiently as you might be.

Keep it real

A proportion of the apparent signs of depression, particularly among younger men, in the Western world today, are down to the goalposts having been moved as regards expectations. Dr Sandra Scott believes that the celebrity lifestyles that dominate so many areas of the media have a great deal to answer for.

"Some of the problem regarding the stress and depressive symptoms which so many people are experiencing at the moment is that young people now have such high expectations of how they should be or what they should achieve. We live in a world where a we're surrounded by media telling us what our aspirations should be, that we can all have and should want these very wealthy lifestyles and we can all do anything we like. The media are good at what they do and the messages get through.

"Unsurprisingly, therefore, many people, again particularly young people, have these huge ideas about who they can be and what they can have. This is fine, up until a point, a realistic point. It is of course important for young people to dream and to want to push themselves to reach their full potential. However there can be a problem when there is a significant gap between the dream and their reality. A recent survey showed a huge aspirational gap in today's youth, and not achieving unrealistic dreams can lead to unwarranted feelings of failure which can make people feel that they're not happy, and this is simply because they don't have what they think they ought to have.

"Ultimately, if you continually feel that you can achieve these artificially high expectations and then you don't, you can end up with this sense of failure, which is entirely unwarranted. But it's dominant feelings of failure that are associated with depression.

"It's as if an artificial pressure has been placed on people, and the first step as far as taking some of the pressure off is to take a good realistic look at what is really achievable for you with your unique set of skills or talents, and not what you just think you should be getting. A lot of people would be a lot happier if they just did that. Being more realistic and grounded will also help you deal or cope with disappointments and knock-backs when they come along – and they always will. It will be easier for you to put them in perspective, to accept that they are as much a part of life as the good stuff and to move on."

There are other ways to complain about the soup

who blow up sometimes – usually they are reliably calm or predictably unpredictable.

Practising yoga and meditation will contribute to you being able to control your emotions in general, as they provide a far better understanding of the mind and how it works in conjunction with the body and its physiological responses. Breathing techniques will also help, as they will put you in a better position to control the changes the emotions are bringing to your body, and so not let them get out of control – the whole notion of taking a deep breath when entering an emotional situation is valid and is based on this.

Anger management

Counting to ten when you feel your anger is about to boil over is not only the most convenient diffusion technique, it's also one of the most effective. Primarily, it will divert your attention from whatever has set your anger off for at least ten seconds. This provides an important interval that will give you time to form rational thoughts as a response to the situation, rather than react purely on emotion. Being able to think may well prove the difference between an impulsive action that may escalate the situation and a considered one that will calm it down.

emotions that have been triggered. Also, the pathway that sends the signals between the two areas may not be strong enough to handle the signals needed to cope with very powerful emotional responses. However, it is very possible to influence how much you are able to regulate your reactions.

Because the degree to which we control emotions is learned behaviour – from when we are children we are taught and in turn practise self-control – this circuitry can be improved upon. The cortex is like any other part of your brain, and will get stronger the more you use it, thus working hard to control your emotions will make it easier the next time, and so on. Having a strengthened cortex will also improve the neurological pathway between it and the amygdala, as the deeper these routes are worn the more efficiently they will carry signals. It's because emotional self-control quickly becomes habit-forming that it is rare to see people

T

Tip: Although it's true that important decisions based purely on emotion will rarely be very good, it's just as correct that if you totally suppress your emotions the human decision-making process becomes seriously impaired as there will be little room for creativity or flexible thinking.

F Fact: To a large degree your brain will be existing in the future, and as regards movement and timing of those actions it will be anticipating things that are about to happen rather than reacting to what has already occurred.

As you count, take a deep breath on each number – exhaling in between, of course. Not only will this slow your counting down, but it will also relax you and offset the fight-or-flight stress triggers.

Just your imagination

Stress as a tangible condition, with identifiable outside causes, was dealt with in detail in Chapter 6, but equally important is internally produced stress and how it affects you. This can often be harder to handle and have a more serious impact, as there will be little apparent logic to how it can come about, and fewer worldly sources that can be addressed.

Your own worst enemy

As adults we are all going to worry at some points in our lives. It's an inherent cognitive activity that causes agitation within our brains and is usually related to something that might or might not happen in the future or that has happened in the past. As such, worry is a major precursor to stress and all that goes with it – sleep disorders, gastric problems and headaches. But also, as you'll have noticed from what it is you worry about

T Tip: Let the Joneses be the Joneses and concentrate on being who you are – trying to keep up with other people simply for the sake of it is one of the most stressful things you can do, as a) you will never be in control of your own destiny; and b) it probably won't be right for you.

Are you insane?

It's highly unlikely, although periods of self-doubt among today's men are increasingly commonplace. This is because of the growing levels of expectations, the constantly changing environment and almost total lack of discernible guidelines. Depression is of growing concern (see p.220) in the twenty-first century, as are thoughts that life is sometimes overwhelming. This isn't madness though, and is relatively easy to treat.

If you are worried about such feelings, it's always best to address them as early as possible, and you shouldn't feel any stigma about seeking professional help. Your first step should be to consult your GP, who may recommend therapy or even prescription drugs to address whatever is causing you problems. The serious signs of madness, such as delusional behaviour, schizophrenia or paranoia will be very obvious to those around you, and, hopefully, they will have persuaded you to get help or gone as far as to get it for you.

Are you eccentric though? Very probably, and it's nothing to worry about because nearly everybody else is too.

most, it's more or less irrational – the past cannot be changed and any future we worry about is usually one we have no control over. Unfortunately though, this lack of logic as regards worrying often serves to become a worry in itself, making us feel worse and hugely increasing potential stress levels.

The good news is that we don't have to worry at all, or if we do at least we have control over how much, because worrying is a learned behaviour not something

T

Tip: If you are a worrier, avoid caffeine and alcohol as both will serve to raise anxiety levels.

that is hard-wired into our systems. It is believed that worrying is cultural in the West because from late childhood onwards, we are subconsciously taught we need to prove we are taking our lives "seriously". The manifestation of this is that those who worry the most somehow have the most gravitas. This is borne out by the fact that the children of carefree parents tend to grow up into pretty chilled-out adults.

Worrying also can be a convenient barricade to hide behind. It can stop you having to make decisions, taking risks, making changes in your life or even doing anything at all. To keep worrying about the component parts of a situation allows you to ignore the big picture, and thus avoid actually advancing things. It can also

Alternative approaches

Reflexology, aromatherapy, acupuncture and massage have all been cited as natural remedies for worry and anxiety, and while they might not work for everybody, one of them might be right for you. After all, because worry is all in your mind, if you think a therapy is doing you good it probably is. Yoga and meditation will help you relax, and assist in controlling your emotions, while breathing exercises help keep you calm in stressful situations.

Recommended complementary medicines for anxiety include celery juice, St John's Wort and kola nut, all of which lift the mood. Kava-kava root suppresses the nervous system to lessen feelings of anxiety – not unlike alcohol except not addictive; and ginkgo and vitamin B complex can sharpen brain activity to make decision-taking less of an overwhelming proposition.

There are also a number of herbal supplements you can take that will relieve conditions that can contribute to your low mood – don't forget, what might seem like depression may be due to an easily treatable set of symptoms. How you feel might be a result of hormonal imbalance, low blood sugar or simply not getting enough sunlight. A general lack of vitamins will contribute to a general mood-lowering, particularly the B vitamins as they are needed to efficiently metabolize the fats that will keep your brain and nervous system in tiptop condition. Omega-3 fatty acids will be vital for the same reason, as your brain is over fifty percent fats, thus you need to keep it topped up. Whole foods containing complex carbohydrates will help regulate your blood sugar, and swapping to them from sugary food will revitalize you by giving you a much more even energy supply.

Getting out in the sunlight genuinely does lift a mood. It supresses the production of melatonin in the pineal gland, which, as the hormone most associated with sleep, can lead to feelings of physical and mental lethargy if levels of it are high during the day. Excess melatonin secretions during the day will also cause the night's production to suffer and sleep will be disrupted. It is believed that sunlight boosts the brain's production of melatonin-inhibiting seratonin, and levels can also be raised by taking a herbal supplement called 5-hydroxy tryptophan. Likewise, the herb rhodiola will help the brain utilize serotonin and thus lift your mood.

Chill out (dude)

Telling people not to worry sounds almost as trite and as irritatingly pointless as telling them to "Cheer up, it might never happen!" However, in order to reduce your levels of self-generated stress it helps to remind yourself of the futility of fretting about the following:

Yesterday
What is in the past has already happened and therefore cannot be changed. Worrying about it will not alter this fact, so concentrate on minimizing any prospective fallout or subsequent events.

Anything you cannot control
The only excuse you have for worrying about the outcome of, say, a football match or board meeting would be if you were playing in it or sitting on it and, therefore, able to directly contribute.

A situation you have already made your contribution to
You've been for the job interview, sat the exam, put the bid in, or made the pitch: now forget about it. Remain secure in the fact you've done the absolute best you can and let the previous point come into play.

Stuff that has no immediate effect or purpose in your life
Although as good, humanitarian people it is natural to worry about things that are removed from our lives, sometimes it's stress we could really do without. Know where to draw a line as to feeling compassion for far flung suffering.

easily become habit-forming, and as well as triggering stress in your system, it will prevent you from getting the most you can out of your life.

Don't worry. Be happy

Having anxieties about major events in your life or a radically changed situation – a job interview, life after death of a spouse, an exam, moving house – is perfectly natural, as you will need to think things through as thoroughly as possible and try and cover all bases. Under these circumstances you are merely motivating yourself into analysing whatever it is facing you, which proves you are taking responsibility. Then if they become the trigger to take positive action, what you are doing is entirely healthy.

Problems occur when worrying becomes counterproductive. It settles in almost as a mental defence mechanism and thus can

B

Best investment: ginkgo biloba

This plant that has been cultivated in China for thousands of years, and is starting to become recognized by conventional medicine as being an effective remedy for lethargy or low moods. It is taken as tablets made out of the extract from the leaves and improves blood circulation in even the smallest capillaries, meaning it increases blood flow to the brain and so aids memory and sharpens concentration.

Tip: Going for a run or doing physical exercise that requires very little conscious thought can help you think clearly as it allows more connective pathways to be formed in the brain for creative thinking.

lead to problems with concentration, chronic indecisiveness, low self-confidence and, in bad cases, obsessive behaviour or panic attacks, as well as the physical manifestations of stress. This is known as mild anxiety, and around twelve percent of men in the UK suffer from it. If you recognize any of these symptoms in yourself it will be worth talking to your GP about how you feel, which in itself will go a long way to stopping you worrying about worrying. There is also a range of self-help techniques:

Keep a diary

Writing down how you feel about various aspects of situations will allow you to more easily identify your own habits and so be careful of allowing them to apply to future events. Also, it will force you to analyze your reactions to things as they are occurring in fine detail and so reach a better understanding of what you need to address.

Talk about things

But only to people you are sure you a) trust; and b) respect the judgement of, as you do not want the additional worries of who they might tell or how they might spin

Tip: When problem-solving, don't start from the obstacle and attempt to work forwards; think of the prospective goal and then work backwards.

Psychologists, psychiatrists & psychotherapy

Both psychologists and psychiatrists treat people with mental problems, and both treat problems that vary in seriousness from occasional anxiety attacks to full-blown schizophrenia, but surprisingly few people can differentiate between the two. The distinction between the professions is all in the suffix: "...iatry" means it is a branch of medicine, while an "...ology" is a science. Thus psychiatry will be the treatment of the mind – the psyche – and its disorders from a medical perspective, while psychology is the study of all aspects of it, not necessarily just the problems.

A psychiatrist will have gone to medical school and will have qualified as a doctor of medicine before specializing in psychiatry. A psychologist will have completed several years of academic training and their doctorate will be a PhD.

Clinical psychologists are those that treat people with mental disorders, but most psychologists doing practical work specialize in a field such as sports or education or occupation, and concentrate on improving performances. The largest proportion of those qualified in psychology work in research into the human mind and behaviour. Because of its medical background, the vast majority of mental problems will be managed by psychiatry, either with prescribed drugs – psychologists cannot prescribe as they have no medical credentials – or psychotherapy. This is the "talking therapy", in which behavioural problems, bad habits, fears, relationship or emotional issues, or stress are overcome by talking through the patient's history to uncover and address the root causes of problems.

The man with a plan

Having clear long-term and short-term plans will always be preferable to drifting aimlessly through life, because knowing what you are going to do puts you in control. It is this being in control that is the key, but you have to be in control of your plan as well, which means it will have to be as fluid as your circumstances. Too often people vastly increase their stress levels and end up achieving far less than they set out to by bending their lives to accommodate their plan.

your problems; also you need to be able to accept their opinions. Don't forget that the purpose of these discussions is your anxieties, so you need to be talking about your reaction to situations rather than the situations themselves – you are looking for help with your worrying rather than career/marriage/whatever advice.

Don't talk about things

This doesn't mean bottle them up, but to talk to all and sundry will mean you will end up with too many conflicting opinions, which is even less help than none at all. Be just as careful about seeking advice purely from people you know will agree with you too. While this may temporarily boost your confidence, that will soon disappear and leave you equally anxious as you will have moved no further forward.

Tackle your demons

Simply do it in a way that gradually introduces you to this new, decisive you. Identify worries you have over seemingly less-than-crucial occurrences – will your team win, how many golf balls will you lose this afternoon, why didn't that woman on the train smile at you yesterday – take a deep breath and shrug them off. Start by willing yourself to go into situations like that without a care and it will spill into other, more important areas of your life.

When to bring in the professionals

If you have tried self-help, or applying the chill out checklist (see p.215) to individual situations and have made such lifestyle changes as eating healthily, exercising and getting plenty of sleep – all of which serve to make you feel less anxious in general – yet feel worry is still inhibiting your life, you should get help.

The first place to go is your family doctor. There is a chance they may prescribe tranquillizers or antidepressants (see box on p.222) but in the first instance they are more likely to advise you to take up some form of talking therapy. This will probably

Five ways to fend off worry

1. Don't get overtired: it's much easier to get irrational about things if you're exhausted.

2. Stay busy: the more time you have on your hands the more likely you are to think up things to worry about, and if you are actually contributing to something you'll worry about it less because you have a degree of control.

3. Learn to delegate: in spite of the previous point don't take on too much as you may feel overwhelmed, which will add to your anxiety levels, and you won't have time to assess situations properly.

4. Be enthusiastic: in all areas of your life, as it's a great deal harder to worry about something if you're excited about where it could be going.

5. Relax: beating yourself up about worrying too much creates a vicious circle that doesn't take long to bring on real stress.

It's alright to mess up… sometimes

root of your behaviour – it is like a milder version of psychoanalysis. In any of these events you may be referred back to your doctor for a prescription to alleviate your symptoms.

The most important thing to remember about mild anxiety is that it can be addressed, whether it is the result of a mental illness or not, and sufferers shouldn't be shy to talk to their GP.

Perfection is overrated

This has been said elsewhere in this book, but it is particularly relevant here, as so much of the stress we put ourselves under when carrying out tasks at home or at work comes from what we tell ourselves is a search for perfection. Too often we are far harder on ourselves than we would be on anybody else, but while there is nothing wrong with setting our internal bars high, this can easily become counterproductive as it means we're either seldom satisfied with anything we achieve or are unable to finish a project.

take one of three forms: cognitive behaviour therapy, which examines the way you think and will look to alter it to confront and conquer your anxieties; counselling to assist your decision-making process so it is no longer overwhelmed; and psychodynamic psychotherapy which delves into the psyche to uncover and confront whatever is at the

Although doing a sloppy job will benefit nobody, least of all yourself, striving to achieve perfection – that is, perfection as you see it – not only seldom brings a worthwhile effort/reward ratio, but can also do you a great deal of damage. Not being able to leave something because you are perpetually dissatisfied with it is an incredibly stressful

Pick your battles

There are things worth getting stressed about, where the fight-or-flight syndrome will probably give you an edge, but there is also a huge amount of stuff that isn't worth worrying about. Be selective about what you are going to be bothered about, and make sure you don't expend mental energy on anything that doesn't merit it or will be taken care of anyway.

Are you paranoid?

Probably not, although smoking massive amounts of weed or a serious crack cocaine or crystal meth habit will point you in that direction.

In the strictest psychiatric terms, paranoia is used to describe the condition in which somebody has delusions of a) being victimized by an individual or group intent on doing him harm; or b) harm actually being inflicted on him by an individual, a group, a disease or a parasite. It also covers the belief that a person's actions are actually being controlled by a force greater than oneself; or that that person is an emissary for a higher, otherworldly power. An irrational fear of something like water or flying or spiders or public speaking is a phobia rather than paranoia.

Although the term is commonly used to describe anybody with apparently exaggerated concerns about people around them – fellow board members, the police, your mother-in-law – doing them harm, it has applications in and outside of psychiatry. They all involve delusions of some sort, and need not be restricted to fear of harm: erotomania, for example, is the paranoid delusion that the sufferer has somebody sexually obsessed with them.

experience, as it means there is no closure and it will always be on your mind.

The chances are it will have a negative effect on those around you too. Quite the opposite from your so-called perfectionism bringing admiration or even appreciation from colleagues, there is a much greater

chance it will irritate them enormously. You will probably be holding others up while you mess about with whatever it is, then at best they will think you are indecisive and at worst anally retentive. Either way it is unlikely to increase your chances of promotion.

T

Tip: Don't always do the best job you can. Instead do the best job you can before six o'clock – it's important to have a life outside of work for no other reason than to be able to put your work in the context in which it will be received.

Doing yourself more harm than good

The fundamental problem with endless tinkering is it says more about how you relate to what you have already done than it does about what you are trying to achieve, and your obvious dissatisfaction speaks of a lack of confidence. The chances are that these fine-tunings will not make or break the final result, if indeed anybody else notices, and a work stopped earlier

Brainstorming works

As the first stage of any problem-solving exercise, throwing out ideas, good and bad, with little or no restraint, has been proved to be one of the most successful methods of coming up with innovative or effective solutions. Brainstorming stimulates brain activity and encourages lateral thinking, and doesn't have to be carried out in a group. Individual brainstorming is equally valuable – just make sure you write down those ideas as soon as they pop into your head.

would still gain the same acceptance or acclaim. It will also do wonders for your confidence when this happens, as it will make you aware that you are intrinsically better at what you are doing than you might realize.

There's also the purely pragmatic aspect, inasmuch as fiddling and fiddling with something because you are not wholly satisfied with it will always come to a point, probably sooner than you think, at which physical and mental fatigue means it starts to become self-defeating. Also, you will always find something else to change or fine-tune, so unless you're a mathematician, there will never be an automatic cut-off point.

Depression: a twenty-first century condition

There are over 1.5 million men in the UK suffering from depression, and as many as

---

The symptoms of depression

Perpetual feelings of sadness or emptiness
You will find very little pleasure in so many of the things you used to enjoy, and will find what is wrong with a situation before you notice the advantages or good points.

Feelings of hopelessness or worthlessness
A pessimistic mood affects your approach to just about everything in life – friends, family, work and so on. You will feel it is better to do nothing about things rather than face the inevitable disappointment of it going wrong.

Inability to concentrate or make decisions
This is linked to the above, as at the back of your mind you are thinking "What's the point?", and therefore not really putting any mental effort into anything. You will also find it difficult to remember details.

Irritability
Because, somewhere deep in your brain, your pre-depressed self knows this state of affairs isn't right, you are continually dissatisfied with how you are feeling and functioning. You just want to be left alone most of the time.

Disrupted sleep patterns
Depressives either can't sleep or sleep fitfully through anxiety, or they oversleep, thinking there is little worth getting up for – this is more common among younger men. Both symptoms contribute to the general fatigue that accompanies depression.

Eating disorders
Weight gain or loss may be noticeable as it's not unusual for a depressive to lose interest in food or to eat too much out of habit or restlessness.

Loss of energy and susceptibility to infection
Your whole system will be functioning well below its best, and therefore it won't be making full use of nutrients being absorbed even if you are eating properly, thereby compromising your metabolism and your immune system.

Thoughts of suicide
The two positive notes here are that it is only the severely depressed that think this way, and far fewer act on it than don't – according to Mental Health America less than fifteen percent of the severely depressed commit suicide, yet over seventy percent admit to thinking about it.

---

ten percent admit to extended periods of feeling down. In the past these men were more likely to be older, as retirement, loss of partners, poor health and daily life becoming progressively more difficult contributed to feelings of loneliness or frustration. These days though growing numbers of young men, from adolescents upwards, are being diagnosed with depression as modern life increases expectations and pressures.

There is, however, a world of difference between going through a bit of a bad patch and full-blown depression.

T *Tip: Be aware that your children could be depressed, as what is usually assumed to be regulation teenage stroppiness may be something far more serious. Look for signs such as loss of interest in social activities, plummeting school performance, neglected appearance and increased drug or alcohol usage.*

What is depression?

Chemical depression accounts for the vast majority of cases of depression. It occurs when the brain does not produce enough of the hormones which lift the mood – serotonin and norepinephrine – and because they work on the nervous system it can trigger any of the symptoms of depression (see box opposite) in any combination. It then quickly becomes a downward spiral of constantly bleak moods, and because the symptoms will make the sufferer feel worse, even the subconscious notion that it might be depression furthers the cycle.

Those suffering from chemical depression are far more susceptible to bad reactions to upsetting occurrences in their lives, but a traumatic event such as the death of a family member or a long-lasting stressful situation can set depression off in those with no hormonal imbalance. This is psychological depression, and more likely to be a temporary situation that is best treated with a talking therapy.

The term "clinical depression" refers to either sort of depression that is serious enough to be sustained and affect every aspect of your day-to-day life. It is not something that clears up in a few days.

B

Best investment: oily fish

Once again your mum knew what she was talking about when she told you to eat your fish because it would make you smarter: a good supply of omega-3 fatty acids is vital to maintain the brain cells' outer membranes and so assist nerve signals, memory and the ability to learn. Beyond that, though, whole grains, pulses, liver, poultry and eggs help the mind to function, as the B vitamins – particularly 1, 3, 6 and 12 – aid the nervous system and mental performance, and work to stabilize emotions. The amino acids found in high-protein foods such as dairy, meat and fish help build neurotransmitters, and carbohydrates aid the absorption of tryptophan, which contributes to the brain's serotonin production.

What can you do about it?

If you feel you are suffering from any sort of lengthy depressive episode, i.e. you are showing the symptoms listed on p.220, you should seek professional help. Start at your GP's surgery, where you will be given an initial diagnosis. That will determine what, if any, further action you should take – you may find it helps a huge amount just to talk to somebody about how you feel.

The prescribing of antidepressant drugs is a common option (see box below). Although the jury's still out on whether these are addictive or not, they work to lift the internal mood, which will either become an end in itself or make the sufferer far more open to talking therapies. The majority of treatment for depression is a combination of drugs and talking therapies, but for anything to have the best chance of working you have to initiate it as soon as possible.

There are also a number of things you can do yourself, which will help alongside any medical treatment or will work to lift your mood if you are merely feeling down.

Stop drinking or taking drugs

Although alcohol may make you livelier in the pub, it's a depressant as it reduces your levels of serotonin so ultimately lowers your mood. The after effects of many recreational drugs will leave you feeling less positive than you were before you got high.

Eat right

Avoid refined sugars and binge eating, as it will send your blood sugar levels into wild fluctuation, and the crashes can have a seriously detrimental affect on your mood. Also the processed fats in junk food will add to any depression by depleting your body's stores of the mood-lightening vitamins B and C.

Get some exercise

Walking or running or working out will help your system function properly, which

F

Fact: As well as the suicide risk, depressives have a higher mortality rate as their physical health and immune systems suffer due to disinterest in their own well-being.

Understanding antidepressants

At the time of writing, debate is raging as to the effectiveness of prescription antidepressants as permanent patient solutions, or as possible causes of long-term damage. Discussion centres around the government-endorsed swing towards talking therapies that is happening in the UK, concerns about over-prescribing in general and the range of alternative treatments on offer. Drug therapy is still widespread though, and in around eighty percent of cases it is successful at rebalancing hormones and chemicals within the body to relieve feelings of depression. The two main types of antidepressant being prescribed are:

Selective serotonin reuptake inhibitors (SSRIs): the most widely used antidepressant, this has very few side effects and works by increasing the levels of serotonin in the brain. Prozac is an SSRI.

Serotonin-norepinephrine reuptake inhibitors (SNRIs): very similar to SSRIs, but as norepinephrine increases the heart rate and triggers glucose release within the muscles, it acts as a stimulant, and therefore is not good for those with insomnia.

Are you depressed?

Once again, probably not. The chances are you are experiencing a temporary depressed mood, rather than any sort of clinical disorder, and it will be the result of an external event or situation making you feel sad or miserable. When that changes or, with time, you come to terms with it, the chances are your mood will lift.

will improve your health and will release endorphins, the "feel good hormone". Exercise helps you sleep better too, while from a psychological point of view, you'll have improved self-confidence and feelings of self-worth as you will look better and feel more vitalized.

Get some sun

If you can do that exercise outdoors it will be doubly beneficial: oxygenating your brain helps it function and sunlight releases melatonin, which makes you feel more alive.

Have a laugh

Read a book or watch a film that you know will be funny, as not only will it serve as a handy distraction, but laughter reduces the levels of the stress hormones cortisol and adrenaline – the idea of laughter therapy as a bona fide treatment is currently gaining ground.

Don't suffer in silence

Nearly three-quarters of all adults suffering from depression are not getting treatment a figure that is much higher for men than women, in spite of more women suffering from depression than men.

Dr Sandra Scott explains why this is and what should be done about it:

"Get help if you need help: if you really believe you've got something wrong. One of the reasons we believe the rates of depression

Talking about it

As you'd probably expect, talking therapies involve exactly that – talking. But talking to somebody who is trained in listening to people with anxieties or troubles, then helping them find the answers within themselves. These listeners could be psychiatrists, psychologists or counsellors, and there are a number of different talking therapies, but what they have in common is they have a much lower relapse rate than medication.

The main reasons why talking therapies are more successful is because they do not simply treat the symptoms and chemically engineer a change of mood, but as the sessions progress will work on the cause of the depression. Some will seek to change patterns of behaviour, others will establish the root cause of your unhappiness and help you to confront and deal with it, and others will simply allow you to talk about stuff to somebody who will listen without judging and then support you as you look for a conclusion to whatever is troubling you.

Even if you're not depressed and are maybe just having a rough time in your life – jobwise, in your marriage, with your sexuality – just being able to talk honestly and openly with somebody can be a huge help.

The British government's Department of Health offers a comprehensive downloadable brochure on talking therapies that is equally relevant on either side of the Atlantic. Visit: dh.gov.uk/en/publicationsandstatistics.

are lower for men than women is that many men are reluctant to talk about emotional problems so their difficulties can go unnoticed by those who can help them. Sometimes it may be going against everything you believe in, but if you think there might be something wrong with you, if you are unhappy and have been for some time and cannot shift it by yourself, then get help.

"There is still a huge feeling among many men that it's not really appropriate to seek that sort of emotional help, thus if they go to a GP they are much more likely to talk about the physical symptoms of depression rather than the psychological ones. They also can present differently from women – they are more likely to try to hide sadness and present with aggression and frustration. Young men tend to deal with their symptoms differently, for example by increases in reckless behaviour such as illicit drug taking and alcohol abuse, and their depression can go unrecognized or be labelled as something else.

"It may be that you will be more comfortable going online at first to try and look up what you are feeling and to get more information about your condition. This is a very good first step, because if you don't understand what your issues are it is much harder to speak about them even if you want to – at least as articulately as you may need to in order to ensure you are understood.

"Write things down too. Sometimes putting it down on paper simply helps you take it seriously, which may spur you on

The best of the web

bacp.co.uk
The British Association for Counselling and Psychotherapy offers a range of services that include finding an accredited psychotherapist, information about counselling and what you should expect from therapy.

nmha.org
Mental Health America (formerly the National Mental Health Association) offers information about care, medication and legal issues, plus a series of downloadable factsheets and easily understood answers to FAQs.

mentalhealth.org.uk
A charity that provides information about mental health, conducts research and campaigns to improve public services and spending in that area. The site features an A-Z of Mental Health, which will explain just about any condition or term.

rcpsych.ac.uk
The Royal College of Psychiatrists offers a vast range of well-researched, up-to-date and readable information on mental health and its treatment, including ten downloadable leaflets on frequently enquired about subjects.

cmha.ca
The Canadian Mental Health Association offers a wide range of advice and information about all aspects of mental health, also a series of DIY tests designed to assess your state of mind.

mhfederation.org
The Mental Health, Addiction and Retardation Organizations of America raises money for the US's mental health charities and organizations, but also offers a vast range of help and information.

mind.org.uk
The UK's leading mental health charity, which works to ensure those with mental health problems are looked after properly and treated with equality and dignity.

to do something about it. Also, it will help you accurately capture it, and what it felt like at the time, because sometimes when you're caught up in whatever moment it was, when you come to recall it you can actually have forgotten how bad things were, or the important details like what triggered your downward spiral.

"The most important thing is for men to realize it's okay to ask for help, and that depression is a biological illness, and there are all sorts of ways they can get help. Clinical depression involves a chemical imbalance and if you had diabetes – another illness caused by a chemical imbalance – you'd treat that. Depression is no different."

Ten top tips for the best mental health

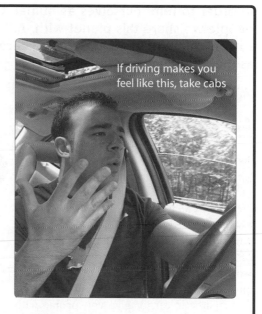
If driving makes you feel like this, take cabs

▶ **Talk to somebody** Do so as soon as you feel you are becoming overwhelmed or that you might be becoming depressed. The earlier you get help the more effective it will be.

▶ **Eat plenty of fish** The omega-3 oils in such fish as salmon or mackerel will nourish your brain, which is over fifty percent fat.

▶ **Be aware of your emotions** Notice how they are making you behave, then practise keeping them under control – some emotional input is healthy, too much can be dangerous.

▶ **Get out more** Sunlight will trigger the release of melatonin, which boosts your whole feeling of well-being.

▶ **Know when to stop** Don't carry on with a project or a job imagining you are a perfectionist and everything has to be exactly right.

▶ **You probably aren't going mad** But it is very healthy to wonder about it from time to time.

▶ **Live your own life** If you are constantly trying to keep up with

somebody else's standards you will be constantly stressed and usually dissatisfied.

▶ **Find out your family history** Depression can be hereditary, and therefore you will be far more susceptible to it if your father or grandfather suffered from it.

▶ **Counting to ten really works** If you feel yourself starting to lose it, start counting and take deep breaths as you do so.

▶ **Don't drink if you feel depressed** It will only make you feel more so.

In a relationship

In order to fulfil ourselves as human beings we need to get along with the people we share this planet with. Although these relationships come on all sorts of different levels, they are all necessary for the good of our health as well as the continuation of the species.

No man is an island

As human beings we are social animals, and throughout your life you will form a series of friendships, which will let you know you are part of a larger community, that you are accepted, cared for, trusted and liked. All of which is hugely important in a man's measure of himself and how he is progressing in the world around him. Friends will also provide an outlet for you when times are bad with a sympathetic ear, or give you people with whom to share your success. They will boost your confidence and provide moral support or physical back-up when you need it, and, perhaps most importantly, will not be slow in letting you know if you are acting like a berk.

And you will trust their judgements as much as you expect them to trust yours.

The remarkable thing about these

T

Tip: Be prepared to learn to communicate. It's not something all men do naturally, but it will be the difference between relationships working or not, so approach it like learning any other skill. Consciously build on your experiences and don't dismiss it as something that should happen by itself or somehow doesn't matter.

Friends are good for your health

Men and women who have friends they are in regular communication with live longer and enjoy better mental and physical health. A recent study at the Harvard Medical School likened the effects of not having friends to the dangers of obesity or smoking, as the subjects with no or few friends had higher cholesterol levels, less-efficient immune systems and greater rates of chronic stress. The study concluded that having people to share situations, ideas and circumstances with left them happier, with higher self-esteem and more likely to look after themselves. This reduced the likelihood of stress, which in turn lowered blood pressure, heart rates and cholesterol levels. It also lessened the likelihood of risky behaviour to the degree that those with friends even drove more carefully.

How it all works: the perfect relationship

The key to successful relationships lies in being able to tick as many of these boxes as possible:

Respect works both ways

Treat others in relationships in exactly the same way as you want them to treat you – this applies to work, marriage, friendship, team-mates, anything. If you treat others carelessly, then you have no right to complain if you are being given a hard time.

Take a hit for the team

What's worth more, your pride or your relationship? Sometimes it will be for the greater good to swallow something you might not be overly happy about – a healthy relationship will never be about winning.

Be honest

Don't bend the truth to try and get your own way as you'll either have to live that lie forever, or it will catch up with you and bite you on the arse.

Wrap things up

Look for closure in any dispute. If you let feuds or fights fester they will never "just go away." In a marriage, try not to go to sleep on an argument.

Give as much as you expect to take

If you are going to bend your friends' ears with your problems and get a considered, caring response, then be prepared to spend as much time playing agony uncle to them; likewise take the wife's problems as seriously as she takes yours.

Don't give up

Just because a relationship has got a little tricky there's no need to walk away from it. Always look to sort things out before you consider dumping somebody.

There shouldn't be anything you can't talk about

If you are keeping secrets then it is not a relationship founded on mutual trust, which means it will be doomed from the start. This isn't quite the same as the "Be honest" point: it's more serious.

Know when to call it a day

The previous point won't always work and sometimes it'll be best for all concerned if you bring an unfulfilling relationship to an end.

Listen up

A dialogue is a two-handed affair, so if you are using the periods when the other person is talking to think up what you are going to say next, your reactions won't have anything to do with their point of view.

Because they got married he's going to live longer, be healthier, have more money and do better at work. Not to mention more sex. No wonder he's smiling

The coupling conundrum

The human race is genetically engineered to keep going – see Chapter 7. To ensure the best chance of survival, at some point most of us are going to form some sort of meaningful personal relationship and one with a view to lasting a long time. Because this is so fundamental to who we are, these relationships can bring the most joy and fulfilment to our lives and can also cause equally enormous problems.

Why get married?

Seeing as 46 percent of all UK marriages will end in divorce, as will 51 percent in the US, and these figures have been rising steadily for the last thirty years, it would seem there is increasingly less point in getting married. Yet recent statistics for weddings in Britain show the figures have been creeping up since an all-

relationships is that while on the surface they may all be wildly different, they are all essentially the same. What you expect from and how you are with, say, your dad or people who work for you or a woman you fancy will, hopefully, be hugely varied, yet each relationship will stand or fall on consideration, mutual respect, a degree of tolerance, unselfishness and the ability to be able to trust within it. These points will lie at the base of every tangible reward that may result from the relationship and form the foundation for whatever longevity it might assume. But it is crucial they be balanced on both sides.

T

Tip: Meeting new people is the gateway to new friendships, but while it might follow that the more people you meet the more friendships you are likely to form and the greater support structure you are likely to enjoy, friendships are about quality rather than quantity, and a few good friends will be much more valuable than dozens of acquaintances.

Expert advice: "Is it natural to have one life partner? I think it's a rarity! However, I wouldn't have got married if I didn't think I was going to spend the rest of my life with the guy, but then I didn't get married until I was 33, so I assume I'd already done the non-monogamous thing. That's definitely the best way to do it."
Sarah Hedley

time low in 2001. And not without good reason either.

There is little in life that, according to every survey ever carried out on the subject, offers as much obvious benefit to a man as getting married. Married men live longer than their single counterparts; they are likely to earn more; get promoted at work earlier and receive more positive assessments; get ill less; have more sex; suffer less depression and are much less likely to top themselves; have far fewer problems with drink or drug addictions; manage their money better; suffer fewer stress-related complaints; and are nearly twice as likely as single men to say they are happy with their lives. Incidentally, these figures are more or less the same for women, and the only negative point thrown up from their half of these surveys is that married women tend to do more housework. However, this is believed to be related more to having children than having a husband.

And this ringing endorsement of being a husband rather than a boyfriend is getting louder, as the percentile gaps between the figures for married men and their single brethren get bigger every year.

Perhaps it should be pointed out that the notion of marriage in this context is about formally committed long-term unions, thus it includes civil partnerships.

Not just a knees-up

The reason why married people do so much better is because marriage satisfies us on two distinct levels – inherent and practical – both of which are pretty straightforward.

As we get older, we invest more in friendships and so expect more in return, thus loyalty, reliability, stability and so on,

T

Tip: If you think you aren't ready to settle down just yet, you probably aren't. Letting circumstances or other people try and convince you otherwise is never a good idea.

Step away from the lingerie department!

According to Sarah Hedley, the worst thing you can buy your other half is underwear.

"Don't buy her underwear. Imagine what it looks like from the other side – 'I bought you this underwear, now can we have sex. Oh yes, and can you put it on first.' You need to be a bit more sophisticated than that.

"Don't buy her shoes either. Regardless of whether she likes the shoes or not, there will be a whole experience attached to shopping for them that you will just have stolen from her. Take her to lunch, go with her shopping for exactly the same pair of shoes, and she'll get the whole experience without having to foot the bill."

play as much of a part as the more immediate reasons to hang out with somebody. It's relevant that friendships made among older people tend to last longer and with a greater degree of trust involved. A good marriage satisfies so much of this innate need for dependable company, to leave us feeling fulfilled on a deep subconscious level. It's why the proportion of married men who claim to be happy with their lives is nearly twice what it is for single men, and why a married man's mental health is considerably better. This feeling of well-being is something they take with them into other aspects of their lives, notably the workplace where it contributes to their greater success levels.

Perhaps even more importantly, it satisfies the propagation of the species aspect. Psychologically, this commitment to settling down with a permanent partner – in spite of the high divorce rate, very few get married assuming it to be temporary – represents

T

Tip: Remain sensitive to whoever you are dealing with. There is nothing dishonest about presenting slightly different facets of yourself in different relationships, and it is vital not to treat everybody you deal with in exactly the same way – it's pretty much a given your wife won't appreciate being called "mate" as she gets punched on the shoulder.

the successful negotiation of some sort of "growing up" watershed, and then becomes a precursor to having children.

Your life will be better

On a far more prosaic level sharing your life with somebody who cares about you as much as you care about them means you look after each other as a matter of course. And look out for each other – married men or women are much less likely to be victims of crime than single people. According to the surveys married men suffer fewer cardiovascular problems, have lower blood pressure and cholesterol levels, and take less time off work sick with niggling little illnesses.

Much of this improved health is down to the Nag Factor of being married. In the nicest possible way, wives nag husbands to watch their weight, get their blood pressure and cholesterol checked, go to the dentist, get that bad back looked at and so on. Then if they do get ill, it's far more likely to be dealt with at the early stages, while care at home should be that much better if it does get serious. All of which contributes as much to the low sick day count as the frequent and scathing accusations of being a "bloody hypochondriac". It's so much harder for

A

Expert advice: "Massage is one of the best things you can do in a relationship – I know it's a cliché, but the reason it's a cliché is because it's true. With so many men, it's a bit of a foreplay tactic, with them just using it to try to get in some woman's pants. But if you appreciate it for what it is, as a way of helping your partner de-stress and having physical closeness of a non-sexual nature, then it really comes into its own. Massage classes for couples are really booming, because it gives people another way to be physical – I don't feel like sex tonight, but how about a massage?"
Sarah Hedley

> **F**
>
> *Fact: Isolated acts of domestic violence – as opposed to sustained spousal abuse – are much more frequent among cohabitees than among married couples.*

married men to shirk their responsibilities if they are hungover, no matter how truly awful they might feel.

However, it's also much less likely they're going to be hungover. Most men's rates of risky behaviour drop significantly once they tie the knot, simply because, according to surveys, they believe that "isn't what life's all about any more". They feel part of something bigger, and while most won't – and shouldn't – completely give up going on the lash, most won't want to nearly so much. Of course this won't be for entirely unselfish reasons – most men will quickly work out it's never a good idea to upset the wife too often.

More than simply a piece of paper

There are, at the time of writing, some five million people in the UK cohabiting, a tenfold increase during the last fifty years.

Around three-quarters of these couples say they are likely to get married, to each other, at some point in the future. They are also very likely to get divorced at some point after that.

Currently, over fifty percent of couples in the UK (the same in the US) live together before getting married, and the divorce rate among them is more than twice what it is among those who didn't. While this statistic is in no way a guarantee of marriage failure –

The marriage rate around the world

US	9.8 per 1000 people
Russia	8.9 per 1000 people
Czech Republic	8.4 per 1000 people
Romania	8.3 per 1000 people
Portugal	7.3 per 1000 people
Israel	7.0 per 1000 people
New Zealand	7.0 per 1000 people
Switzerland	6.9 per 1000 people
Australia	6.9 per 1000 people
United Kingdom	6.8 per 1000 people
Globally	6.5 per 1000 people

Source: UN 2007

The Bridget Jones myth

Contrary to popular belief, men are far more likely to live by themselves than women. In 2007 sixteen percent of men between the ages of 25 and 45 lived alone, compared with eight percent of women. However, among men it is far more likely to be a temporary condition yet women seem more at ease with long-term singledom. This is believed to be because men get lonelier more easily, get more stressed at work and need somebody to talk to who isn't in a pub, and put simply, they just like being looked after – the One Mum To Another Syndrome. Women, on the other hand, are far more inclined to relish the ability to run their own lives exactly how they want, thus are more reluctant to give it up.

D.I.V.O.R.C.E.

Regardless of how much better it will be for most people to remain married or in a relationship, there will be many for whom getting out of it would be far better for their health. Because the home is traditionally a place of safety, away from the stresses of the world as well as the dangers, the effects of living in a relationship gone bad can be more damaging than having a miserable time at work. It will have a lower profile though, as the resulting senses of shame or failure or disappointment at a marriage going wrong are, for many men, far more difficult to talk about than problems at work.

In cases in which a single unforgivable act, such as infidelity or violence, has caused all vestiges of trust or respect to have disappeared, it will be clear cut, but in other instances where the reasons for the breakdown are less easily identifiable, setting proceedings in motion will be far less straightforward. Because divorce is such a drastic step and rarely one that ends in happiness for both parties, before you reach for m'learned friends, ask yourself these six questions. And make sure you get well-considered, satisfactory answers.

Why do you want to get divorced?	If you are just having a row, then realize that is what it is and as an isolated incident it can surely be resolved. However, if it's one more manifestation of deep-seated differences that you can no longer live with and you are certain can never be sorted out, that's a whole other matter.
Did you ever get married to start off with?	Are you together for the purely practical reasons of servicing the needs of two individuals – mortgage, bills, sex, company? Then you should probably call it a day without making yourselves miserable in the process. But if you're a genuine one-half-complements-the-other couple, think twice.
Are you simply bored?	The chances are your partner is too, therefore, if you sit down together and talk about it, it will be relatively easy to do something about. Be prepared to take a bit of stick though, and you might have to give up your right to the bacon always being on the left-hand side of the eggs.
Is it that the grass seems greener outside of your marriage?	If you're contemplating getting out of your marriage not because there's anything too wrong with it but because what's going on elsewhere seems so much more exciting, be warned – it rarely is. The chances are you will soon get tired of whatever it is you're coveting at the moment. (See previous point.)
Are you just threatening divorce to get your own way?	Ironically, if you have no intention of going through with it then you absolutely should. Any relationship that is being held together with that sort of threat is already finished.
Do you still love your partner?	If you do, then divorce is going to be doubly difficult.

T

Tip: Adulterers will very probably do it again. If you are planning on settling down with somebody who left their partner after cheating with you, there is a very good chance they will cheat on you further down the road.

33 percent won't get divorced – it rather flies in the face of the modern belief that getting to know one another properly before tying the knot will build a stronger union. In fact, pre-marital cohabiting is believed to signify an underlying selfishness on both sides – neither party is prepared to fully commit, creating an "If you pass this audition then maybe I'll marry you" state of affairs. Often, for men rather than women, there will be

more pragmatic reasons for living together – it's cheaper, more sex and having somebody to talk to after a bad day at work being the most persuasive arguments – but none of them are indicative of lasting commitment. Another significant factor is that those who lived together first don't take marriage as seriously as those who didn't. Therefore, they are far more likely to see divorce as a solution to problems that could be worked out.

Of couples living together that do not have the intention of getting married, the chances of them staying together are even less optimistic. According to statistics, just under twelve percent will stay together longer than ten years. And, crucially, cohabiting couples are just as likely to have children together as married couples, yet the statistic for them splitting up shows the same rate for those with and without children.

It seems, regardless of how un-twenty-first century the institution of marriage may

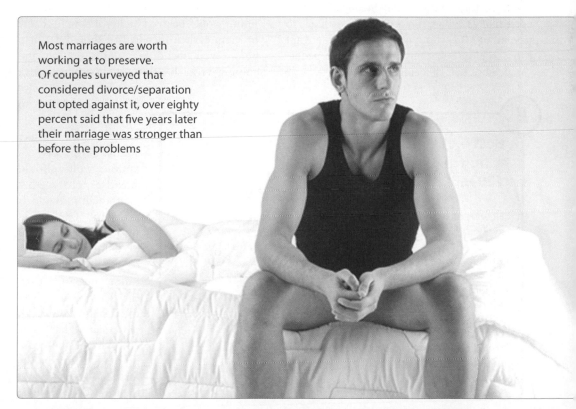

Most marriages are worth working at to preserve. Of couples surveyed that considered divorce/separation but opted against it, over eighty percent said that five years later their marriage was stronger than before the problems

Why get divorced?

There are thousands of unique reasons for divorce, but the most common triggers are (in order):

1. Financial disagreements
2. Infidelity
3. Sexual problems
4. Career frustration
5. Life changes
6. Abandonment
7. Drug or alcohol addiction

T

Tip: The more equal the relationship the happier and more fulfilled the marriage, so only take charge when she wants you to.

Should you get counselling?

appear, the act of going through a formal wedding ceremony in front of your family and friends elevates the level of commitment to a degree that simply moving in together can't. Although, once again, there is no scientific evidence to support this, research has shown that, in spite of being outwardly dedicated to the relationship, cohabitees set greater store on their independence. They are less likely to share finances and more likely to be unfaithful – both men and women are apt to carry on behaving like two single people instead of half of a couple.

For many couples relationship counselling is the absolute last resort. This is because, traditionally, outside help in something as personal as a marriage is seen as unnecessary intrusion. Yet the success rates are very high and over eighty percent of couples in Britain who have received counselling say it put their relationship back on track. Relate, the UK's biggest counselling service, believe this figure would be even higher if couples came to them earlier. Ideally, you should get help before you spend years of resenting and sniping at each other, otherwise you may both be too defensive to allow a solution to be found.

If you take counselling as an option you should attend sessions together – although individuals can still be helped – and be prepared to tell the full story of your relationship. From hearing that, the counsellor will then help you both understand that story and pick out significant points and habits formed. As a result, the three of you will be

B

Best investment: a bunch of flowers, £20–£50 ($50–$100)

Flowers work. Practically everybody loves getting a bunch of flowers – men and women. And after they've been given, they'll cheer up a room to such a degree that everybody who comes into it will smile. Also, next time you buy a bunch for somebody check out the looks you're getting from women as you walk along carrying them.

Why is the divorce rate so high?

According to our relationships expert Sarah Hedley, it's a matter of social evolution and, post-feminism, it was inevitable.

"There's so much more divorce around now because divorce is a lot more acceptable – there used to be a stigma attached to being a divorcee, even as recently as the 1970s, but that stigma has gone now, which, in a way, is a good thing.

"Also, although men and women have more in common than they've ever had, they don't need each other as much as they used to and I think that's the key thing. Feminism happened, and although women still earn 17.5 percent less than men, across the board, they are part of the workforce now, so when they marry they do so out of choice rather than necessity. These days the average person is marrying out of love, rather than because you've got pregnant or you want to move out of the parental home and all the reasons our parents got married. So if they fall out of love, they get divorced."

able to identify the strengths and weaknesses of the relationship and start to redefine how it can go forward by emphasizing the former and accommodating the latter.

Usually the results are very straightforward, and any redirecting is easy to absorb into your lives. This is because, so often, those in the relationship are so wrapped up in its minutiae they cannot see aspects that are very obvious to outsiders. Also, the chance for both parties to talk openly to somebody other than each other can bring to light things that have never been mentioned before.

T

Tip: Perfection is overrated. If you want to find that life partner before both of you are dead then let go of that checklist of what they need to be. Learn to see past their "flaws" just as you'll hope they will accept yours.

Fit for divorce

There is a good chance that the divorce you are contemplating will be a liberating state of affairs and becoming single once again will hugely enrich your life. But then again it might not. Like more or less everything else in this book getting divorced will be a great deal easier if you are ready for it, although

Battered husbands: the reality

A recent American survey concluded that 27 percent of adult men had been the victims of domestic abuse, and, as men in their twenties and thirties suffered far more than their older counterparts, this is set to be an escalating trend. The health firm that conducted the survey also believed the actual figure was far higher, but many men were too embarrassed to admit they get bullied.

The definition of abuse in the survey included assault (with or without weapons), sex against their will and "non-physical abuse" which covered threats, controlling or manipulating behaviour and persistent disparaging remarks.

T

Tip: Ex-girlfriends are generally bad news as far as your present relationship goes. In spite of you being very sure that they have been securely consigned to your history, and therefore less of a threat than new acquaintances, the chances are your other half won't see it that way.

these preparations will be mental rather than physical. Initially you have to be steely enough to face the pain this divorce is going to cause to the spouse, children, parents, in-laws, friends… it's going to affect all of them, and none of them well, and children particularly acutely.

It will mean a bigger disruption to your life than getting married or even having children did. Then you were eased into

those situations with a great deal of positive preparation, and those experiences were adding to your life. Divorce will only be taking away. You will have to rethink finances, accommodation, domestic arrangements and habits, and probably face a degree of loneliness as a result. It will seriously affect your state of mind too. There is the sheer stress brought on by all of the above, added to which there may well be the unpleasant prospect of a messy legal battle with somebody you used to share a bed with. The act of splitting up a partnership you have invested so much in over the years will also put a serious dent in your self-esteem, but it is important to remember this will not last forever.

It's not just about you

Then there's the collateral damage. Getting divorced will mean the world looks at you differently to when you were Mr Family Man. Just as married men tend to do better at work, divorced men's careers can slow down suddenly, and in social situations be prepared for it to be the only thing that defines you to some people.

Friendships vs partnerships

There's no reason at all why this should be a conflict. It's healthy for both you and your partner to have friendships outside of your relationship – that is, your own friends, that you hang out with by yourself,

The divorce rate around the world

US	4.95 per 1000 people
Puerto Rico	4.47 per 1000 people
Russia	3.36 per 1000 people
United Kingdom	3.08 per 1000 people
Denmark	2.81 per 1000 people
New Zealand	2.63 per 1000 people
Australia	2.52 per 1000 people
Canada	2.46 per 1000 people
Finland	1.85 per 1000 people
Barbados	1.21 per 1000 people
Globally	1.3 per 1000 people

Source: UN 2007

F

Fact: For the last 35 years men have been getting married older. In 1972 the average age of a UK bridegroom was nearly 25; in 2007 it was just under 29.

rather than other couples. Even if your partner is, as should be, your best friend, these extra-marital friendships are vital for more than just the chance to moan about your other half. Because human beings are complex individuals, it's highly unlikely that most of them are going to be satisfied with the relatively tunnel-visioned approach to existence that would be offered by no life outside a domestic relationship. Provided, of course, you remember what your priorities have to be and they don't interfere with your life at home.

A wider view of life

Primarily, outside friendships bring an all-important different perspective on life, an angle other than within the household. Such peripheral opinion can be a huge advantage

T

Tip: If you are about to embark on a big, potentially stressful situation, one with plenty of scope for arguments – like extensive building work, launching a business, emigrating – it is a good idea to go for some counselling sessions beforehand. Even if you know you have a rock-solid relationship, it will help to be able to understand each other that bit better.

when it comes to discussing problems, just as they can be an important pressure-release

The longer you stay married the longer you are likely to stay married – over fifty percent of all divorces happen during the first ten years of the marriage. If you make it beyond that, the rate dips below thirty percent; and past twenty it will be lower than fifteen percent

Foreplay vs choreplay

Men who do housework get more sex, and not merely as a reward. Sarah Hedley explains:

"Buy her time. Work out what is taking up a huge amount of her time and buy her that time back. That's what being in a partnership is about – you've tuned in to what she needs and you've made it happen to give her back an hour or so for herself, her life. Now see where that takes you.

"We are all very, very time poor at the moment and if you can give your partner back some time then she will have time to feel more free to relax and de-stress, to feel sexy. Because there are only so many hours in the day, if a woman is left to take care of the responsibilities of running the house, then she runs out of time and energy at the end of the day to do anything else. Do the hoovering, or whatever, then there will be more time left at the end of the day for you to be with each other. It's called choreplay, and it really works."

valve for thoughts you perhaps couldn't express at home. These friendships offer the chance to behave in ways that might not be entirely appropriate at home – providing, of course, you don't forget your responsibilities to your domestic situation. Also they may allow the chance to pursue activities that do not interest your partner but mean a great deal to you.

For men, these friendships will often mean people they were friends with before they met their partner, as close male friendships tend to be more enduring than women's. Be careful, however, that this doesn't lead to problems in itself. These will be people who will know you as well as your partner does, if not better, and such friendships can lead to jealousies or feelings of exclusion. Think about it very carefully if these long-standing friends are women.

Women have egos too

The male ego is a much talked about state of affairs, but it's worth remembering that women have self-esteem as well. We've already

The best of the web

Relate.org.uk
The UK's largest provider of relationship and family counselling services offers support either at face-to-face sessions, over the telephone or online. The site features a directory of Relate locations, and explains how you will be asked to pay "what you can afford" for a session, usually between £5 and £40.

Counsel-search.com
An American site devoted to accredited marriage and family counsellors, providing a nationwide directory and series of articles discussing such topics as how to choose a counsellor, what is involved in a session and what the different services are.

Cccs.co.uk
The Consumer Credit Counselling Service, a charitable organization offering free, confidential counselling on money matters, and financial management services for those with money troubles.

Bacp.co.uk
The British Council for Counselling and Psychotherapy offers advice on how to find a reputable psychotherapist or counsellor.

discussed treating your partner as an equal in all things – except getting spiders out of the bath, obviously – but more importantly than that your partner will have an ego every bit as sensitive as yours. Constantly reminding her of her failings or refusing to appreciate what is being done, even if it's everyday stuff, is enough to erode anybody's feelings of self-worth and will result in a breakdown of the relationship and a loss of any respect for you.

Ten top tips for good relationships

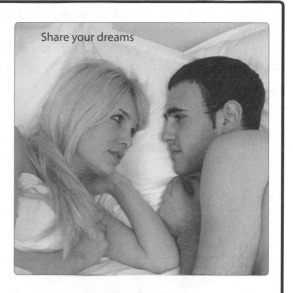

Share your dreams

▶ **Getting married is good for your health** And your wallet and your career.

▶ **Choose your friends for quality rather than quantity** The last thing you need in your life is a bunch of pointless acquaintances.

▶ **Relationships are about giving and taking** Treat others as you expect to be treated yourself.

▶ **Adulterers will probably do it again** They will always be difficult to trust.

▶ **Don't ever threaten to divorce your wife if you've no intention of going through with it** Not only is this wrong on so many levels but one day she'll call your bluff.

▶ **Try not to tell too many lies** Unless they're little ones and you're doing it for the greater good and not just to save your own skin.

▶ **Relationship counselling works** It's successful in over three-quarters of cases.

▶ **Do more than your "fair share" of the housework** You'll end up getting more than your "fair share" of sex.

▶ **Enjoy being nagged** If it's about things like looking after yourself a bit better, it really is for your own good.

▶ **Divorce is far more traumatic than getting married** You will feel like it is a step backwards.

On holiday

A good holiday a couple of times a year is one of the best cures known to man for stress, overwork, boredom and even low-level, niggling illnesses. Two weeks away somewhere sunny or spectacular – or both – is as good for the body as it is for the soul, provided you stay healthy while you're away.

The not so friendly skies

Quite apart from the stress caused by the eye-watering cost, sometimes unhelpful staff and almost compulsory delays, air travel can be physically bad for you. The main culprits are dehydration, poor air quality and reduced oxygen availability, immobility and bodily expansion.

Hydration, hydration, hydration (Part 1)

Humidity levels in the main cabins of commercial airliners will vary, but, uniformly, they will be lower than is good for you at take-off and will continue to fall as the flight progresses – put simply, the longer the haul the drier the air around you. Potentially, you could dry out far quicker than on the ground and your equilibrium will suffer as a) oxygen levels in cabin air are lower than air you'd normally breathe; and b) cabin pressure reduces oxygen saturation in the bloodstream. Should you start to dehydrate, your blood will thicken and transport oxygen around the body and brain with less efficiency – and with less oxygen to utilize, an uncomfortable fatigue

and drowsiness can result, which could also increase stress levels.

Approach any flight of over a couple of hours like a marathon runner and begin your hydration process beforehand. During those two or three hours between check-in and boarding drink at least 500ml of water, topping up with a further 250ml at the gate. Avoid vast quantities of coffee or alcohol both before and during the flight, as they will serve as diuretics – although something to relax you or a drink after a meal is perfectly acceptable. Once in flight, you need to be drinking 250ml of water each hour to stay hydrated and if you experience a dry mouth, itchy eyes, dull headache or general discomfort, you are on the way to

T

> *Tip: Take your own bottle of water on board, as the galley will not always be open and the cups of water handed out can be small. Don't bring bottled water from home as current airline security measures mean liquids over 100ml are confiscated at check-in, so buy your bottle in the departure lounge.*

How it all works: ear popping

The ear is split up into three parts: the outer ear – the part you can see, which leads down to the eardrum; the middle ear – comprising the eardrum and the air-filled cavity behind it; and the inner ear – which contains the nerve endings that transmit signals for hearing and balance. Sound is processed as the sound waves come down the ear canal of the outer ear to vibrate the fan-like membrane of the eardrum in the middle ear, and register in the inner ear. For this to happen efficiently, the air pressure on both sides of the eardrum must remain the same, and it will be constantly readjusting itself in the middle ear with air brought in through the Eustachian tube, a tiny tube that connects the back of the nose with the middle ear. If changes in pressure on the outside of the eardrum are swift, the Eustachian tube cannot equalize it within the chamber behind the drum and a vacuum is caused. This will suck the eardrum inwards, stretching it and preventing it from vibrating properly, hence the muffled hearing and discomfort inside the ear when cabin pressure changes. The same state can occur if nasal blockages from a head cold prevent air from reaching the Eustachian tube.

Yawning and swallowing can relieve the situation, as it activates the muscles that open the Eustachian tube and pushes a small bubble of air into it from the nose – you may need to do it several times though. If that doesn't work, increase the pressure through the Eustachian tube by taking in a mouthful of air, holding your nose shut and trying to push the air out through your blocked nose. Do this gently though, because to blow too hard without clearing the blockage

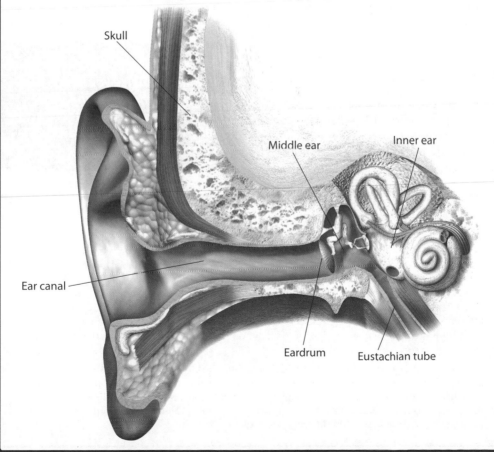

Skull

Middle ear

Inner ear

Ear canal

Eardrum

Eustachian tube

T

Tip: No matter how thirsty you are, never drink tap water on aircraft, as there are no set standards for in-flight water purity, and also you will have no idea in which country the tanks were filled.

dehydration. Wetting your face with a spray or a dampened handkerchief can help, and you should continue to rehydrate for a couple of hours after the flight has landed.

Pressure situation

At cruising altitude the air pressure in commercial airliners' cabins will be lower than on the ground, meaning your blood oxygen saturation will be lower than normal, by as much as ten percent. This shouldn't affect anyone in good health – although it may contribute to drowsiness or lack of concentration – but if you have cardiovascular problems or are very overweight, seek advice before you fly. If you experience aching lungs, clammy skin, dull headache, nausea, lack of

focus or impaired vision, the chances are you're becoming oxygen deprived. Explain to the cabin crew that you are having difficulty breathing and ask if the oxygen can be turned up; this should get you back on course.

Air quality in aeroplanes is a questionable issue. Airlines maintain it is perfectly adequate – better than most office blocks, they claim – while so much anecdotal evidence suggests otherwise. Never be too surprised if you pick up a low-level bug on a long-haul flight and if you are particularly susceptible to bugs, or are of a nervous disposition, breathe through a water-saturated handkerchief.

Don't sit still

For most of us, air travel means being squashed into a confined space in uncomfortable position, and as seat pitch – the distance

T

Tip: As soon as possible after landing immerse yourself in water – bath, swimming pool, sea – as this will assist the rehydration process and help you to relax.

Deep vein thrombosis

As the name suggests, this is a blood clot or thrombus that occurs in the large veins, such as the femoral, deep within your legs. DVT has become so associated with long-haul flying because the extended stretches of inactivity in the constrictive position of aircraft seating are ideal conditions for blood clotting. With large veins come some sizeable blood clots, and while they may not do much damage in your legs, substantial pieces can break off and work their way up to the veins that feed into the heart and lungs to cause serious problems. The effects of DVT may not be felt until some time after the flight as the blood needs to flow freely once more for the clot to start moving through the veins.

The chances of a healthy person getting deep vein thrombosis are slim, but those odds increase greatly among smokers, the overweight or those with a family history of blood clotting complaints. The same precautions for swollen feet should be taken to avoid possible DVT, but if you are susceptible to blood clots, it is recommended you wear calf-length compression socks to keep the blood flowing smoothly in your lower legs.

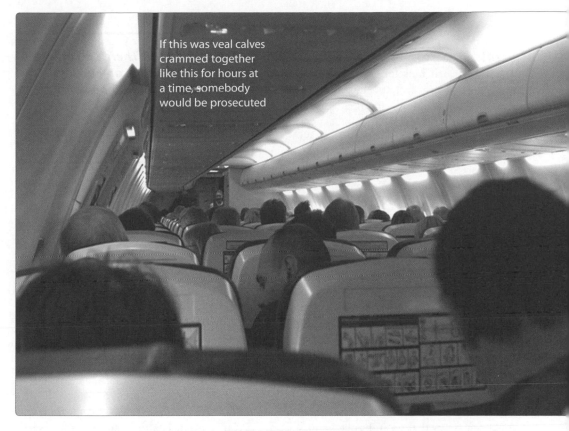

If this was veal calves crammed together like this for hours at a time, somebody would be prosecuted

between the front of your seat and the back of the one in front – seems to be getting shorter, this situation won't be improving. Such constriction of movement and pressure on parts of the body can cause a serious restriction in blood flow, which brings on big problems.

The most immediate effect is a swelling of the feet and ankles. This is commonly assumed to be down to cabin pressure, but it's simply a gravitational pooling of blood in the veins in those areas due to sitting with your feet on the floor for a long period of time. The dispersal of blood from these areas will also be hindered by pressure on the legs and waist from sitting, which constricts veins.

T

Tip: During your flight, cabin pressure will cause the gases in your stomach to expand by as much as twenty percent, therefore avoid gas-producing foods such as cabbage or broccoli, or beer or fizzy drinks. Wear trousers that can be discreetly expanded and be thoughtful of fellow passengers should internal pressures get too much to bear.

F

Fact: The air quality on the flight decks of most commercial airliners will be of a much better quality than in the main cabin, as higher oxygen levels serve to keep the pilots sharp.

As elevating your feet will not always be practical, sit with your legs out as straight as possible, rotate your ankles frequently and stretch your calf muscles every half hour or so by drawing your feet up and pointing your toes. Get up and walk about at least once every hour, as the contraction and expansion of the muscles in your lower legs will pump the blood away from where it is collecting. This exercise will also ease constriction all over your body and stimulate your heart rate to assist blood flow.

Keep healthy and fit on holiday

The best way to keep fit on holiday, if there's no chance for swimming, is to pack running shoes and get out on the road on a few early mornings. It can benefit more than your health, as being out and about in the area you're staying when it's waking up is a great way to discover some of its true character. You'll see views that go unnoticed and spot landmarks or sites that may be worth going back to when you've got more time.

A

Expert advice: "There's no excuse for not keeping fit on holiday; take your running shoes with you and anywhere you're going the road's just out there."
Gideon Remfry

Watch what you're eating – especially if you're drinking a great deal – as it's easy to pile on the calories through two weeks of rich hotel/restaurant food. Don't neglect breakfast, but don't turn it into a bagel/croissant-heavy carb-fest. Instead opt for cereals, fresh fruit and yoghurt and don't overdo that caffeine if you're going out in the sun, as it will speed dehydration. Go for fruit or fruit juice at lunchtime to keep your blood sugar levels up, and visit a local supermarket, street or farmers market to stock up on fruit, nuts or other healthy snacks. Treat yourself to a decent dinner, as if you've eaten healthily all day you deserve it – you are on holiday, after all – and it's important to get something in your stomach

Have a good flight

• Make sure you've informed the airline in advance about any dietary or health requirements, then, when you check in, make sure these requests have been registered.

• Don't let airline staff stress you out, no matter how awkward they are appearing to be - console yourself by remembering you're going somewhere exciting and they're not.

• Be prepared for delays, carry any medicine you may need along with an MP3 player, reading material, carbohydrate snacks and plenty of water.

• If you are delayed and it can affect a condition you suffer with, make sure you inform airline staff at the earliest opportunity.

• Don't get drunk; relax with a drink or two, but don't overdo it as alcohol will have a more acute effect when you are in the air and will serve to dehydrate you more quickly.

• Remember to avoid excess tea and coffee as these are also diuretics.

• Move around the cabin if you can, without getting on fellow travellers' nerves, obviously.

• Keep hydrated, drinking plenty of water before and during the flight.

before a night on the town (see p.187).

Really, all healthy eating abroad requires is to follow the same rules as you would at home, and if your holiday offers the bonuses of really fresh fish and poultry or locally grown fruit and vegetables, take full advantage of them.

Health insurance

Many budget tour operators make more money selling travel insurance than they do selling holidays, hence the pressure on you to buy it, but while you should definitely have medical/travel insurance before you fly, make sure it's got what you need. A general rule of thumb with insurance policies is that you get what you pay for, and the less expensive the

T Tip: Just because you see local people drinking the water don't assume it will be safe; for you, they may well have built up immunity to bacteria contained within.

policy the flimsier your coverage. Make sure yours not only covers you for having to go to hospital, but will pay all medical bills abroad – this is because items like ambulances, drugs, surgery, convalescence, meals in hospital and follow-up visits to outpatient clinics or GPs may all be billed as separate items. Also, if it

A hotel room workout

If your hotel doesn't have a gym, the following schedule works most of your major muscles and should help keep you trim until you get home. Do as many reps as you feel are beneficial.

Press ups – works arms, shoulders and upper back
Employing a selection of different styles, such as clapping, arms spread wide, raising feet off the floor, etc, will utilize different muscles.

The lunge – quadriceps
Stand with feet slightly apart and hands on hips; step forward with right leg, until knee is bent at right angles, left knee is almost touching the floor and your back remains straight; step back with right leg to starting position. Repeat with left leg.

Donkey kicks – hamstrings and hips
Get down on your hands and knees; lift left leg up to bring the knee to the chest then kick back with it as far and as high as you can; bring it back to chest and return to the floor. Repeat with the right leg.

The crunch – abdominal muscles
Lie with back flat on floor and feet raised so knees are at right angles, shins are parallel with floor and arms are crossed over chest; raise upper body to crunch ribcage towards the pelvis. Lower shoulders back to floor and repeat.

Of course there's no reason why you should be stuck in your hotel room to work out

Jet lag

There is no real cure for the discomfort and tiredness that can be brought on by crossing into different time zones and having to readjust your body clock. The best you can do is prepare by being rested, well nourished and properly hydrated before you travel, then when you arrive set your watch to the new time immediately and throw yourself into the new schedule. Avoid big, carbohydrate-heavy, drowsiness-inducing meals, drink lots of water and carry on as normally as possible for the time zone you are in. If you feel you will be too tired to make it through the evening, have a short nap during the afternoon then stay up at night.

covers your getting flown home, check that it includes your partner or family.

Water, water, everywhere

You have to be much more careful than merely drinking the water in many countries, and a common cause of water-related food poisoning is ice. Tempting as it may seem, if you are not sure it has been made with sterilized or chlorinated water, don't load that rum and coke with ice, make do with chilled mixers instead. Also, salad items

that have been washed under taps could be contaminated – and this applies to all food items that will not be cooked. Finally, do remember to peel all fruit before you eat it.

Most of the larger hotels practically anywhere will be safe in this regard. Water

T

Tip: As restaurants in many other countries offer huge portions, don't be shy about asking for a doggy bag – it could take care of your next meal.

The fat of the land

Local cuisine might be more damaging than you are used to – unless, of course, you're American. The fattest popular holiday destinations are as follows, with figures given as a percentage of the adult population who are overweight.

USA	74.1
Barbados	69.7
Argentina	69.4
Egypt	69.4
Malta	68.7
Greece	68.5
Trinidad & Tobago	67.9
Seychelles	64.6
United Kingdom	63.8
Canada	61.1

Source: World Health Organization

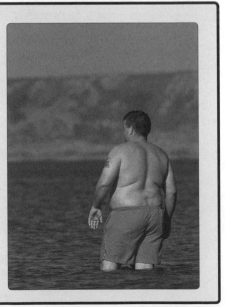

You don't have to drink the water to get sick

Over two million Britons contracted food poisoning abroad last year, and although most of that wasn't life-threatening, it's more than enough to ruin a holiday. The most likely complaints are described on page 107, and in hotter countries such things as dairy products and seafood will be particularly susceptible to spoiling if not kept properly, as will cooked food that is not refrigerated as soon as possible.

Be well prepared for an increased likelihood of bacterial infections by getting as fit and healthy as possible beforehand, and that should include tiptop gastric health. If you take on as many nutrients as you can in the lead-up to your holiday, your immune system will be as ready as it can be to ward off attack. Likewise, if you are going to a very high-risk area, a course of probiotics (see p.105) in the weeks before you fly out will make sure the good bacteria will be prevalent in your gut, no matter what.

will be treated to make sure it is good for use in the kitchen or ice machine, but it's still not advisable to drink it as it won't be quite what you are used to and may upset you. In all cases it's best to steer clear of roadside food vendors, unless what you're about to eat is well cooked and still sizzling hot.

Be careful of swimming in contaminated water too - raw sewage is the most common pollutant and, however careful you think you are being, some of it will enter your system and it can bring on extreme forms of gastroenteritis. Dirty water can cause rashes and infections in your bodily orifices as it seeps into ears, nose, eyes and the penis. This is a very real problem in the waters around the UK, as floods in 2007 led to overflowing sewers and long-term contamination of many parts of the coastline. Never swim in water where a dead animal or bird has been found; this will be a breeding ground for botulism, especially if the water temperature is very warm.

A place in the sun

In search of a suntan is the reason so many people go on holiday, yet it is also the reason why there are currently so many cases of skin cancer being diagnosed – over seventy-five thousand new cases diagnosed in the UK last year, a rise of four hundred percent in the last thirty years. In spite of it being widely accepted that the notion of a "healthy tan" is an oxymoron, you can still get away with doing it in the traditional manner... as long as you're never less than very careful.

B

Best investment: a box of drinking straws, £2.00 ($3.00)

Carry it with you at all times as it will allow you to buy drinks from street vendors and enjoy them without the risk of picking up any bacteria because your mouth won't have to touch the bottle or can.

How it all works: tanning and burning

A suntan is the darkening of the skin through exposure to the UVA and UVB waves of the sun's ultraviolet rays. It occurs because the melanocyte cells in the epidermis, or outer layer of the skin, are stimulated into producing extra melanin to protect against potential DNA damage by the ultraviolet rays. Melanin is the pigment that provides the skin with colour and protects against the sun by dissipating UV rays as harmless heat. This is why people from hotter climates have dark skin, as large amounts of natural melanin are protecting them from the sun, and why suntans fade after a holiday as protection is no longer required. During the protection process, UVA radiation produces an oxidizing effect in the melanocytes, darkening both the pre-formed and existing melanin, while the UVB rays cause the increase in production. The initial effects of the darkening will be immediate, increasing in intensity – the deep tan – after a couple of days.

Sunburn happens when living tissue is overexposed to UV rays (both UVA and UVB radiation) and the production of extra melanin either isn't sufficient or hasn't happened quickly enough to prevent some DNA damage occurring. Once this happens, the body sets off a series of defence mechanisms, depending on how serious the sunburn is. The painful redness and inflammation is a result of the epidermis releasing protective chemicals, which trigger a swelling of the blood vessels nearest the skin surface. If the burn is more serious, blisters form as the blood vessels leak a fluid that protects the skin as it recovers, and they shouldn't be burst. Peeling occurs when the damaged skin cells are jettisoned en masse as because their DNA make-up is no longer what it should be, the brain has deemed them "out of control", presenting a big risk of turning cancerous. However, it is very important to remember that just because you've peeled, the risk of skin cancer hasn't gone away – there is a high chance the UV rays have penetrated deeper, causing problems that will reveal themselves at some time in the future.

Top layer of skin, mostly dead cells

Epidermis

First stage of burning:
Redness on the top layer of skin

Second stage of burning:
Blistering in the epidermis

Third stage of burning:
Possibly cancerous cell damage in the lower dermis layer

Different wavelengths

UVA has a long wavelength – between 400 and 315 nanometres – is less easily blocked by sunscreen and is the cause of melanoma, which is the starting point of 75 percent of all skin cancer deaths. UVA penetrates deeper into the skin, adversely affecting collagen and elastin, thus ageing the skin.

UVB has a medium wavelength – between 315 and 280 nanometres – is more likely to cause sunburn but more efficiently filtered out by sunscreen. It is believed to cause moles and some skin cancers, but UVB contact with skin also can produce beneficial vitamin D in the body.

Tanning types

Because tanning is a reaction to damage already being inflicted, how well you will tan depends on your skin's ability to produce enough melanin to protect you from being burned (see box opposite). In this respect, everybody's skin will respond differently, depending on how much melanin a person has to start with. There are a number of categories of skin type that need to be considered.

Very fair

A skin type which will burn very quickly,

F

Fact: Although exposure to sunlight stimulates vitamin D production in the body, it only takes twenty minutes or so, a couple of times a week, of going about your regular business in the sun to get the maximum effect from this. A longer period, or increased intensity, will not add any more vitamin D but will leave you open to all the risks of UV radiation.

T

Tip: If, as a fair or very fair-skinned person, you are determined to get an al fresco suntan, start it off before you go away with a rigidly monitored course of sunbed sessions. Although sunbed tanning is becoming increasingly disapproved of by the medical profession, at least that way you will have kick-started what melanin you are able to produce. But do not make a habit of sunbed tanning and it is never recommended for teenagers.

probably not tanning at all as exposure can only be for very limited periods – the incidents of skin cancer in Scandinavia are nearly twice the EU average. This group should apply sunscreen of Factor 30 and upward.

Freckles or numerous moles

Those with this type of skin have a much greater likelihood of skin cancer, thus should also use above Factor 30.

Fair

Will burn easily, thus only a light, golden brown-ish tan will be possible. Sunscreen should be between Factor 15 and 30.

The European Health Insurance card

This UK government issue card entitles the bearer to access to whatever state-provided medical care is available in whatever European Union country they are visiting, and is also valid in Iceland, Liechtenstein, Norway and Switzerland. Many travel insurances will be invalid if you are not carrying one of these cards, but they are not a substitute for health insurance when away as there could be many expenses incurred that are not covered by that country's state healthcare.

No such service exists for Europeans travelling to the US, or for Americans travelling anywhere in the world, and private travel health insurance should be purchased.

European Union citizens in the UK can apply for a European Health Insurance card in any Post Office, by telephone at 0845 606 2030 or online at ehic.org.uk.

Light

As burning will take a while to happen, a mid-brown tan is possible, provided it's achieved gradually. Sunscreen Factor 8 to 15.

Dark or olive

Thanks to a large degree of inherent melanin, this skin type will not readily burn and so will tan profusely. Sunscreen Factor between 4 and 8.

Very dark

Although black people can sunburn, it is rare and takes a long time. UV rays can still be harmful, so a Factor 1 to 4 is still recommended for entire days in the sun, especially for those not used to it.

A sunscreen summary

The SPF rating of sunscreen is the degree of protection it offers the user – it stands for Sunburn Protection Factor – and the higher the number the longer, not the stronger, the protection offered. What the number signifies is a multiplication factor of the amount of time you can spend in the sun before you'll burn: if, with no protection, it takes you twenty minutes to burn, then applying Factor 5 will extend that to one hundred minutes, while Factor 2 would

A

Expert advice: "When on holiday, try and eat as much fresh local produce as possible. It can be very easy not to disturb any healthy eating plan you might have if you are somewhere with fresh fish and fruit and olives. But if you are in a city or living purely on processed hotel food for two weeks you will have to make an extra effort to find some whole food to make sure you keep your bowels moving."
Dr Sarah Schenker

T

Tip: If your shadow is shorter than you are, the sun's rays will be dangerously intense and extra care needs to be taken.

For the frequent flyer

If regular business trips are playing havoc with your fitness regime, follow these guidelines:

• Carry your own snacks, so that the two hours between check-in and flight time isn't spent grazing high-carb convenience food.

• Air travel causes fatigue through dehydration and poor air quality, which leads to feelings of hunger, so drink plenty of water and carry your own healthy food.

• Stay away from the room service menu, especially outside of restaurant hours. It's too easy to be tempted and the chances are it will offer quick-fix calorific stodge.

• Two or three extra beers a day will soon make themselves known on your waistline, so don't drink either for business bonding or out of sheer boredom.

• Set a time to work out or run and stick to it, either getting up early or blocking out an hour of your schedule.

mean you could stay out in the sun merely twice as long than you could without protection.

However, it is not magic bulletand these timings are simply guidelines don't take into account the intensity of the sun you'll be under. Also, be wary of those offering all-day protection – Factor 50 and upwards – as they will still need regular re-application: they willwear off or sweat off or wash off while you are swimming.

Remember to reapply sunscreen every couple of hours, regardless of what time limit the Factor calculation gives you. This is because that time will be how long your skin will be safe in the sun for, under sufficient application, not how long each application lasts. Sweating, moving about, lying down, putting on and taking off clothes all contribute to it wearing too thin to be of any use after a couple of hours. Always reapply after swimming, even if yours is of a waterproof variety, and if playing sports make sure it is one of the specially formulated sweatproof, performance types.

Never forget that on the slopes, because the air is so thin, the sun can be as intense as the action

T

Tip: When you get to your destination, invest in a small, inexpensive cool box; it will keep fruit fresh and drinks cold on the go or in your hotel room and you can donate it to the room's next visitor when you go home.

If you've still managed to get burned

There is no "cure" for sunburn, and the best you can hope for is to manage the symptoms with a minimum of discomfort and without increasing the damage already done.

The first thing to do is get out of the sun immediately – this is important

T

Tip: The aloe plant grows abundantly in tropical climes - recognizable by thick, spiky, fleshy leaves and tubular flower shafts rising from their centre. Cut one of the leaves open to release a thick liquid that will cool, soothe and moisturize irritated skin.

because in some cases sunburn may not become apparent for several hours, meaning significant damage has already occurred. Sunburn symptoms are partially the result of the body trying to cool itself down, so help it by applying cooling gel or après sun lotion. Compresses made from towels soaked in iced water can be particularly effective, but avoid thick creams as they may prevent the skin from dissipating the heat and so intensify your condition.

Anti-inflammatory medicine – a brand containing aspirin or ibuprofen – will help ease the pain and bring the swelling down.

Sun safety

The sun will be at its most intense between 10am and 2pm
Restrict your sunbathing to much shorter stretches during this period.

Just because you're not hot, it doesn't mean you're not burning
Out on a boat or on the golf course, for instance, the wind may well be keeping you cool, but the UV rays will still be getting through.

Check your sunscreen is of the "broad spectrum" variety and filters out both UVA and UVB radiation
It is not unusual for less expensive sunscreens to only block UVB rays, leading the user to believe they are better protected than they are: although UVB rays cause proportionately more damage, the UVA rays will still burn you if you are overexposed to them.

Make sure you apply enough sunscreen
It's not at all uncommon for people to under-apply sunscreen and thus compromise its protection capabilities. If you don't want to put on a great deal then switch to a higher SPF, but remember to reduce the time limit accordingly.

Reflective surfaces like sand, water or snow will intensify the sun's rays
This not only increases the amount of UV radiation hitting the skin, but also means it will be coming at you from a different direction as well – whitewashed walls or pale patios will have the same effect.

Be careful of those bits of you not used to the sun
Areas of your body usually exposed will have a more protective level of melanin than the bits that only see the light of day on holiday or when sunbathing.

The sun's rays will be more intense the higher up you are
And not just because you're closer to it either, but because the thinner air provides less resistance to UV radiation.

Wear a hat – even if you've got a full head of hair
The head is particularly sensitive to heat, thus leaving it uncovered greatly increases the risk of sunstroke. Opt for one with a wide, all-round brim, as that will provide sunburn protection for the nose, ears and neck.

After that, apply a moisturizing cream, something with aloe will soothe, or a cream containing between 0.5 and one percent hydrocortisone will boost the healing process. Don't burst any blisters as these will be protecting the new skin that is forming, and drink plenty of water as it's likely you'll be dehydrated from your time in the sun.

It usually takes between twelve and twenty-four hours, from the time it started, for sunburn to peak, therefore it is important you stay out of the sun, or keep the burned area covered, for the next two days. Seek professional help if the symptoms persist after two days, if you are feverish, or if over half your body is covered with blisters.

Keep your cool

Heat stroke, or sunstroke, is the name given to the extreme end of a condition called hyperthermia, during which the body is absorbing, or producing, more heat than it can dissipate. It's the opposite of hypothermia, when the body is losing more heat than it can produce or absorb.

If you have reached the point of heat stroke, your body temperature will be dangerously elevated as your internal thermostat will have been overloaded and can no longer function properly. This occurs because the cooling mechanisms have been overwhelmed by any of the following: high external temperature, intense or prolonged physical exertion or dehydration. As a result the body's temperature rises from between 36 and 37°C to 40°C or above, at which heat exhaustion causes collapse, and any further rise becomes potentially life-threatening as systems shut down. This, however, is the end product of a relatively lengthy process that will give plenty of warning signs that you are overheating or dehydrating.

Hydration, hydration, hydration (Part 2)

Starting to sweat when you get hot is perfectly normal, as, on the droplets of perspiration, it draws heat from inside the body to deposit it on the outside of the skin where it dissipates through evaporation. However, the body needs to be sufficiently hydrated to allow it to sweat enough to keep cool under intense conditions, so it is vital to drink more water as the mercury rises.

Your traveller's first aid kit

It should be kept it in a cool place and contain:

A variety of plasters
Antiseptic wipes
Antiseptic cream
Various-sized gauze dressings
Rolled crepe bandage and safety pins
Disposable sterile gloves
Scissors
Tweezers
Painkillers
Insect bite cream/spray
Digital thermometer
Distilled water for cleaning wounds or eyes

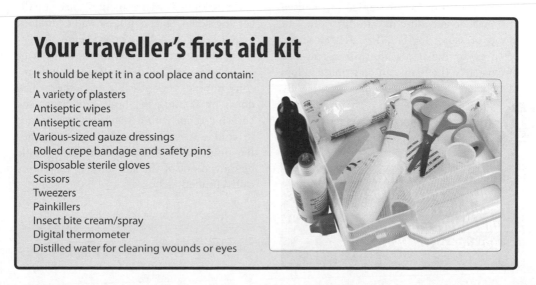

Hangover hell

The main component of a hangover is dehydration, thus the morning after the night before is never going to be a good time to be out in the sun. Make sure you are adequately rehydrated after drinking at night, and be aware that hard boozing in a hot climate will dry you out quicker than it would back home. For this reason, all day drinking is not such a good idea and you ought to give your system a chance to recover – and rehydrate – during the day.

Dehydration comes on very quickly – if you feel thirsty, it's already started because your body is letting you know – and once you've lost up to five percent of your body weight through fluid depletion you will experience all-over discomfort, muscle cramps and headaches. While this would impair an athlete's performance, it won't, at that point, be too dangerous. Any further loss of fluid though, and sweating will become so difficult that the body's internal temperature starts to rise drastically. If physical effort or high external temperature are continued it will increase massively, bringing progressively dangerous warning sings.

First, breathing becomes difficult as the heart beats faster to try to get enough oxygen around the system in the bloodstream. The skin reddens because blood vessels dilate to assist this movement of oxygen, but that causes blood pressure to fall and dizziness can result, often accompanied by nausea and headaches. Reacting to this drop in blood pressure, the blood vessels close up, often giving the skin a bluish tint, and lack of oxygen to the brain can contribute to loss of balance and impaired concentration. By now the blood is thickening through lack of oxygen and the rising core temperature is brings on hot flushes, counteracted by chills.

If lack of water continues to allow the body to get hotter, breathing will become very shallow and confusion, impaired vision and overall weakness will set in. Then you will pass out. Worryingly, among older people, fainting can be the first obvious sign of heat stroke, as other symptoms may not appear too unusual or will pass quickly.

If heat stroke strikes

Heat stroke can be avoided by keeping hydrated and not getting too hot – wearing a hat is vital as, just as your head loses heat easily in the cold, so it absorbs heat if exposed to the sun. If you feel any of the symptoms leading up to heat stroke, get out of the sun straightaway, preferably into an air-conditioned environment to speed up the cooling down. Start drinking water, but don't gulp it down: take it on board gently.

If the situation is advanced to the stage of feeling weak and disoriented and air-conditioning is not possible, assist the cooling down by fanning the body and head, and covering them with a sheet or towel soaked in cold water. Once anybody has reached the point of heat exhaustion, they should be moved out of the sun and an ambulance called immediately.

T

Tip: The better condition your skin is in before you hit the beach, the more even your tan will be as there will be fewer dead skin cells and less dirt on the surface interfering with the passage of the UV rays.

Skin cancer's spreading

Around 2500 people died of skin cancer in the UK in 2007 and in the same year in the US that figure was 11,000 – three percent of the total diagnosed for the former, and in the latter, just over one percent. Although the fatality rates for skin cancer are relatively low, it is the fastest rising form of cancer with the number of new cases having tripled during the last twenty years. And the reason the percentage of people dying from it in the US is so much smaller than in the UK is because they are a great deal better educated about its dangers.

What is skin cancer?

The vast majority of skin cancer is caused by cumulative overexposure to UV radiation over a period of time, which is why skin cancers are more prevalent among older

T

Tip: Those of African or African-Caribbean descent or from the Indian subcontinent should also check regularly for skin blemishes that could be cancerous. While the melanoma rate amongst Caucasians is twenty-two percent compared with one percent among black people, the fatality rates are considerably higher among the latter because, frequently, tumours will be allowed to progress further without being noticed for what they are.

F

Fact: The highest incidents of skin cancer can be found in New Zealand, Australia and South Africa, countries with high levels of sunshine and large Caucasian populations.

people and usually appear on exposed areas of skin such as hands, forearms, necks and faces. In these cases, it is due to DNA damage to the epidermis cells, which start growing out of control of the usual cell construction instructions and can become cancerous. The risk of contracting skin cancer increases hugely if you have suffered bad sunburn – sufficient to blister – at any time in your life, as this may have caused DNA damage.

Skin cancer falls into two main categories, non-melanoma and malignant melanoma, with the former being the less serious and easiest to treat, and the latter the cause of the majority of all skin cancer

The ABCD of moles

Cancer Research UK advises examining your body on at least a monthly basis, to look for new or altered blemishes. It recommends this alphabetically inspired checklist:

Asymmetry: do two halves of an existing mole no longer look the same?

Border: have the edges of a mole started to become ragged, irregular or faded?

Colour: has a mole changed colour or is no longer a uniform hue?

Diameter: has it grown?

If the answer to any of the above is yes, you should go and see your doctor.
For more information visit info.cancerresearchuk.org/healthyliving/sunsmart.

Fact: The highest rates of melanoma are among white men over the age of fifty. This is believed to be linked to findings that men in their forties spend more time outdoors than any other demographic, and therefore have the greatest exposure to UV radiation.

growths on your chest or back. The other type is squamous cell carcinoma (SCC), which is more likely to spread, but is just as easily treated if detected early. Symptoms are small, hard red bumps, or red, scaly, scab-like patches or crusty sores that refuse to heal on skin usually exposed to the sun.

Melanoma is the most dangerous form of skin cancer, with malignant melanomas accounting for around three-quarters of all skin cancer fatalities. Although the risks increase with age, this is one of the few cancers that can affect young people – melanoma is not uncommon in the 15–40-year-old age group. It is highly noticeable and if caught early is 99 percent curable; visible warning signs are new moles (dark or black spots or patches on the skin) appearing, existing moles changing colour or

deaths. Non-melanoma skin cancer comes in two varieties. Basal cell carcinoma (BCC) is the most common form of skin cancer, the easiest treated and the least likely to spread.

Warning signs are small waxy nodules on your face, ears or neck, or flat, scar-like

What happens in Ibiza stays in Ibiza

Although losing a few inhibitions and carrying on in ways you wouldn't dream of at home is often the whole point of going on holiday, it's important to bear in mind that risky behaviour abroad could always be that bit more hazardous.

Drinking

Lower duty means cheaper prices and, as is very often the case abroad, the measures will be larger and the beer stronger, making it possible to drink much more than you are used to or indeed meant to. You could unwittingly become perilously drunk, affecting not only your health but also your personal safety and that of those around you. Never forget all the same dangers discussed in Chapter 9 will still apply, but problems can increase exponentially in an unfamiliar environment and with a police force who don't or won't speak English.

Sex

With a drunken situation comes the same likelihood of spontaneous and unprotected sex that there could be at home – just possibly more of it. Pack more condoms than even the biggest optimist could imagine to need as you don't know how easily available they will be where you are going. Make sure you carry them with you at all times.

And while partying with the locals, be aware of the increased rates of STDs and HIV in some parts of the world, see box opposite and on p.259. Then be reminded that prostitutes somewhere else are going to be no less dicey a proposition than prostitutes at home, no matter how enticing they might appear.

Drugs

Don't take anything if you're not sure what it is and be aware that local varieties may be much stronger than you are used to. Also, just because drugs appear to be "part of the culture" – i.e. sold and used seemingly openly – this doesn't mean the local police and judiciary will be in any way tolerant if they choose to haul you in. Be sure of the local laws and do not flout them.

AIDS/HIV around the world

Sub-Saharan Africa	5.0 percent of population living with AIDS/HIV	22.5 million people living with AIDS/HIV
Caribbean	1.0 percent of population living with AIDS/HIV	230,000 people living with AIDS/HIV
Eastern Europe & Central Asia	0.9 percent of population living with AIDS/HIV	1.6 million people living with AIDS/HIV
USA & Canada	0.6 percent of population living with AIDS/HIV	1.3 million people living with AIDS/HIV
South America	0.5 percent of population living with AIDS/HIV	1.6 million people living with AIDS/HIV
Australasia	0.4 percent of population living with AIDS/HIV	75,000 people living with AIDS/HIV
South & Southeast Asia	0.3 percent of population living with AIDS/HIV	4 million people living with AIDS/HIV
Western & Central Europe	0.3 percent of population living with AIDS/HIV	760,000 people living with AIDS/HIV
North Africa & Middle East	0.3 percent of population living with AIDS/HIV	380,000 people living with AIDS/HIV
East Asia	0.1 percent of population living with AIDS/HIV	800,000 people living with AIDS/HIV
Globally	0.8 percent of population living with AIDS/HIV	33.2 million people living with AIDS/HIV

Source: UNAIDS/WHO 2007

shape, a mole that suddenly starts persistently itching or hurting, or a mole that starts bleeding or seeping.

T

Tip: Between dusk and dawn it is even more important to wear plenty of insect repellent, or to cover up, as during this time the malarial mosquitoes will be feeding.

A suitable case for treatment

Any of the above warning signs should prompt a visit to the healthcare professionals, at which point you will either be referred to a specialist or told it is nothing to worry about. If it does need treatment, there are several different choices and the success rate is high – provided it is diagnosed early enough. It is impossible to overstress that anything on your skin you suspect might be cancerous should be properly investigated at the first viable opportunity.

Tip: Before swimming in the sea check what time tides are; if it turns while you are out and you don't notice you could get into serious trouble.

Get the needle

The majority of holiday-makers will not need to get vaccinated before they travel, but as destinations become ever more far-flung, so the diseases on offer will be equally exotic, and need to be protected against. Although requirements and advice can alter as health concerns change within different countries, a general principle is that anywhere outside of Northern and Western Europe, North America, Australia and New Zealand can pose a health risk, so seek advice from your travel agent or GP or check the NHS Direct website (nhsdirect.nhs.uk).

In these health risk countries, the need for vaccination will be far less pressing if you are merely going away on a brief business trip, during which your time will be spent in air-conditioned, five-star luxury with minimal contact with the country you are visiting. Even then, however, you should take advice before deciding to get vaccinated, and those

rules will not apply if you are vacationing at even the highest end holiday resort. You will still be spending time in the open air, the sea, the swimming pool or on the beach, leaving you susceptible to a range of viruses.

Also, bear in mind that some tropical countries will ask for evidence of certain immunizations as an entry requirement and this will be worth you checking out if you are not booking through a travel agent.

It will also be vital to make sure your childhood vaccinations – diphtheria, tetanus, whooping cough, polio, Hib (influenzae type B), meningitis C, MMR and pneumococcal – are up to date, and this may mean a booster shot. Your GP will advise on this, and arrange for the jabs should you need them.

A

Expert advice: "If you are going to hammer it while you're on holiday, it will help you if you do some sort of exercise and try and eat as well as possible, because it will give your body the best possible chance of recovering from all those nights on the town. And it would do you a lot of good to take one off every few days."
Gideon Remfry

How it all works: vaccinations

Inoculations against specific diseases stimulate the body's immune system into producing the required antibodies by introducing controlled doses of the disease to be protected against into the system. When the body is attacked by hostile or unknown viruses or bacteria, the system produces the relevant protective antibodies to fight it off, and in the case of a genuine infection often the infection takes hold due to lack of antibodies. Vaccination brings in a small quantity of potentially hostile bacteria or viruses, causing the system to produce the right antibodies, but the biologically altered invaders will not actually inflict the diseases themselves. Once these antibodies have been produced, they remain in the body for years, allowing the immune system to recognise the disease in its real form and to wipe it out before it takes hold. Each separate vaccinable disease requires its own individual injection.

Treatable STDs around the world

Sub-Saharan Africa	11.9 percent of adult population infected	53.5 million people infected at any one time
Caribbean	7.1 percent infected adult population	1.63 million people infected at any one time
South & Southeast Asia	5.0 percent infected adult population	6.6 million people infected at any one time
Eastern Europe & Central Asia	2.9 percent infected adult population	5.13 million people infected at any one time
Australasia	2.7 percent infected adult population	506,250 people infected at any one time
USA & Canada	2.4 percent infected adult population	5.19 million people infected at any one time
North Africa & Middle East	2.1 percent infected adult population	2.6 million people infected at any one time
Western & Central Europe	2.0 percent infected adult population	5.06 million people infected at any one time
South America	1.9 percent infected adult population	6.08 million people infected at any one time
Globally	3.8 percent infected adult population	82.296 million people infected at any one time

Source: UNAIDS/WHO 2007

From whom and for what?

If you believe you may need vaccinations, the first place you should go is to your GP – this is vital if you are already on medication, as you will need to make sure the vaccine you are about to take will not have any adverse effects. At the surgery you may be able to get the immunization you require on the spot, especially if it is merely boosters to the British childhood schedule. However, many surgeries will not keep stocks of the less commonly called for vaccines, and you may be asked to come back at a later date or referred to a specialist holiday health centre, which are usually situated in larger branches of pharmacy chains.

F

Fact: Sunbed tans contribute to skin cancer as much as the sun's rays, as in both cases UV radiation is involved.

T

Tip: Apply insect repellent over your sunscreen to ensure effectiveness, and reapply after every reapplication of sunscreen, or after every couple of hours.

You will be charged by the surgery both for the vaccine and the act of injecting it because vaccinations for travel are not provided for on the NHS – it is to specifically protect against disease you won't get in Britain, so why should they? The cost of holiday vaccinations is around £15 per jab.

Timing your jabs

Don't leave it too late to find out if you need vaccinations. Many take time to produce antibodies so six weeks before you travel should be the minimum. Be mindful that vaccines can require two or more shots given with an interval of at least four weeks in between each one. Also, in the case of some multiple inoculations, while they can all be administered at the same time to different parts of the body, if that is not possible there must be a gap of three weeks between shots.

T

Tip: If your travel agent tells you vaccinations are not required for a certain destination, make sure they are not referring to a vaccination certificate, while inoculations themselves may still be recommended.

The best of the web

mscuk.org
The website of the Marine Conservation Society, where you can find up-to-the-minute information about the levels of pollution on beaches around the UK.

fitfortravel.scot.nhs.uk
Part of the NHS Scotland and a comprehensive advice site for travellers' health, it has up-to-date details of which countries require what immunization.

masta.org
The Medical Advisory Service for Travellers Abroad, was founded by the London School of Hygiene and Tropical Medicine. It has a network of travel clinics all over the country and much useful advice on immunization.

traveldoctor.co.uk
How to prepare before going abroad, what to do if you become ill and many useful travel tips.

skincancer.org
Comprehensive American site, dedicated to advice about all aspects of skin cancer from clear explanations of what it is to facts and figures to precautions to be taken if heading for the sun.

airlinequality.com
An impartial guide to the world's major airlines, including those all-important leg room and seat pitch surveys.

who.int
The World Health Organization has all the facts and figures about the state of health or risk of disease all over the world.

Ten top tips for travelling healthily

Looks like the UV rays message is finally getting through

▸ **Pack more condoms than you think you'll need** Then make sure you've got a couple with you when you go out.

▸ **Never drink water in an aircraft bathroom** Quite literally, you don't know where it's been.

▸ **Double your regular water intake when flying** Then make sure you are properly hydrated before boarding, as cabin humidity and lower oxygen levels will dry you out much faster.

▸ **Get out of your seat and move around** Do so for a minute at least once an hour on a long haul flight, and rotate your feet at the ankles as often as you remember.

▸ **Make the most of local cuisine** Provided it includes locally grown fruit and vegetables and genuinely fresh meat and fish, but not if you're in Las Vegas, obviously.

▸ **Any sort of risky behaviour you indulge in at home will be even riskier abroad** You won't know what the local attitude is, you may not be able to speak the language and, surprisingly, people might be all too willing to take advantage of tourists.

▸ **Get vaccinated early** Many of them will take a few weeks to become fully effective.

▸ **The sand, snow or sea will intensify the sun's rays** Take extra care when out in it under these conditions.

▸ **Don't turn breakfast into a carb fest** Followed by a morning of inactivity it will send you home considerably wider around the waist.

▸ **Hangovers are always worse in a hot country** This is because of the ease of dehydration.

In later life 13

According to medical science, on the physical side it's downhill for us from our mid-twenties onwards. Worst of all, although we get smarter we get progressively less able to do anything about all these good ideas we might have. While this book won't make you live forever, it can help you put off the effects of ageing until the last possible moment.

Youth is wasted on the young

As time passes so you will start to wear out, much like everything else in life. Alarmingly, as a man living in the developed world you are liable to reach your peak of physical condition a full fifty years before you finally fall off the end of your mortal coil. Which means, because the average life span is seventy-plus years, for at least two-thirds of your life it will never get any better than it is right now.

This is a great shame because with age comes experience and increased mental powers, but even all that won't be much use against the inevitable march of time.

Structural alterations

Why you start wearing out is because from the moment you are born your body is in a constant state of regeneration with cells dying all the time and getting replaced with

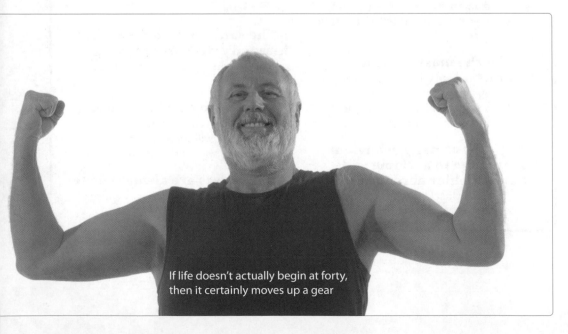

If life doesn't actually begin at forty, then it certainly moves up a gear

F

Fact: Due to changes in posture, compression of vertebrae and shrinkage of connective tissue, a man can lose up to two inches in height between the ages of forty and seventy.

new ones. As you get on in years, the rate with which you can manufacture new cells slows and eventually they begin to die out faster than they can be restored. This rate of steady cell degeneration increases with each passing summer, and will affect different aspects of your body in different ways.

Osteoporosis, as the result of a reduction in bone density, is probably the primary effect of ageing, and affects as many as one in ten men over the age of sixty. It occurs gradually, and comes about when the bones are not getting enough calcium and phosphate to keep building them. This means they are brittle and increasingly prone to fracture. Dietary intake of these minerals may need to be stepped up, because, as you age, your body will actually start reabsorbing them from your bones back into your system. It may be necessary to take calcium supplements, especially if you are lactose intolerant and don't drink milk. Regular exercise – running and walking, in particular – will also help preserve bone density, as the system adapts to cope with the rigours of impact and retains more minerals in the bones.

The tissues connecting the bones will suffer too, because the slowing down of the body's cell production means what it is making will be larger and, therefore, less flexible, in the joints and this can result in a painful stiffening. Time-induced wear and tear is also a big factor, and the cartilage that sits in between the joints' moving parts will wear thin over time, meaning it provides less protection from friction and impact. This can lead to arthritis through inflammation

How it all works: middle-aged spread

How did that get there? That spare tyre "suddenly" appearing around the midriff seems almost inescapable to most men in their forties and comes about as the result of an unfortunate double-double whammy. Because they are less active, older men need less food than they used to, but habit probably means they are still eating the same amounts, thus they are taking on surplus calories which will be stored as fat. A slowed-down metabolism means what is being used will be burned less efficiently, thus more of that will be converted to fat too. Then, as you are a man, this fat will be distributed attractively around your waist, and once it gets there the muscles that might hold it a bit more upright are starting to lose density and strength, therefore will be more likely to let it sag.

Perhaps the worst thing about middle-aged spread, though, is it has no respect for age – it can start to show itself as soon as your lifestyle becomes less energetic, which might be as early as your twenties.

The only fail-safe way to keep it at bay is to eat healthily and make sure you continue exercising, so as to burn off as many calories as you take in. Once it's there though, a combined schedule of strength and aerobic training should see some reduction (see Chapter 4), but don't be fooled into thinking endless repetitions of sit-ups or crunches will get rid of it. Although firmer abs will help your posture as your gut will be less able to drag you down, and that will save your lower back, as previously discussed you can't spot reduce through targeted exercise. If you start to lose weight all over, eventually that spare tyre will start to deflate.

Being fat, smoking and getting old earlier

Although smoker's skin will make you look much older than you are, it is obesity that will actually age you quicker. Tests conducted in London recently revealed that men with casual smoking habits – less than ten per day – had a bodily age of, on average, 4.6 years older than their non-smoking counterparts. After a forty-year, twenty-per-day smoking habit a man's body would be 7.6 years older than his actual age. However, a man who has been obese for over ten years will have a bodily age of 8.8 years older than a slim fellow who was born in the same year. Put smoking and obesity together, though, and it adds up to 10.2 years of additional ageing.

It is the obesity aspect of these figures the World Health Organization is finding particularly worrying, as while smoking figures have gone up and down over the years, obesity is increasing relentlessly, especially among young people. There is currently a growing number of overweight children and adolescents who are experiencing such adult-related conditions as heart disease and type 2 diabetes much earlier than previous generations. It is being perceived in medical circles as a dangerous "advanced ageing", leading to fears that, as their conditions put greater strains on their systems for longer, their life spans will be reduced.

It is accepted that while advances in modern medicine are already reducing the impact of obesity and its derivative conditions, nobody is yet sure what knock on effect such childhood ill health will have in later life. There is a growing fear that this current generation of young people may be the first to have a shorter life expectancy than their parents.

and stiffness and can be further aggravated by a reduction in synovial fluid – the joint's internal lubrication. Stretching exercises will help keep joints mobile, while it is important to maintain fluid levels with fish oil supplements.

Loss of muscle tissue can start occurring naturally as early as your thirties, and exercise will become increasingly important to maintain mass and strength. Muscles may also lose density as their regeneration slows and the body deposits fat within them. They might also stiffen as the regenerated tissue is tough and stringy due to larger cells. Maintaining muscles to provide support and protection as bones degenerate will become increasingly important, just as strength will be needed for balance, mobility and coordination.

Age and the organs

The vital organs start to decrease in efficiency as they get older, but this is gradual and in the cases of a healthy liver and kidneys, not really dangerous. They are rarely used to maximum capacity, thus any decline will be taken up by their natural reserves.

Ageing affects the heart in a number of ways. The muscles within it decline and the walls become less elastic, meaning it beats slower, with a shorter pumping stroke, and

The eyes have it, or probably not

Sight diminishes after about the age of forty because the cornea and the lens of the eye start to become opaque and the pupil gets smaller, contracting the field of vision. The most obvious effect is an almost universal problem with reading that requires either magnification or more light to cope with small text. Also, shifting focus from one object to another will take longer and some green/blue colour blindness may occur.

Are you getting enough?

It may not be possible to get enough nutrients from your diet, especially as you will naturally be eating less, so these supplements will be particularly important:

What it is	What it does	What you need
Calcium & vitamin D	Maintains bone strength and density; vitamin D allows the calcium to be absorbed efficiently; aids the nervous system	800 milligrams & 5.0 micrograms
Beta-carotene (vitamin A)	Helps build bones; prevents eyes drying out	1000 milligrams
Vitamins C & E	Prevents lipid oxidation, thus aids blood flow and reduces plaque formation and blood pressure	60 milligrams & 10 micrograms
Folic acid	Promotes alertness	400 micrograms
Vitamin B complex	Assists cell growth; aids the nervous system; helps guard against macular degeneration (age-related blindness)	B1 1.2 milligrams B2 1.4 milligrams B3 16 milligrams B12 3.0 micrograms
Zinc	Boosts the immune system	10 milligrams

calcification can occur in heart valves, as the body absorbs calcium from the bones (see above). These factors restrict blood flow, as does the hardening of artery walls in and outside the heart. It increases the chances of congestive heart failure, heart attacks or strokes, and raises blood pressure to put more strain on your pump. Reduced blood flow will slow the response to stress or danger and impede healing abilities, while decreased oxygen to the muscles adds to fatigue.

This reduced oxygen delivery will not be helped by lung capacity getting smaller as you get older, because the muscles that control breathing are weaker and the ribcage becomes stiffer and less able to expand and contract. This means more air remains in the lungs after exhaling, leaving less space for what the next breath ought to be bringing in.

Men who have exercised throughout their lives will reach their senior years with

T

Tip: As you age your body will not be able to regulate its internal temperature so efficiently, thus you will need to be much more careful about exposure to extreme temperatures.

A

Expert advice: "Don't judge it all by the bathroom scales and think that just because you aren't putting on weight you aren't getting fat. Muscle weighs more than fat, thus as your body starts exchanging the former for the latter your weight will stay around the same or even go down."
Gideon Remfry

much stronger cardiovascular systems, but those taking up exercise in later life will need to start slowly because of these limitations.

Snow on the roof but a fire in the hearth

Although the numbers of living sperm per emission goes down with the passing of time, there will be very little change in a man's fertility as he gets older; indeed it is not uncommon for men to father children above the age of sixty. Sex drive can decrease slightly, as some testicular mass may be lost meaning testosterone levels can decline, and it might take a little more to get you aroused as responses will be slower. Repeat performances could be confined to memory too, as it will take longer to replenish seminal

F

Fact: Although hearing will be diminished, your ears will keep getting bigger – men's ears continue to grow at approximately 0.22mm per year for their entire lives.

fluid reservoirs and to get another erection.

In spite of erectile dysfunction being more common among older men, this is not a natural result of the ageing process. It comes about because of other medical conditions that will be more prevalent among this age group, such as diabetes or high blood pressure. Older men get fewer erections than their youthful counterparts, though, and that's just a fact of life.

Eating late

Because very little will change as regards your digestive system as you get older, other than a slowing down of your metabolism, dietary requirements for a healthy later life aren't actually that much different from what you've always been eating. To achieve the necessary nutrition you'll need to maintain a good balance of fresh fruit and vegetables, protein, fibre and carbohydrate, but there will be certain things you should avoid. Foods high in cholesterol should be given the swerve; no more than 25 percent of your calorific intake should come from fats and as little of that as possible should be saturated; and sugar needs to be limited, because of the increased risk of diabetes.

It will benefit you to eat less more often – five or six small meals a day – and to make sure you keep up your water intake, even if it does mean visiting the gents more often than you might like.

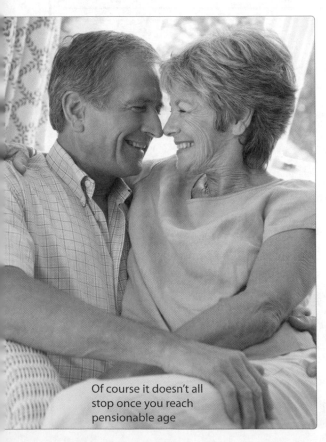

Of course it doesn't all stop once you reach pensionable age

Don't stop now

As middle-aged spread starts to creep up on you, it's easy just to surrender and watch it accelerate. But you could do something about it. Even if you've never exercised before it's never too late to start with this relatively easy programme – you don't even need any special equipment. Do as many repetitions of each exercise as you feel is giving you a good workout.

Sit and stand

Exactly what it says on the tin: sit on a straight backed chair with feet flat on the floor and knees bent at right angles; with your hands dangling loose by your sides, stand up straight; sit down again, slowly; repeat. To make it a little more difficult, hold your arms straight out in front of you.

Standing press-ups

Stand about one metre away from a wall, and put your hands flat on it, each about 20cm outside your shoulders, with your arms straight; keeping body and legs rigid, bend your elbows so your face is brought towards the wall; stop when your elbows are bent at right angles; press back until your arms are once again straight; repeat.

Step-ups

Stand at the bottom of a flight of stairs or in front of something that is at least 25cm high and will support your weight; step up on to the first step with left foot then bring right foot up to alongside it; step down with left foot then bring right foot down next to it; to complete one exercise, repeat movement starting with right foot; repeat for each foot.

Hamstring curls

Stand straight with feet about 30cm apart, holding the back of a chair if you need to balance; bring left heel up towards left buttock by bending knee; slowly lower foot back to the floor; bring right heel up to right buttock; slowly lower foot back to the floor; repeat with each foot.

Reverse crunches (see right)

Lie on your back with hands by your sides or behind your head; bend knees to right angles and lift feet 15cm off the floor; keeping knees bent at right angles and using abdominal muscles, lift feet until shins are parallel with the floor; lower slowly to 15cm above the floor; repeat.

Knee lifts

Stand straight with feet about 30cm apart, holding the back of a chair to the side of you if you need to balance; lift left knee straight up in front of you, until it is bent at right angles with thigh parallel with floor; lower foot slowly to the floor; lift right knee to right angles; lower slowly to floor; repeat with each leg.

Holding back the years

Life expectancy around the world varies enormously, except in one region: the bottom 39 countries are all African – Swaziland is the lowest with a life expectancy of 31.84 years for men and 32.62 for women. The UK ranks at number 24 with 76.23 (men) and 81.3 (women); the US is at 29 with 75.15 and 80.97.

	Country	Men	Women
1	Andorra	80.62 years	86.23
2	Iceland	78.83	82.62
3	Japan	78.67	85.56
4	Sweden	78.39	83.00
5	Australia	77.8	83.59
6	Switzerland	77.75	83.63
7	France	77.35	84.00
8	Italy	77.01	83.07
9	Canada	76.98	83.86
10	Spain	76.46	83.32
	World average	63.89	67.84

Source: US Census Bureau

How long can you go on?

It is believed that the upper age limit for the human body is around 120 years, and to get there you will need an ongoing lifestyle that promotes health, fitness, low levels of stress and strong emotional support. It is far from unusual for the people of the islands of Okinawa in Japan to live past one hundred years old, and their lifestyle couldn't be further removed from so much of the Western world. Their diet is low in fat, refined sugar and processed foods, yet high in fibre through fresh fruit and vegetables. Everybody, regardless of age, exercises, and a strong sense of spirituality, family and community eases stress levels. The rates of prostate and colon cancer in that region is eighty percent lower than in the US.

Age and IQ

Any reductions in brain power as you get older will be the result of a disease rather than an inevitable occurrence. This has long been a popular scientific theory, but it wasn't until the last century, in Scotland, that long-term tests were completed to provide evidence.

A thorough IQ and mental alacrity test was given to a group of nearly 100,000 11-year-olds in 1932, then 66 years later, in 1998, 101 of that group – which represented a random cross-section – sat exactly the same test under exactly the same conditions. The 77-year-olds fared considerably better than they did aged 11. The most interesting finding was that the levels of improvement were more or less the same across the whole group, meaning everybody seemed to have acquired more intelligence. The IQ levels had remained constant over that time too, and the brighter-than-their-peers kids were still the sharpest tools in the box as pensioners.

Sorry, I've forgotten your name

Researchers at the University of Toronto recently found that older people have difficulty remembering isolated facts like names or telephone numbers, because the older brain has a wider focus. This means when being introduced to somebody in a room full of people, rather than concentrate on a single fact – the name, for instance – they will be taking in the wider aspect and will have to sort through a jumble of information if they want to immediately retrieve that one name.

While this may lead to what appears to

be slowness of thought and distractibility, it is why the tests proved older people to be better at analysing situations, making broader-based judgments and being more mentally flexible if circumstances change. This happens because the extraneous information the older mind has been absorbing will be processed and sorted, allowing for a wider spectrum of knowledge to be called upon when considering the situation at a later date. Although much of the information absorbed appears trivial when taken as individual aspects, it meant the older people knew more about every situation than their more tightly focused younger contemporaries, thus were better equipped to work out what needed to be done.

The downside was that this was thought to be why older people seemed to have problems making instant decisions or thinking on the hoof – fluid intelligence. Interestingly, though, they were far more

T

Tip: To aid memory and sharpen concentration take ginkgo biloba in daily doses of between 50 and 500mg per day. It increases blood flow within the brain and it protects against oxidative damage from free radicals.

likely to say they didn't feel ready to make a decision, rather than take a guess and try and pass it off as "gut reaction" like many of the younger test subjects did.

Staying sharp

The notion of the brain as some sort of muscle that will function much better if it is regularly exercised has been gaining credence

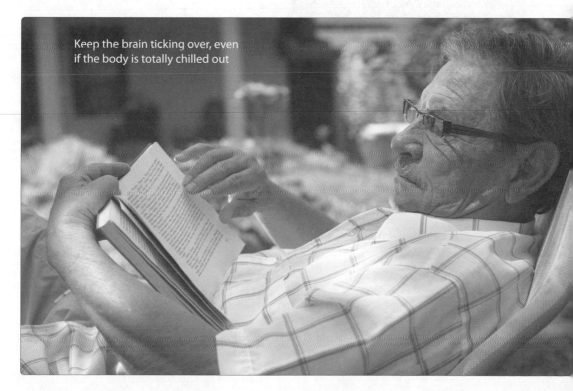

Keep the brain ticking over, even if the body is totally chilled out

M

Mythbuster: you can't teach an old dog new tricks

Although it is a long-standing comedy notion that old people are unable to come to grips with anything that hasn't been made out of wood, there is actually no natural decrease in mental capacity as you get older. The number of nerve cells in the brain (neurons) do not go into decline with age, and they continue to make the new connections needed for learning and memory.

for some time now, as older people with smart spouses or intellectually challenging working environments tend to stay sharper later in life. A long-term study of healthy adults over the age of 65 in the US has proved thisi

Cognitive training sessions of two hours in length, once a week for five weeks, were enough to bring on marked improvements in memory, concentration, problem solving and numeracy skills and these were improvements that remained in place five years after the training sessions ended. Cognitive training is anything that stretches the brain by pushing it to solve puzzles or problems on the hoof – sudokus, crosswords, Rubik cubes, word searches, mental arithmetic are cognitive exercises.

The conclusion of the experiments was that if people regularly challenge themselves with short bursts of mental workouts, their brains' abilities will develop to maximum potential. "Tapping in to your cognitive reserve" is how scientists are describing it.

Don't wait until you're over sixty either. The younger you start these exercises

T

Tip: The older you are the longer vaccinations will need in the body before they become effective, so be sure to leave plenty of time if getting jabbed to travel abroad.

What's the point?

This century, for the first time, the number of sixty-year-olds alive in the UK was greater than the number of sixteen-year-olds, signifying an expected average life span that has nearly doubled since 1900. While this represents a huge achievement for medicine and science, it also begs the question: is this curve heading further than is actually good for the human body?

Although keeping fit and healthy and active can offset the physical demands of ageing, it seems less can be done to reduce the likelihood of Alzheimer's (see opposite) and senile dementia. Because the percentage of Alzheimer's sufferers rises so steeply as people get into their eighties – there are currently around 700,000 sufferers in the UK – with people living longer this figure is expected to more than double in the next twenty years, then double again in the following twenty. This is leading to concerns over the creation of a large number of people with a very low quality of life and who are in need of constant care.

At the moment, this situation is not helped by the fact the levels of spending on research into Alzheimer's is less than ten percent of that spent on finding cures for cancer.

B

Best investment: *Brain Age 2*

This brain training game, to be played on the portable Nintendo DS, was designed in collaboration with prominent Japanese neuroscientist Dr Ryuta Kawashima. It works as a portable cognitive training device, and features a series of numerate, verbal and logical skills workouts, which culminate in examinations of your mental prowess. It then assesses the results as something called your "brain age", against which you will be able to measure future progress. The Nintendo DS console is priced around £120 ($200); the *Brain Age 2* game around £25 ($40).

the more benefit they will have and the same research showed the importance of entering those twilight years with the sharpest faculties possible.

Fading to grey

Alzheimer's disease is the leading cause of senile dementia in the developed world, and around three percent of those over sixty-five and forty percent of those over eighty will be sufferers. It is a progressive degenerative condition that attacks the cells in all areas of the brain to destroy the memory, the ability to function and emotional control. Symptoms include forgetfulness, loss of memory, mood swings, confusion and a noticeable lack of purpose in speech and action.

At the time of writing Alzheimer's is incurable, with even very little evidence as to what might be preventative. Very little is known as to whether it is caused by anything other than old age too, although it is believed to be hereditary with children of sufferers having a fifteen percent chance of getting it themselves.

Age and immunity

The immune system will also function progressively less efficiently as the years roll by, and when you reach your sixties it won't be much more than forty percent of what it was in your thirties. This will happen on two different levels. Initially the central nervous system reacts slower and less sensitively to signals that infections are invading the body, and secondly the cells

T

Tip: If you have time on your hands and you want to keep the old grey matter turning over, look no further than your local evening institute. Learning a foreign language or a musical instrument or something that requires dexterity – pottery, woodwork, upholstery – are ideal brain trainers.

F

Fact: Once the body passes the age of seventy it is likely to produce something called autoantibodies, which can attack the system to trigger rheumatoid arthritis and a hardening of the arteries (atherosclerosis). Making sure you are getting enough vitamins B3 and C will help fight against this.

older people are far more prone to viral and bacterial infections and need to take extra precautions.

Remaining well nourished is key to keeping your immune system working as well as possible, although staying fit is also important as it will help those nutrients get metabolized. Healthy eating will become far more significant at this stage in your life, as you will be eating less but require more or less the same amount of nutrients, so you will need to make sure you are getting everything possible from the food. You may need to add to what you are getting from your food with supplements. B vitamins are imperative as they boost the immune system and maintain the nervous system; and make sure you are eating plenty of whole grains, pulses, nuts, eggs and dairy.

that will then be produced to fight infection will be less dynamic than they would have been when you were younger. This means

The best of the web

alzheimers.org.uk
The website of the Alzheimer's Society, a charity dedicated to raising awareness and funds for the fight against the disease. The first stop for anybody who wants to find out more about Alzheimer's or make a donation.

laterlife.com
Health, travel, fitness, relationships, courses, insurance, health farms… in fact all human life is covered here with the older person in mind.

healthscotland.com
From Scotland's NHS website, pages that deal comprehensively with all health-related aspects of getting old.

senior.com
Where the US senior community find out about health, travel, the law, care-giving, stay in touch or just hang out.

runningforfitness.org/faq/agegrading.php
Where to go to calculate how your running times compare with world records, as relative to your age.

50plus.org
The home of the Lifelong Fitness Alliance, an American organization dedicated to seniors' health and fitness, offering advice, tips and events.

Any inherent inefficiency of the immune system means that vaccinations will be less effective, but they are still wholly worthwhile. Inoculations against flu, streptococcal pneumonia, tuberculosis and hepatitis B should be obtained, and the UK vaccination schedule should be maintained with whatever booster shots are necessary – at the very least, you will need to be vaccinated against tetanus and diphtheria.

Ten top tips for growing old gracefully

▶ **Eat more smaller meals per day** Your digestive system may be functioning less efficiently and should not be over worked.

▶ **Make sure you get enough nutrients** You should be eating less than you did as a young man but you will still need the same vitamin and mineral intake.

▶ **Go swimming instead of running** It is a non-impact exercise, therefore, it will put no undue strain on your joints.

▶ **Get vaccinated earlier** Especially if it's for foreign travel as it will take longer for the vaccine to become absorbed into your system.

▶ **Just about everybody needs reading glasses by the age of fifty** Don't be shy about whipping yours out.

▶ **Don't be scared of keeping fit** It will actually get easier as you get older because your muscles start to function more efficiently.

▶ **Drink plenty of water** This is particularly important as older men are more prone to constipation, which can lead to hernias.

▶ **Stay sharp with some form of brain activity on a daily basis** Do sudoku or crosswords for instance, as this will keep the old grey matter functioning as well as it ever did.

▶ **Dress your age** Mutton dressed as lamb will rarely look any more impressive than mutton dressed as mutton.

▶ **Don't believe the hype** When you were a young person, you may have been brainwashed into thinking there's no fun to be had once you get past forty – this simply isn't true.

Part 2
Fit for life

A man for all seasons (14)

As you go through life, what is "normal" for you – as regards your health and fitness – will change. From decade to decade your requirements, the risks and how you need to handle things will be very different. But it's far from downhill all the way: each period has as many plus points as it does negatives.

Man in his twenties

It is at this time that a man can expect to have the most fun. A lack of familial responsibilities combines with relatively high earning potential, the anticipation of possibilities, loads of energy and peak levels of testosterone and this turns life into an exhilarating prospect. But it can also be the most potentially damaging time too. Male suicide rates are high among this age group; depression is a common problem and often undiagnosed; and young men in their late teens and twenties are far more likely to be victims of violence. Beyond that, this time of life is made even more confusing and contradictory by the continually teetering balance between what you and people around you feel you should be doing, and what your capabilities and experience actually allows.

However, the advantages of being twentysomething vastly outweigh the downside. At this point you should be at your naturally healthiest and fittest, as so much of your system peaks during these years. Your metabolism will be operating at its most efficient, thus in spite of you eating so much because you are still growing, there is relatively little danger of you getting fat, also you should have masses of energy. This doesn't mean you shouldn't watch what you eat though, and your need for almost constant feeding ought to be sated with complex carbohydrates (whole grains, fruit and vegetables), rather than fat and sugar.

Technically you will be at your manliest, as testosterone levels and sperm counts will

F *Fact: The biggest cause of death among men aged between seventeen and thirty in the UK is road accidents: 6.1 per 100,000 of the population per year.*

All-over medical checkup (heart, lungs, blood pressure, cholesterol, diabetes, liver, kidneys and overall fitness): every two years.

be at their all-time high. This means not only are men of this age at their most sexually potent but macho-type behaviour among them is most widespread – hence the disproportionate statistics for violence. Any feelings of invulnerability will be further increased by the fact that your immune system is working better than it ever has, or will do so again, so fighting off infection will be relatively straightforward.

Mind games

Apart from the fighting and the predisposition for STDs, the biggest problems of being in your twenties will be psychological, as in

T

Tip: If you wear glasses, get your sight tested every six months as your eyes will still be changing.

F

Fact: This age group has the highest proportion of smokers, and it is now that a lifetime habit is most likely to start.

spite of the testosterone surge it is unlikely your self-confidence is keeping up with the macho public face.

What will seem to be expected of you by family, friends, bosses, teachers or yourself, as you start out in the world, can often put undue pressure on a young man, while decision-making will not be easy due to the limited amount of worldly experience you have. Confusion about sexuality is most common at this time, and love lives will be further complicated by what young men perceive they should be doing. Hormone levels and the rest of the world in general – lad's mags, music videos, TV – will be

What's good about being twentysomething	What sucks about being twentysomething
Your high testosterone levels mean you will be full of confidence	The amount of new life experiences you will encounter will often cause self-doubt
Suicides among this age group are falling	Incidents of self-harm are rising
Your muscles are at their strongest; your potency is at its highest; you have the least chance of putting on weight	You are the most confused about your appearance, your sexuality and your attractiveness
You will be meeting new people all the time	There is relatively little emotional connection between men of this age, thus loneliness can be a problem
Your metabolism is so fast you can eat what you like without putting on weight	You will need almost twice as many calories as your dad does, thus will need to be eating fairly constantly
Apparent lack of responsibilities	Pressure to get started on "life's ladder"
Your system will best be able to cope with the excesses of drink and drugs	You are far more likely to dangerously overdo it with drink and drugs
Your immune system will be operating at its peak and you will feel invincible	Because you feel invincible you are less likely to look after your health, thus serious conditions are often allowed to develop unchecked

Be careful of:

STDs and AIDS
Not because your system is any more susceptible, but simply because statistics say your behaviour is likely to put you at much greater risk.

Testicular cancer
Monthly self-examination is vital, as not only are you most vulnerable to it at the moment but it is the type of cancer most likely to affect you at this age.

Weight gain
You are still growing and you will need to eat heartily, but be careful of getting fat at this point as it could become a habit. Now is the time to get into an exercise routine.

Anaemia
Iron deficiency, causing general fatigue, isn't uncommon in men of this age so eat plenty of leafy green vegetables.

Random acts of violence
The vast majority of assaults in the UK are committed by young men aged between fifteen and thirty on other young men aged between fifteen and thirty.

telling you that you should either be coupled up or out sowing abundant amounts of wild oats, yet a genuine lack of self-confidence

Twentysomethings are fitter, faster and with very little to worry about

about appearance, sophistication and all-round manliness makes this a huge task.

It all amounts to the difficulties men have in passing from childhood into adulthood without the support system that women seem to have. Females are far more likely to talk about things among themselves or with their mothers, and have all manner of media offering them advice. Men could get through this difficult period if they talked about what was going on in their lives and admitted to fears and insecurities, to each other, to their dads, to teachers or – before things get really bleak – counsellors. If they did more of that their biggest worries would be exactly how much fun to have that particular night.

Man in his thirties

By now, if you've made it out of your twenties without being stabbed to death or getting killed in a car accident, you should be a much more stable individual. Statistically you are likely to be either settled down in a relationship and starting a family or, at the very least, aware of the value of doing so. This is a completely natural result of a man's inherent programming for procreation and you are following through now because you have become self-confident enough to form close personal relationships. Also, you are grown up enough to be far less selfish than you were ten years ago.

This is a serious change of lifestyle that will allow you to get something a bit more meaningful from your leisure time than a skinful and a bit of a scrap, and many men will be rather grateful for this. But although the risky behaviour of your previous decade will be far less frequent it's unlikely such shenanigans have been consigned completely to history. It will still be necessary and not altogether unhealthy for you to prove there's occasional life in the old dog. The big difference about going on the town at this age, though, is that you will exercise more restraint as you have more to lose. Now, if you do get into trouble, your life experience is far more likely to get you out of it without a trip to casualty.

Career-wise, things should be taking

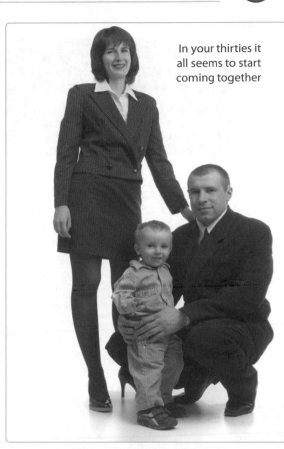

In your thirties it all seems to start coming together

What's good about being thirtysomething	What sucks about being thirtysomething
You are much more confident than when you were in your twenties	Dissatisfaction is replacing insecurity and male suicides peak during this decade
You will probably be married or in a stable relationship	You'll have to adjust to a whole new way of life as half of a couple
Your propensity for risky behaviour will have decreased massively	You will be a trifle envious of your single friends still whooping it up
Your immune system will still be working well but less efficiently than when you were in your twenties	Your metabolism will have slowed noticeably, so it will suddenly become much easier to put on weight
Your earnings will have increased	Your financial commitments will have multiplied
You will be much better equipped to take big decisions	You will have many, many more big decisions to take
You are still young enough and by now experienced enough to get a huge amount out of your life	Trying to do too much, career-wise, leisure-wise and family-wise is a major cause of frustration

F

Fact: If you are still smoking at this age, you are probably smoking a great deal more than you were when you were in your twenties.

off for you. You'll be in that unique position of having the energy of a young man, but with enough experience gained to know how to channel it. Also you shouldn't have got cynical about things yet, thus will still have a huge enthusiasm for life. However, while your potential for earnings and promotion prospects are looking healthy, your work-related stress levels will be increasing, added to which may well be the pressures of a newly growing family. It's little wonder the male suicide rate peaks among thirtysomethings and incidences of impotence are higher than at any age below eighty.

In spite of it being a period of high pressure, as a great deal will be expected of you by a growing number of people, you are actually far better equipped to deal with whatever life throws at you.

Stress and the thirtysomething man

It is now being recognized that men are suffering from stress at a much younger age, and it is over the past couple of decades that potential triggers for it have increased dramatically. A fundamental cause is the changes in social convention that have happened since their fathers were their age and for which so few contemporary life models exist. A generation ago a man lived with his mum until he got married, then he lived with his wife until one of them died. Nowadays the wealth of choice of domestic arrangements means there are so many that haven't existed long enough to have rules, and many require a great deal more effort to make them work.

Likewise men "growing up" later and later and often persisting with the carefree

All over medical checkup (heart, lungs, blood pressure, cholesterol, diabetes, liver, kidneys and overall fitness): annually.

Be careful of:

STDs and AIDS
Although you are not at as high a risk as you were ten years ago, this is still a dangerous time for the many single thirtysomething men.

Drink and drug addictions
This is when habits start to gain a hold, as you are less likely to binge drink but more likely to drink every night, and will have more money to afford more and better substances.

Prostate problems
This is when you need to get examined twice a year for trouble with your prostate gland – not necessarily for cancer, but for lower-level infections and inflammations such as prostatitis.

Weight gain
Be warned, middle-aged spread starts now. Especially if you've recently achieved the enviable domestic situation of having at least two meals a day cooked for you.

T

> *Tip: Although many men will have settled on their career by this time, it is never too late to change tack – just make sure any life changes don't have an adverse effect on those around you.*

behaviour of their twenties well into their thirties and forties – adultescence, anybody? – conflicts with genetics and many of those around him will be urging him to settle down, start a family and get on at work. Once again this leads to stress because there are no cut and dried ways of doing things, and the more decisions that need to be made, the greater the pressure on the man making them.

Work and financial pressures have increased too, as, once again, the world they are making their way in will be very different to their father's. There is no such thing as a job for life any more; employment laws have been eroded to the degree that you may not be particularly well looked after if you do keep your job; and international outsourcing means there is always somebody in a far-flung country who will do your job for less. Yet the financial pressures of this life stage remain at least as heavy as they always were, and your inherent need to be working (see Chapter 6, p.114) will be unchanged.

It is vital that men of this age talk to people, to ease whatever pressure situations they might be feeling. If that stress is domestic-related, then you have to share it with your partner. Even if the problem is your partner.

Man in his forties

Astonishingly, forty is the cut-off age at which young people (those under thirty) think you become officially "old", a fact which seems to say more about them (the youngsters) than their grizzled counterparts. Furthermore, in recent studies the most

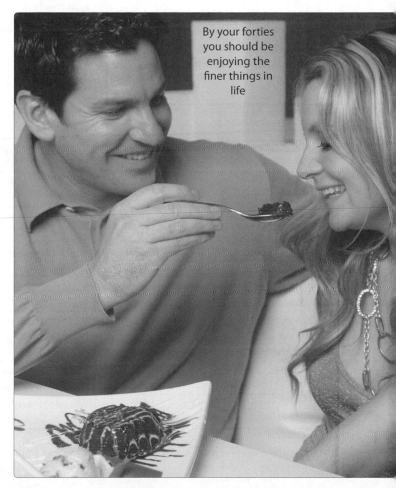

By your forties you should be enjoying the finer things in life

popular reason young people gave for their hedonistic behaviour was that they believed they had to whoop it up to the absolute max at that age because there is no fun to be had later. They also believed that not being "young" any more makes people inherently miserable and perpetually resentful of those who still have their youth.

Little do they know. Whoever thought up the title of that old Will Rogers movie, *Life Begins at Forty*, had it exactly right: as you ease into your fourth decade your quality of life is set to drastically improve.

You will have developed enough understanding of the world and the people

> *All over medical checkup (heart, lungs, blood pressure, cholesterol, diabetes, liver, kidneys and overall fitness): annually.*

T *Tip: Make sure you are drinking enough water, as it's now your face will start to show wrinkles.*

in it to be scared of nothing, and this self-confidence will help you get the best out of whatever you are doing because people will see the best side of you. At work, you should be able to cope with increased responsibility without your stress levels rising, and you should be earning enough to have eased any financial worries you might have had during the previous decade. Many men are starting to reach their career goals at this time of life, which can be very fulfilling.

Fortysomething men have become more health conscious than at any previous time in their lives – maybe this is a result of being nagged by their partners, but at least

What's good about being fortysomething	What sucks about being fortysomething
You accept the fact you're not indestructible and take your health far more seriously	There are many more potential problems to be aware of
You are more likely now to want to get fit than at any other time	The highest number of exercise-related injuries is among this age group
Your earnings will be high	Your expenditure will be peaking as your family grows
You will rarely indulge in risky behaviour, and you will have considered the consequences	You may be tempted to buy a big motorbike or a sports car
Your family should have settled into a tight, trusted unit with children that no longer need constant attention	Single men in their forties are a notoriously broody bunch
You should be achieving your career goals	If you haven't, work-related frustration may be starting to boil over
You will be starting to enjoy the good life	You will be much more susceptible to gastric disorders and peptic ulcers
You will be much more confident about discussing feelings and problems with other people – notably your partner	Because your responsibilities have increased – both at work and at home – you will have more potential problems to talk about

Be careful of:

Failing eyesight
It's around now you will need reading glasses, even if you've had perfect eyesight up until now.

Weight gain
Your metabolism is performing less efficiently than it has been, yet you are probably still eating as much as you were ten years ago.

Blood sugar levels
Although it is being increasingly diagnosed among younger men, the most likely time for type 2 or adult onset diabetes to appear is in your forties. Men of Indian, African or African-Caribbean heritage need to be particularly vigilant.

Skin cancer
Because it can be a cumulative condition, it is much more prevalent among men of forty and above.

they are doing something about their well-being. Worries about cholesterol levels, heart disease and middle-aged spread mean that, at this age, men are very likely to start a keep fit programme and begin watching what they eat. Also, it's far from unusual for fortysomething men to quit smoking and cut back a bit on the drink. Not a moment too soon, either.

Your family life should, by now, be everything you hoped it would. Time will have developed a relationship between you and your partner that thrives on trust and closeness, while your children will be developing into people that you can actually have a conversation with, although you will still be very much in charge of them. You should have more leisure time, and

T

Tip: Start dressing your age. Although you may look in the mirror and see the same lithe twentysomething looking back at you, the chances are the rest of the world sees a middle-aged bloke who for some reason is wearing his son's clothes.

either taking up hobbies or sports or just chilling out will help keep you healthy as it keeps your brain active and lowers your stress levels.

Really, the only downside of being fortysomething is you will start to notice you're not as young as you used to be, and the physical decline that started ten years ago is gathering pace. However, with your new fitness regime you'll easily be able to slow it back down again.

Getting fit at forty

It is at this point in their lives that men start worrying about their fitness levels and weight gain, and more men in their forties embark on exercise-for-fitness programmes (as opposed to sport-related) than at any other age. And they will need to be very careful about it.

Warming up will be even more important for them, as the unexercised cardiovascular system needs to be eased into it gradually to avoid harmful stress, and a heart rate monitor will be money well spent (see p.165). Stretching and ballistic joint looseners are also necessary, as your tendons and ligaments will be tight and more prone to sprains and strains. An unbreakable rule must be to stop if you feel

In your fifties your life should be a pretty straight fairway – literally as well as metaphorically

pain, and don't push yourself too hard in the beginning of your programme.

Man in his fifties

The main thing about your fifties is that, if you're in good shape, they won't be very different from your forties. The kids will be a bit older, your home life will still be steady, you will be safer than you have ever been – you are very likely to be buying sensible, safety-oriented cars; generally take less risks; and be at low risk as a victim of assault. The career path will probably have started to flatten out, but you will have a bit more spare cash in your pocket – if the mortgage isn't paid off there can't be much left of it – which is just as well as there are few things in life more expensive than teenage children. But the good side of your kids growing up is that, unless they need money, you'll hardly ever see them which can be very liberating inasmuch as it allows you and your partner far more time to have fun. Together.

Although you won't be as strong as you once were as muscle density and size will

Be careful of:

Weight gain
Your metabolism has slowed considerably.

Type 2 diabetes
The risks have gone up considerably, so watch your diet and get your blood sugar and cholesterol levels checked at least once a year.

Cancers
Skin, bowel, stomach and lung. If any moles start changing appearance, get them looked at immediately, and if you are a smoker get checked at least four times a year. Or better still, give up.

Declining eyesight
You may need stronger reading glasses.

Stress fractures or joint damage
This particularly applies to those who do impact exercise, like runners.

Digestive complaints
Your system will have got even less efficient as your production of stomach acid will have slowed.

> *All over medical checkup
> (heart, lungs, blood pressure,
> cholesterol, diabetes, liver,
> kidneys and overall fitness):
> bi-annually.*

The hangovers don't get worse, but...

The actual dehydration and depletion of nutrients will hit you in more or less the same way it always has and you will have the same wretched morning after. Why it will seem progressively worse as you get older is because the disrupted sleep patterns will have a greater effect – although you will actually need less sleep, what you should be getting is more crucial and missing it far more noticeable. Not that you've got any business being out on the lash.

Man in his sixties (and beyond)

The chances are that as you celebrate your sixtieth, you'll have another twenty birthdays still to come, and that those coming decades can be pretty much pure unadulterated "me time". Welcome to the world of retirement and the chance to take a crack at pretty much

have been in decline for a while now, if you started an exercise regime in your forties this will have minimal detrimental effect. Also, being very fit will mean you have a much better chance of staving off the heart disease, type 2 diabetes and high blood pressure to which you will have become increasingly prone. It will help you keep your weight in check as well, which takes more effort now as your metabolism continues to slow down.

You are starting to wear out by now, and your declining immune system means you are more susceptible to infection. If you eat right, stay fit and put a bit more effort into looking after yourself though, there's no reason why your fifties should hold you back from anything.

What's good about being fiftysomething	What sucks about being fiftysomething
You are very chilled out about things in general	You've got the highest chance of being laid off at work
You will have more money and an appreciation for the finer things in life	Susceptibility to type 2 diabetes and noticeable weight gain
The likelihood of testicular cancer is by now very low	Cancers of the bowel, skin, stomach and prostate are most likely now
You are less likely to smoke	If you have been smoking all your adult life it is now that it will be doing you obvious and possibly fatal damage
You are in the decade when you are least likely to get injured in a road accident	You are three times as likely to suffer cardiovascular disease than you were a decade ago
The health and fitness regime you adopted ten years ago is really starting to pay off	Your muscles will be naturally much less strong than in the previous decade
You probably spend less time and money in the barbers	Greying male pattern baldness

anything you've ever had a hankering for. Within reason, of course. Provided you've kept yourself in reasonable shape, you will still be able to do pretty much everything you did before, albeit a bit more carefully.

The biggest barrier to a full and active life as a senior is that senior himself – if you think you're too old to partake in what's going on around you then you probably will be. Follow the example of places like Florida or continental Europe where being old simply means you've lived a little bit

> *All over medical checkup (heart, lungs, blood pressure, cholesterol, diabetes, liver, kidneys and overall fitness): every three months.*

T

> *Tip: Don't be shy about checking out the holidays specifically offered to the over-sixties. They are often far more exciting than what's generally on offer and will also cater to the standards of comfort you need and expect.*

longer, and it's no reason not to get involved in anything. People there are fit, sharp and often difficult to keep up with, and quality of life is something of a self-maintaining spiral – because the demand for activities is there, the range on offer is enormous.

Of course everything will be a bit more of an effort, and your declining hearing and eyesight will be testament to your noticeably wearing out. However, if you are keeping fit then although your muscles are naturally losing density and strength, you will be able to maintain them more efficiently at this age to retain strength. You should be continuing to work out too, because at this age you will

Be careful of:

Rapidly declining eyesight
A hardening of the eye's lens and a weakening of the muscles behind it will mean focusing becomes progressively more difficult, starting with the closest field of vision.

Cancers
Get checked regularly for bowel, stomach and lung cancer (especially if you are still smoking) and keep a close lookout for signs of skin cancer.

Low-level infections
Your immune system becomes increasingly less efficient as you get older, meaning you have to make sure you keep it well nourished.

Boredom
Now you've got all this time on your hands there are loads of things you can be getting on with. Have a look online or in your local library to find out what's on offer.

Osteoporosis
Your bones will become progressively less dense than they were, so you need to make sure you keep your calcium intake up – but don't overdo it as that could cause constipation.

What you eat
Your system will be able to cope with junk food less easily, and because you will be naturally eating less you have to make sure your food is as nutrient-loaded as possible.

What's good about being sixtysomething	What sucks about being sixtysomething
People expect less of you	You will find yourself being patronized
You will be smarter than your younger counterparts thanks to greater experience and a "big picture" way of assessing situations	Your chances of Alzheimer's increases rapidly once you pass 65
Less stress in your life because, once you retire, you have far fewer schedules to keep	Higher potential for boredom and inactivity
Unexpected weight gain or loss will be a reliable early indicator that something is wrong	You will have to work harder to control your weight as your metabolism is still getting slower
You should be free from such money worries as a big mortgage or school fees	Living on a fixed income can cause financial problems
You become less susceptible to heart disease once you get past seventy	Your sixties are the decade in which you are most likely to suffer a heart attack or a stroke
Keeping fit becomes easier because your muscles will work more efficiently	Your muscles are decreasing in mass, density and strength
You understand life to a much better degree and therefore still have an enormous amount to contribute	Ageism is increasing dramatically

also be susceptible to high blood pressure, strokes and heart attacks. However, it may be easier for you to switch to a non-impact exercise such as cycling or swimming to reduce stress on your bones and joints. A good level of nutrition is vital too, as you will need to work that bit more to maintain your immune system.

Mentally you will be as sharp as you ever were, with greater analytical abilities, but again this will be down to you as you'll need to give your brain daily workouts to keep it fit. A downside of this, though, is that Alzheimer's and senile dementia become a very real prospect after the age of 65.

It really is still all there for you in your last two or three decades, providing you're willing to put a bit of effort in – both physically and mentally.

T

Tip: It may be advisable for runners to alternate their runs with non-impact exercise.

It's never too late

Four months after a double heart bypass and at the age of 59, Sir Ranulph Fiennes completed the Land Rover 7x7x7 Challenge, and between 26 October and 1 November 2003 he ran seven marathons on seven continents in seven days. Two years later he climbed 8690 metres (28,500 feet) up Mount Everest, then in 2007 scaled the notorious north face of Switzerland's 3970 metre (13,025 feet) Mount Eiger.

Looking after Number One

You could exercise, eat nutritiously, avoid risky situations, get and stay married, do everything within your power to keep yourself fit and healthy, but the chances are, at some time in your life, you are going to have to get professional healthcare. Whatever the reason, and whatever aspect of the service you will be dealing with, it will help if you know how to get the absolute best out of it.

Don't be afraid of the doc

Although this book will be your best bet for staying healthy, it can't do everything. No matter how well you're taking care of yourself, the law of averages dictates that at some point in your life you're going to have to visit your doctor or go to hospital. And, as you are a man, the chances are you should have done it a while ago.

The vast majority of men only go so far as to visit the doctor when they feel they are so sick they can no longer do all the things they usually do – work, sport, socializing etc – without actually collapsing or throwing up. And then this condition will have had to have persisted for several days and so there will be virtually no chance of preventative healthcare or regular check-ups.

"Men do not go to the doctor's early enough," maintains our resident family doctor Liliana Risi. "They tend to let a complaint fester until it starts to actually stop them from doing something. It is almost becoming accepted among men that modern

life puts so many time pressures on them, it is precluding something as good for them as looking after their health, but it has definitely slipped down the list of priorities.

"That said, nobody wants people to turn up at the doctor's surgery every time they cough. There has to be a balance, and at the moment that balance has shifted away from looking after themselves."

The reasons are manifold, (see box on p.293), and although it is usually explained away as the inherent stoicism involved with "being a man", part of which dictates there will be something honourable in "not making a fuss", underneath it all is a mixture of embarrassment, machismo and fear – mostly fear. According to the American Society of Family Physicians, and widespread anecdotal evidence among British healthcare professionals, there are several different types of fear involved.

Fear of the unknown is the biggest, as the doctor's surgery or a medical centre is a world that is totally alien to most people, like nothing else they are likely to come into contact with and it even has its own language. This means a feeling of being out of control of the situation, which makes many men very uncomfortable; indeed even the anticipation of such a state of affairs can be intimidating. Then there is the likelihood that you are going to be told something you won't be overly happy about, which is never a situation most men rush to embrace. Ironically, the mere fact your complaint *might* be serious, should give you far greater impetus to get it looked at sooner rather than later.

Of course, any feelings of apprehension will be made more so by the fact that the reason you've decided to go to the doctor is that you aren't very well, therefore you will feel even more vulnerable. Thus, it takes even

greater effort to make that appointment.

This last point deftly illustrates the self-perpetuating cycle of not getting yourself looked at when you should, and there is a widespread view among healthcare organizations on both sides of the Atlantic that this reluctance is contributing to so many men feeling stressed or chronically fatigued. Again, it's not without irony that the aspects of their lives that get taken much more seriously – work, sport, socializing etc – would be much more enjoyable, effective or efficient if they kept themselves in tip-top condition. But on a more serious level, considering the current widespread levels of cholesterol, diabetes, obesity and sub-optimal nutrition,

If you can't face all this patient friendly cheeriness UK readers can phone NHS Direct 0845 4647 (24 hours) for front line medical advice (see p.371)

there is a worry that dangerous conditions are being allowed to develop unchecked.

Although it will take some mental effort on your part to initially break what has probably become a habit, there are a number of steps you can take to make your visit to the doctor easier and far more satisfying.

It probably isn't how you remember it

The days of the horribly decorated, depressing-smelling, badly lit doctor's waiting room, decorated with yellowing posters of skeletons and presided over by a fire-breathing receptionist are, mostly, a thing of the past. In both the UK and the US there has been a revolution in how healthcare presents itself. Clinics and larger practices increasingly have purpose-built reception areas, designed to put patients at ease and to be as inviting as possible – even the smaller operations have been urged to make their premises more welcoming. Also, now it is accepted that it may take some time to get seen, waiting areas are being designed and decorated to be as soothing as possible.

In spite of these sartorial improvements actually leading to their own specific set of problems (see box below), the overhaul has increased the functionality of health centre reception areas, inasmuch as the use of space will be designed around patients' needs. Designs take into account patients' desires to move quickly through the entrance to a point at which they can be spoken to, as early contact with a healthcare professional puts a nervous visitor at ease. Receptions are now

F

Fact: According to the American Academy of Family Physicians, women visit healthcare facilities 2.5 times more often than men, and the reason behind this imbalance was found to be lack of habit-forming education – as girls, women are taught the importance of good personal health and it becomes ingrained. Boys rarely receive such teaching and as a result, from an early age, men believe healthcare is something that isn't for them.

Healthcare facilities aren't just for women

There has been a growing feeling among men that they have been marginalized by modern healthcare organizations, as many believe the services on offer have become increasingly female-centric. This is particularly prevalent in the US, where a survey conducted by the *American Journal of Public Health* found that nearly one-third of men surveyed claimed they were put off seeking help because they thought health services had become "feminized" in terms of decor, presentation, reading materials and information on offer. The remarkable thing is this apparent gender bias came as the result of campaigns, on both sides of the Atlantic, to make hospital and health centre reception areas more welcoming and patient-friendly across the board.

However, this might just be an excuse. In 2000, in Seattle, to widespread media fanfare, a specifically men-oriented healthcare centre opened under the name The Garage, using motoring metaphors for different areas of healthcare – "fuel injection" (prostate), "tune-ups" (check-ups), "spark plugs" (Viagra) and so on. After six months and only seven patients, it shut down.

Meanwhile, Dr Risi assures us that healthcare facilities are *not* geared up in favour of women and that men will receive equally thorough and sympathetic treatment.

Why men put off going to the doctor

Reason/excuse	The professionals say	How to get over it
Embarrassment	Doctors and health centre staff now have a much higher level of training as regards communication, discretion and putting patients at ease	Take your partner with you, and remember there is very little a twenty-first century GP won't have seen before
It's some sort of reflection on their masculinity	Everybody gets sick, regardless of how macho they are and no doctor would assume there is any shame attached to it	Bear in mind that looking after yourself will help maintain your manliness for longer
Don't have the time	Most health centres and surgeries now have opening hours extended beyond the traditional working day	Find a practice that offers a greater choice of access
Don't want to bother the doctor	That's what doctors are there for, and you will be a great deal more "bother" if you allow yourself to get very sick	Don't worry about imposing on a doctor's time – they haven't got anything else to do during surgery hours
Whinging is generally frowned upon	Looking after yourself is common sense, and would be applauded by a doctor, never thought of as whinging	Don't whinge; conduct a grown-up discussion with the doctor about what might be wrong
Not in men's nature to discuss problems	This is a big hurdle for a lot of men, and it often helps if they take somebody else with them	Take your partner, who will probably be able to explain your symptoms better than you can
Whatever is wrong will probably go away by itself	Although nobody wants to run to the doctor every time they cough, it is always best to go sooner rather than later	In the long term, be more aware of your own body so you can tell the difference between something minor and a potentially serious complaint
Scared of what they might be told	Whatever you are going to be told will definitely not be any less worrying if you are told it in a month's time	If this is the case, you must be thinking something could be wrong: therefore it is best to get it checked out as soon as possible
Don't like being out of control of the situation – i.e. the doctor is talking at them	Healthcare professionals are now encouraged to involve the patient as much as possible, because it is vital they feel involved in their consultancy and any resultant treatment	Prepare yourself as well as you can before you go, so you can hold a conversation with your doctor

being designed to respect a patient's privacy and wherever possible reception desks are positioned in a way that conversations cannot be overheard in the waiting area. Also private reception rooms are becoming standard in larger operations, so visitors can discuss their conditions with far less likelihood of embarrassment.

These improvements shouldn't really come as a surprise, because, as Dr Risi reminds us, "Doctors want to help people too!" She continues, "there has been a great deal of effort put into doctors' waiting areas and the reception areas of larger practices, because it was realized they had to work a bit harder to allow us to give the best healthcare

F

Fact: The most common reason people in the UK have given for switching to private healthcare is that they feel the doctor has much more time for them.

we can. It was realized that if the patient feels alienated at the point of entry to a healthcare facility then that feeling won't get any better while they are waiting, and the consultancy is far less likely to be a satisfactory one.

"Reception staff are being purpose-trained too, to respond to people sympathetically and discreetly and to be aware that they could be putting people off. The addition of private areas at reception is making a difference, because people are finding out they can discuss sensitive or potentially embarrassing issues with total discretion."

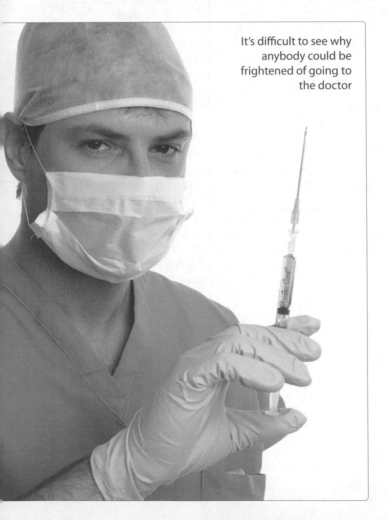

It's difficult to see why anybody could be frightened of going to the doctor

Time for health

Three of the biggest barriers standing in between men and their pursuit of good health involve time: they haven't got enough to be able to go to the doctor; health centre opening hours are inconvenient; the doctor has such a limited amount of time with each consultation, would-be patients don't feel like they're getting anything done. In today's healthcare climate, these are far from insurmountable.

As regards the first point, it comes down to time management and priorities, as

There's no need to go it alone

If you are particularly nervous, or you think it might help you better understand what you are being told, take somebody with you when you visit your healthcare professional. If it is your partner who knows your state of health as well as you do, this could be particularly useful as he/she may be able to bring up points you have forgotten or even be aware of some things you are not. Also, it will make it much easier to discuss and analyse what you were told when you get home. There is no reason whatsoever why a doctor should object to you bringing somebody else to a consultation, but it is always good manners to ask before you do.

was discussed in Chapter 8. If you're thinking you don't have time to keep fit, it's a matter of sitting down and plotting out how you actually spend the hours in your week, and you'd be surprised at how much spare time you actually have. Or if you are really doing things every waking minute of your day, then it's all about weighing up the importance of keeping yourself well against other activities you might be pursuing. According to Dr Risi, men need to move "keeping healthy" much higher up the list of things they could not see themselves doing without. "So many men simply don't take looking after themselves seriously enough – it's why married men tend to have much better health," she says.

Health centre opening hours, on both sides of the Atlantic, have taken into account the pressures on people's time during working hours and are now making great moves to facilitate this. Many establishments now operate shift systems so people can be seen in the evening or early in the morning, or they are being far more flexible within limited opening times.

The amount of time a doctor will have to see you is a problem that, unfortunately, has not got any better recently, but this isn't his or her fault and they will still try to do their very best in the limited time they have – in the UK, among GPs, the average time for a consultation is down to six minutes. There is no point in putting off a visit, or getting frustrated because of this. It is an unfortunate fact of life and the best thing you can do is follow the guidelines below

and be as well prepared as possible before you get there.

Help them help you

When you go to visit a doctor, you know they won't have much time and you will want to get the best possible result from your consultation – the latter point is equally important to lengthier private consultations, as you don't want to waste money or need to go back for more repeat visits than you might have to.

Before you go

Make up your mind what it is you are going to see your doctor about – it may help to write it down – and be sure of what it is you are going to tell them. As Dr Risi says, "Take a checklist with you of things you want answered, don't allow yourself to get knocked off focus and make sure you get across the point that you came there for in the first place. Otherwise you'll have to go back and that won't be the best use of your time or the doctor's."

This may involve diagnosing yourself at home first, and, contrary to popular wisdom, doctors are not averse to this; indeed they actively encourage it as it shows you are taking responsibility for your health, therefore taking it seriously. Then on a far more immediate level, any information you can give them about your condition, or the more specific symptoms you can describe, will help them reach a judgement in a shorter space of time. Dr Risi's view on this, which she believes is prevalent among the medical profession, is that with so much access to health information available online it would be odd if somebody didn't try and find out what was wrong with him/herself first. Especially if he/she is of a group that is reluctant to seek professional help in the first place.

When you are at the surgery

As well as taking a list of points you want answered, take a list of points you want asked. This may seem a little odd, but what will help your doctor more than anything is knowing everything he/she can about you. "We need," explains Dr Risi, "as complete a picture as we can get of a patient – are you married, what sort of job do you do and so

on. This will all help to assess your state of mind, which will have a bearing on your state of health and what, if any, remedies should be prescribed to you."

This will mean that you will need to be prepared to give all sorts of information you might not have considered relevant, and if not asked for a rounded description of your life you should volunteer one. As Dr Risi stresses, a consultation should be more like a conversation and not simply a matter of you sitting down and having somebody with a stethoscope around his/her neck talking at you, and this will go a long way towards alleviating feelings of powerlessness the situation might be causing.

Take notes while you are talking. This will have a twofold advantage: it will help you remember points you want to bring up for further clarification and it will help you remember things when you get home. However, you need to listen. When you are nervous to start off with, and dealing with things you are unfamiliar with, it is very easy

What you should get checked for and how often

Age	Checkup should include	Frequency
Twenty-something	Heart, lungs, blood pressure, cholesterol, testicular cancer, liver function, kidneys, diabetes, weight/fat, overall fitness	Every two years
Thirty-something	Heart, lungs, blood pressure, cholesterol, prostate problems, testicular cancer, liver function, kidneys, diabetes, weight/fat, overall fitness	Annually
Forty-something	Heart, lungs, blood pressure, cholesterol, blood sugar levels, skin cancer, liver function, kidneys, weight/fat, overall fitness	Annually
Fifty-something	Heart, lungs, blood pressure, cholesterol, blood sugar levels, skin cancer, thyroid problems, liver function, kidneys, weight/fat, overall fitness	Twice a year
Sixty-something and beyond	Heart, lungs, blood pressure, cholesterol, blood sugar levels, skin cancer, thyroid problems, liver function, kidneys, weight/fat, overall fitness	Every three months

to fixate on ticking off the points on your list to such a degree you forget to listen to the answers you are getting.

At the end of your consultation

Although your time with the doctor will be limited – and he/she will have an internal clock that will wind things up at a certain point – try not to allow yourself to feel rushed. When you are asked if there is anything you didn't understand or anything that wasn't covered, consult your notes and make sure they go over anything you are not clear about or didn't get answered. It will save time for both of you in the long run if you get everything sorted out now.

Once you get out of there

Get any prescriptions filled out immediately, complete any courses of tablets and make sure you follow any instructions you have been given. While the modern healthcare professional may be keener on you playing doctor and self-diagnosing, he/she will not be so happy if you start making unilateral decisions as regards your treatment.

A feeling of false security

According to recent surveys in both the UK and the US, there is a wide gap between how men feel about their own health and what their state of health actually is – far wider than it is with women who tend to have a far more realistic idea of how healthy they actually are. The vast majority of men said they felt their general health was either good or very good, regardless of their weight or eating habits or exercise regimes. What

---

Get the most from your doctor

Prepare well beforehand, so you are sure what your symptoms are.

Write a list of what you want to ask and what you expect to be asked.

Take somebody with you, if it makes you feel more confident.

Volunteer information and hold a conversation with your doctor.

Listen to what he or she is saying.

Write things down.

Don't be afraid to admit you didn't understand something or need it explained again.

Try not to be rushed, but appreciate your doctor has time pressures too.

Follow the advice given and courses of medicine prescribed.

---

is worrying healthcare professionals is that these feelings of well-being are based on little other than there not seeming to be anything wrong, and this could be storing up serious problems for the future.

Many chronic or creeping conditions such as coronary artery disease, high cholesterol levels or vitamin or mineral deficiency do not necessarily involve feeling bad, or will be adapted to as a new norm. The concern is that left unchecked, potential problems

F

Fact: Unsurprisingly, married men are far more likely to go to the doctor earlier than single men, as their wives tend to take their health more seriously than they do.

Alternative healthcare on the the web

nccam.nih.gov
The National Center for Complementary and Alternative Medicine in the US, will help you find a local practitioner.

icmedicine.co.uk
he Institute for Complementary Medicine will do much the same job in the UK, as they keep registers of approved healers.

who.int/mediacentre
The World Health Organization has general background and factsheets on alternative medicine at its media centre.

will not be addressed until they make a drastic or life-threatening impact. It is widely believed that far more men should feel far less confident about their state of health and, while not necessarily assuming something is wrong, be very aware that everything might not be as it should and to get checked over by their doctor on a regular basis. At the risk of sounding like a failed Seattle healthcare practice (see box on p.290), it's kind of like an MOT.

Natural alternatives

Currently, all across the Western world people are turning away from conventional healthcare and opting for an alternative approach. According to the World Health Organization, over fifty percent of the populations of Europe and North America have tried complementary or alternative medicines at least once, and in the UK and the US the annual spend on them is £120 million and $17 billion.

But are they any good?

Debate rages all around the world as to the value of alternative remedies, and as their effectiveness isn't backed up by the sort of clinical trials that would surround a pharmaceutical development, there is very little hard evidence to say whether they work or not. Although in many examples, there is a logic to some of these cures and

GP's surgery vs Accident & Emergency

According to Dr Risi, going to A&E will not only put extra strain on an already stretched system, but will not do you the most good either.

"Don't go to casualty with anything other than an emergency or unless you've had an accident. This is very important, because those departments have a role to play, which is to patch up casualties and deal with accidents and emergencies – hence the name. They don't need their premises cluttered up with people who just aren't feeling very well.

"Also, they don't specialize in that sort of stuff – illnesses – so if there is anything seriously wrong with you they will have to pass you on to somebody else. That means your treatment will then involve a lot more people and mean coming back for all sorts of appointments. If you're not feeling well, go and see your GP."

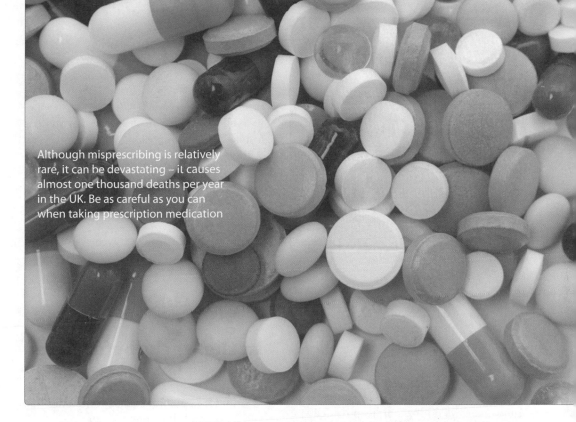

Although misprescribing is relatively rare, it can be devastating – it causes almost one thousand deaths per year in the UK. Be as careful as you can when taking prescription medication

it's possible to make sense of how they might work, people tend to arrive at them with a pre-formed viewpoint and are either very black or very white about the whole issue. Personally I will always try something natural first and only if it doesn't seem to be having any effect will I "go chemical", but many people I know and respect wouldn't touch iridology or acupuncture or suchlike with a pole. It is also believed there is a considerable psychological aspect to this and if patients believe whatever they are trying is doing them good, it will be. And there isn't anything wrong with that, either.

Although it might not seem like too much help, the best advice you can get as regards alternative or complementary medicine is to suck it and see. Talk to an established complementary medicine practitioner or establishment, and get recommended as to what might be most suitable for you (see box on previous page), then give it a go. Although it might not do you much good, it's unlikely to do you any harm.

Not tablets of stone

When you are given a prescription by your healthcare professional, it's highly unlikely you're going to be able to read what it says, and no more probable that you would know what it meant anyway. But it will always be in your interest to know what it is you are being expected to take and how you should be taking it. Follow this easy checklist and you won't get it far wrong.

1. Ask what you are taking. Not just the genre of drugs, but the specific medication –

Tip: If you change your mind about going into hospital or want to change the date, use the contact number on your admission letter to let them know as soon as possible. That way you stand the best chance of getting the alternative date you want or a convenient outpatient appointment, and it will allow the hospital the most time to reallocate your bed.

4. Get clear details of the course. This should include how long you need to take them for, how many per day and when they should be taken, for example, after meals or before you go to bed. The pharmacist should supply all this information, but you can never be too prepared.

5. Establish what you should do if you miss a dose. This is important, as there probably will be times when you don't take one, and you need to know what to do to make sure they remain effective or you are not putting yourself in danger.

How to go into hospital

In the weeks beforehand

You should have already received an admission letter, stating the time and date of your admission, the name of the ward you will be on and the name of your consultant. Get this photocopied so you can leave a copy with somebody responsible and you can take the original with you when you go.

get it written out legibly – and find out what brand name you are likely to be given by the pharmacist and if any should be avoided.

2. Find out what they will do and how they should make you feel. You want to be able to tell if they are working or not, and if there are liable to be any unpleasant side effects. You can always do this online, provided you know exactly what it is you are researching.

3. Make sure there is nothing you shouldn't be doing while taking them. Like driving or drinking.

What to leave at home

Mobile phone Use of these is strictly taboo in most areas of nearly every hospital, and there's little point in having it there if you're not going to use it.

Watch You shouldn't be wearing it; every ward should have a clock and time will be far less relevant than usual.

Wallet and credit cards Why put temptation on offer?

Cigarettes and lighter Nearly every hospital in the UK and the US now operates smoking bans that extend throughout their grounds and outside areas.

Although you should be allocated a reasonably safe locker, there is no point in filling it with valuables that will not be of any use to you during your stay. Most hospitals will offer a service to keep items in an office safe, but space will be limited and they will not accept any responsibility for loss.

Private vs public – in the UK

According to Dr Risi, there are very few reasons for us Brits to go private when it comes to healthcare.

"Unless you have a comprehensive private healthcare plan – which will be very costly in itself if you want to be covered for everything – then you are better off with the National Health Service. It does practically everything very, very well, and while it might take a little while longer than in the private sector, the job that gets done will be of the highest standard.

"The only time I would recommend somebody to go private is if they have muscular-skeletal problems: the NHS doesn't do them very well. So if you need a long course of physiotherapy for something like a sports injury, you will be better looked after outside the Health Service, but it will be expensive."

Two days before

Check the time and date you are due in, and call the contact number on your letter to confirm you are coming in. Make sure, at this point, that they are aware of any special dietary, religious or other requirements you might have.

Read the letter to see if the hospital has given any special instructions, such as not eating or drinking for a certain period or not taking medication.

24 hours before

Prepare what you will need to take with you:
1. **Clean pyjamas.** If you don't usually use them, buy a pair. You may well be spending all day in them and most hospitals don't take kindly to patients kitted out in their underpants or, worse still, even less than that.
2. **Dressing gown and slippers.**
3. **Any medication you are taking.**
4. **Regular clothes.** Under some circumstances you might not have to stay in your pyjamas, and you will need something to wear when you go home.
5. **Washing and shaving kit, including a towel.** Unless you're in a very swanky private set-up, you will hugely appreciate the relative fluffiness of your own towel.
6. **Books and magazines.**
7. **MP3 player.** If you're not a regular MP3 user, buy an inexpensive one specially and load it up with your favourite tunes. It will greatly lift your spirits and block out the general commotion of the ward.
8. **Tissues and wet wipes.** These will allow you much more independence if you are unable to get out of bed for a bit.
9. **A few quid, some of it in change.** Don't take too much money with you – it's pointless and big hospitals are far from free of petty crime – but you will need something for purchases from the trolley or shop and phone calls.

On the day

1. **Leave time.** Leave more time than you think you are going to need to get there by your appointed admission time.
2. **Don't drive yourself.** There probably won't be anywhere for you to leave your car and you may not be in a fit state to drive when you are discharged.
3. **Take a friend or your partner with you.** It will be a pretty stressful experience and a reassuring presence will be valuable.
4. **Take water.** Buy a two-litre bottle of mineral water to take in with you. It will taste better than hospital water and save you having to keep asking for a drink. Unless, of course, you've been instructed not to eat and drink.

If you're not happy with how you've been treated

In the UK, the first action you should take is to write to the doctor concerned and clearly and rationally express your dissatisfaction. Dr Risi says, "Write a constructive letter explaining what was wrong to the GP concerned. They will welcome such communication as it helps them to help a patient further and to address something they might have been doing wrong. It shouldn't be assumed that if you complain about a GP then you will get bad treatment in the future."

Beyond that in the UK, the Patient and Advice Liaison Services, which will be based in your local Hospital Trust or Primary Care Trust, exists for more serious grievances. Then if you still do not get satisfaction from them, the General Medical Council, the British medical profession's governing body, has a complaints procedure that is outlined on their website gmc-uk.org.

In the US, you should start by writing to the doctor concerned, for the same reasons as in the UK, and they should accept it in the same spirit. If that doesn't work, complain in writing to the facility where the doctor practises, and as a final step contact the state medical board, as US doctors are licensed on a state-by-state basis. Whatever board you might require can be found by Googling, "medical board" and the relevant state.

On your arrival

1. At the ward's reception make sure the staff are aware of any special requirements you might have.
2. If you have any medication give it to the staff at that point, with instructions on how you should be taking it.
3. Establish visiting hours and if they come with any restrictions attached and make a note of them for whoever you are with – many hospitals provide a booklet for patients' friends and relatives.
4. If you are proposing to bring any electrical items in with you, check at this point that it will be permitted.
5. Make sure you wear your identification wristband at all times.

On your discharge

1. Have somebody come and meet you – even if you are going home in a cab.
2. Make sure you fully understand any instructions, medication courses or further treatment schedule you have been given – don't be shy about asking questions or taking notes.
3. Take all your belongings with you from the ward.
4. If you have to pick up a prescription from the hospital pharmacy be prepared to wait a while, so try and time it so you don't keep a cab waiting or make somebody have to find somewhere to park.

Just try to relax. You really are in the best possible hands

Improve your performance

If you've got this far with this book, then you'll be very aware of two basic things: getting fit and improving how your body functions are going to vastly improve your quality of life in every respect; and doing them isn't exactly rocket science. So why are we in the grip of an obesity crisis, with heart disease and type 2 diabetes so sharply on the rise? Because even when faced with so many overwhelming positives, a vast number of people just can't be arsed.

Think fit

Think of yourself, but as more fit and healthy. Better looking, with more energy, sharper thinking, better tempered, maybe even more popular, certainly more attractive, getting more out of practically every aspect of your life, and if not getting more sex then definitely enjoying it more, as will your partner. To get fit you have to think fit, and while this will involve a bit more than merely thinking about it, it is the first step anybody has to take, whatever level of fitness they're starting from or hope to reach. And it's often the biggest stumbling block.

Habitually healthy

One of the recurring themes of this book, both in the text and from the panel of experts, has been how changing your habits will be the foundation of getting fit and healthy. This is because to adopt any sort of healthy eating plan or exercise regime on the surface – i.e. to do it when you remember, or just when you fancy it – won't in the longterm do you any good, as it won't be coming naturally to you. Which means, on a psychological level, it will remain something you don't really want to do and see as an imposition on your life. If you change your habits, then it actually *becomes* your life and anything else will be what you have to go out of your way to do.

The first thing you have to do is break the old habits, because the chances are it was a bunch of essentially self-destructive habits that led you to getting into such a state to start off with. Eating badly is the most prevalent bad habit. As Dr Sarah Schenker explained back in Chapter 4, the fast food

T

Tip: Keep a bowl of fresh fruit at your workstation. It will be on hand for when you do require a snack, and you will be amazed at how popular you suddenly become, especially with your female co-workers.

Get a drink habit

If you measure your water consumption over the course of, say, a week, you'll be surprised at how little you do in fact drink. To actually take on board the required two to three litres of water a day, you really do have to consciously work to turn it into a habit. Keep a litre bottle of water with you all of the time, and perpetually swig from it in idle moments or while you are thinking about something. Eventually this will become like a nervous tic, in the same way as a smoker might spark up under the same circumstances, and that will be how you will genuinely keep yourself properly hydrated. Also, getting through a bottle with a predetermined amount in it will allow you to judge what you are drinking far more accurately than by filling glasses from the tap.

industry is such a powerfully marketed affair it's impossible to avoid unhealthy eating opportunities – note her terminology: what were once called meals and we had three square ones a day, have now been relegated to "eating opportunities".

It's this widespread habit of grazing and snacking throughout the day that should be where you start and while you will need to think yourself out of reaching for the crisps or the chocolate bar or the fizzy drink, you can make it easier on yourself by avoiding certain situations that encourage bad eating. Don't go down to the shop when you have a break; get out of the office rather than sit at your desk with a sandwich; change your walk home from the pub so you no longer pass that kebab shop where they know you by name; hang with a different lunchtime crowd so you're no longer in that pattern of pub on Monday, McDonalds on Tuesday, fish and chips on Friday and so on. The time when you'll have to steel yourself the most is when you put your head down and ignore that very attractive display of Danish pastries when you get your early morning coffee in Starbucks – if you can't think yourself past it then get your coffee elsewhere, preferably an establishment where the staff aren't trained to try and sell you cakes.

It's once you've broken these bad habits that you can start replacing them with good ones. As you remove the nutrient-free snack food you will still need to fuel your body, but now you can replace it with healthy food.

Fruit, salads or yoghurt make convenient snack food, and get into the habit of drinking water, as not only will this keep your stomach full and remove the temptation to pop a can of soda, you really do have to work to keep yourself properly hydrated (see box above). Then, if you start to regulate the chaos out of

There's no need for your mid-morning snack to be crisps or chocolate

Often, it will be easier to keep motivated if you take up a sport rather than just work out

avoid big supermarkets, as they spend fortunes on creating environments in which you will buy pretty much what they want you to buy, rather than what is actually good for you, and until you are sure about your new shopping list (see pp.32–33) don't let them manipulate you as well. This may initially be slightly inconvenient, but you will thank yourself for it in the long run and you can always go back once you're confident in what you want.

Start at small shops – butcher, greengrocer, fishmonger etc – or market stalls, where the choice will be much greater and whoever is serving you will be able to give you advice on storing, preparing and cooking what you are about to buy. Just try to avoid their very busy periods and you will be surprised at how much benefit there is to be had from striking up a relationship with a shopkeeper or stallholder.

Routine fitness

As regards getting and keeping fit, it is equally important that this becomes a habit; in fact your exercise routine needs to become as much a part of your regular routine as brushing your teeth or putting your phone in your pocket before you leave the house. Our

our eating opportunities and turn them back into "proper" meals at "proper" mealtimes, you will feel physically less inclined to snack. Also, your metabolic memory will make sure you actually like what is going to do you good and will set you off wanting more. After this, it could only be force of habit that keeps you grazing and you'll just have to think yourself through it.

Supermarket sweep

You will need to change your shopping habits too. Earlier in the book, Dr Schenker identified the problem of many men being unable to shop or unable to do so on a budget, and changing your eating habits will probably involve changing your shopping habits at the same time. In the beginning,

T

Tip: Turn your routine into exercise and buy a bike or start walking places, or buy a runner's backpack (see box on p.307) to put your regular clothes in and run home from work a couple of evenings a week. Then, for new fathers out there, invest in a runner's baby buggy so you and the nipper can get some fresh air together.

resident fitness expert Gideon Remfry spoke earlier about everybody being able to find half an hour three times a week to get fit, and that will pay genuine dividends if it becomes a habit. Rather than look for random thirty-minute periods during your week, set aside specific times and adhere to them rigidly. Then make yourself stick to them in exactly the same way as you wouldn't miss the kick-off of a match, or not bother to turn up to a lecture or to work.

In the beginning this may take some mental effort, especially if it involves getting out of a warm bed an hour or so earlier, but if you carry on then very soon it will become, simply, something you do, rather than something you have to go out of your way to do. You'll know when you've hit that level, because you will be adjusting other stuff in your life – like not staying out late or on the lash – to fit around what has become an immovable fixture.

Fairly soon after that, you will get to a point where if you do skip a session your body lets you know because it's so used to expending increased energy at a particular time it was looking forward to it. This might mean that you will become a bit restless or feel frustrated, but it also means that, because you now truly have the exercise habit, unless you are physically laid up you will definitely not miss the next session.

Motivational difficulties

One of the reasons getting started might be a problem is why do you want to do it in the first place? This isn't as straightforward a question as it might seem. One of the problems with how we live today is so often we need to have an apparently valid reason for everything, and it has to be a reason that would stand up to scrutiny from those around us. This is an aspect of the Busy Life Syndrome, whereby it's not unusual for people to believe that unless there is a tangible and fairly immediate justification for doing something, it must somehow be a waste of time.

It's a situation not unlike the state of affairs Dr Sandra Scott talked about in Chapter 6 when she spoke of people not wanting to do nothing and requiring

Six quick fixes to get you off your sofa

Treat yourself to some brand new, hi-tech exercise kit You won't want to feel you've wasted the money, and if you look like somebody who ought to be working out, you'll feel much more like somebody who ought to be working out.

Get changed into those same hi-tech exercise clothes Eventually you'll get fed up with people asking you, "Are you going for a workout then?"

Have your gym buddy come and call for you If you can't nag yourself into getting started, then arrange for somebody else to do it.

Have a stretch You'll release endorphins, and so immediately feel so much livelier, and your loosened, increased-blood-flowing-through-them muscles will start urging you to use them.

Tell yourself you're not going to do too much Opt for your most basic workout, then once you get started it's pretty much guaranteed you'll want to increase it.

Have a look at the TV schedules Repeats, reality and rubbish: there is probably no better motivation for getting out of the house.

constant stimulation, and in this case just doing something, apparently for the sake of it, is often viewed as downtime. Then add to that, the most common reasons for getting fit and healthy are usually vanity-based, and also involve admitting you'd been getting something wrong in the first place.

This is why so many young(ish) men's only physical exercise is playing sports,: because it makes obvious sense as to why they are doing it. Or they go running, because aiming to do a 10K or a marathon or something has a far greater sense of purpose to it and there's absolutely nothing vain or

How to keep going once you've started

Keep a record While this is an incredibly obvious thing to do, you would be surprised at how many people don't keep a long-term training log or record of what they have been doing. There are numerous fitness websites that will offer an interactive log – although the majority are dedicated to running or triathlon, **progresslog.com** and **activelog.com** are good for all-round fitness records – or you could just do it old-school, with an exercise book and a pen. Either way, looking back at how much progress you have made is a powerful force to make sure you carry on.

Keep a record in photographs Everybody's got some sort of digital camera, so keep a week-by-week series of snapshots of yourself and how your body shape and general appearance have been changing since you started your regime. A good idea with this is to store it on your computer as a slide show and use it for your screensaver as a constant reminder of what you have achieved.

Set a target Having a tangible goal to reach in a certain amount of time is the other side of the keeping-a-record coin. Moving steadily towards a specific target is the best way for so many people to keep motivated however, be aware of the next point.

Don't set a target (or don't set the wrong target) For some people, targets can become a massive de-motivator as they put an unnecessary stress on your exercise/healthy eating plan and turn it into a chore rather than something you should look forward to. Then targets that are too ambitious can have the same effect, while if you set your bar too low you won't get any benefit, thus won't see any improvement and will be much less inclined to continue.

Reward yourself Put a pre-decided amount of money in a jar for every inch you lose around the middle or put on around your chest, or kilogram you drop on the scales, and then after a couple of months use that cash to treat yourself. Ideally to something not necessarily good for you (see next point).

Enjoy a blowout or a few drinks or a fine cigar There's no reason at all why you shouldn't do this every so often, because you will be able to do so without feeling guilty and secure in the knowledge that your newly tuned body can handle it. Being able to cut loose occasionally will stop your fitness regime turning into a sentence – or at least make sure it's one with time off for good behaviour.

Put on a suit you haven't worn since last year. Again this is a really simple tip, but it works because it will make you feel doubly good about yourself – for losing the inches off your gut and cancelling out one of the most miserable things about putting on weight, that clothes you really like no longer fit you.

Buy some new clothes This will help you see yet another benefit to your newly toned body, and if you take your other half with you to help you choose, you'll be doing yourself another favour.

Go and see somebody you haven't seen for ages – preferably a woman Because you've been getting in shape gradually, people around you won't really have noticed, but to look up somebody who hasn't seen any of it should really ramp up your compliment intake.

girly about it, thus, it can be talked about without becoming the butt of anybody's jokes. It is, as Gideon Remfrey said, men in their thirties and forties who take up fitness for fitness sake, because, by that age, they are more aware of what is happening to them and are far less concerned with what is being said about them. Also, practically all of their peers are in the same state.

Again, it's a matter of mind over body, and it is important to acknowledge that although the motivation may be essentially superficial, what you will be achieving is one of the most important things you can do in your life. In other words, it has to be realized that there is no better way to spend your time than getting fit and healthy, if for no other reason than it will ultimately give you more time to spend on the "important" things in life.

Effua Baker – a personal trainer colleague of Gideon's, who was fitness consultant on the *Rough Guide to Running* – talks of most people's motivation being essentially superficial, but that shouldn't be allowed to get in the way of anything:

"I don't get people coming to me and saying they want to raise their VO^2 max or

T *Tip: For those of you who have given up smoking, approach giving up junk food or habitually grazing in the same way – stop dead, don't try to cut down gradually; stay away from snacking opportunities or places where you do so without thinking, as there will be powerful subconscious connections; and do it one day at a time until the desire has faded.*

B

Best investment: runner's backpack: £60–£100 ($100–$200)
These marvellous pieces of kit will have extra, cleverly positioned straps that will hold it tight to your back, meaning a minimum of movement while you run, and cutaway sides will allow your arms to pump unhindered. As a result, you can run to or from work and either have clothes to change into or not have to leave your regular clothes on the back of your chair. The better models should be waterproof, sturdily constructed with plenty of closable internal compartments to stop the contents shifting around, an easily accessible pocket for a water bottle and be made from breathable fabric where it will be held against your body. Although these will cost around three times the price of an everyday backpack, you will soon claw that back with the amount you save in fares, or even if

you are not a runner, having a rucksack this figure-hugging will be much easier on your back than a regular model.

Sometimes it's best to forget the modern world for an afternoon or so, and appreciate life for what it really is

while modern times aren't killing us, they are making it much easier for us to kill ourselves. Or at the very least make us unhealthy, overweight and miserable.

The problem is, we've evolved beyond our needs and unlike every other animal we share the planet with, we can adapt our surroundings rather than adapt to fit what happens to be there. Which means although we are still fairly instinctive creatures, we are creating environments that are at odds with those instincts and what is actually best for us. So much of how we live today is because of the world we have created and we are almost serving *it* instead of the other way around.

There are straightforward physical elements to this, and the most obvious manifestation is in our recent eating habits, and how they were developed to save us time rather than to nourish ourselves. Then there is the lack of the exercise we need to keep ourselves functioning efficiently. It's been evolved out because nobody walks anywhere any more and physical labour is being progressively replaced with jobs in call centres, all in the name of progress. Then those of us sitting at computer screens all day are dehydrating and going down with several different RSIs.

These physical states of affairs can be dealt with, as the last three hundred or so pages have been explaining, but less palpable is the effect they are having on us mentally, and this is even more insidious as it stops us

they want to improve how their heart beats; they just want a better body. That's primarily why people suddenly decide to get fit when they're into their thirties or forties. So many of them don't even want to know how it all works, just as long as they're losing the pounds.

"Which is fine. It doesn't really matter why they're doing it to start off with, because once they start looking better they also realize how they feel better too and they'll probably have got into the habit by then and will keep it up. It shouldn't matter why you start as long as you do."

Will evolution be the end of us?

The idea that the twenty-first century is killing us has been discussed throughout this book in different lifestyle situations, and this one recurring theme seems to involve the words "these days" or "as part of the modern lifestyle". But it's not really that simple –

performing in the way we need to, if we are going to do anything about the former.

Being sad is okay

One of the reasons so few of us are getting everything we can out of life is because we have worked so hard to manage our moods that much of what we need to personally progress is lacking, and our appreciation of the lives we are creating is suffering. Dr Sandra Scott believes this is due to our obsession with engineering out anything we might not like, and refusing to feel unhappy about anything.

"It's alright to feel sad," she explains. "In fact you're supposed to. Having a low mood is a perfectly normal experience – if something bad happens, you feel bad about it. In fact, if something bad happens and you don't feel bad about it, that's when something can be wrong.

"Western societies today encourage a quick fix attitude. We are surrounded by techniques, pills, or gadgets to remove negative stimuli as quickly as possible. Thus, the subliminal message is we should not have to put up with it, we should not even try to and this has led many people to have a very low tolerance of negative stimuli of any sort, when the correct response is, actually, we should tolerate it. More than that, we should accept it and learn to cope.

"Because we can always get instant gratification for hunger or pain or whatever, we don't have to put up with them any more and now we have that sort of response to our sadness: 'I don't want to go through it, I don't want to tolerate it, I want it to go away *right now*.' We want a quick fix for it, but this is storing up problems for the future, as when sad things happen the normal response is to be sad. You have to endure that sadness, learn to live with it, accept it and it will pass. And that's an important part of the human

Sort your life out

Get fit simply for the sake of it and don't view it as time wasted, because although there might not seem to be any immediate gain, it will affect every aspect of your life because you will feel so much more energized.

Accept you are going to have to work at changing some of your habits, and this might include the ones you may not even have realized are doing you so much harm.

Don't always take the easy option because cooking real food from real ingredients or walking to work rather than getting the bus may seem like an imposition to start off with but stick with them and they will become interesting and fun in themselves.

Think positive and check out mindfulness, a method of living in the moment at the expense of outside influences and giving yourself the best chance to find something good in every situation.

Act your age and you will get on in life much better and ultimately be much happier.

Remember that anything worth having is worth waiting for. Therefore, with something as worthwhile as getting fit and healthy it is definitely going to be about the long game.

Don't forget it's not going to be alright all the time because things will go wrong and then you'll just have to roll with it and carry on.

Realize you might not be paying your partner quite enough attention and when you put it in perspective of the rest of your life, this will probably become obvious.

Cheer up.

> **T**
>
> *Tip: Stop worrying what other people think of you and do what you know is right, regardless of what those around you might have to say.*

condition. And we need to learn these coping skills, as without this inner resilience we can become dependent on external escape routes such as illicit drugs, legal drugs, alcohol, television etc and find ourselves turning to them automatically every time we are a bit blue. All of these escape routes invariably come with a negative price tag, which gets greater with time and usage.

"Also, experiencing sadness is important for your state of happiness – you can't fully appreciate the good parts of your life unless you accept and experience the bad parts. If you're really thirsty and somebody gives you an ice-cold drink you appreciate it much more than if you've never been thirsty; eating after working up a ravenous appetite with a taxing workout, the sense of achievement of finally completing a difficult and exacting task: the list is endless… Sadness is happiness's twin, they're yin and yang. It's by experiencing the negatives that you fully appreciate the positives, and if you refuse those bad experiences, it actually reduces your ability to fully experience happiness. People would generally feel a lot better if they went along with their emotions a bit more and stopped trying to shut them off."

Reasons to be cheerful

GP Dr Liliana Risi reckons that so many people that come to see her would be so much better off and in her surgery less if they just cheered up. One of the overwhelming assumptions about modern living is that it is guaranteed to be stressful and we all have so many pressures on us and things to worry about. This isn't really the case, according to Dr Risi, who believes we are no better or worse off now than we ever were, and this state of mind is contributing to a general feeling of malaise.

"It would be naïve to say that everybody's lives were perfect, and there was nothing to worry about, but so many people don't look at the positives and what they have to be happy about. Too often this state of unhappiness or the so-called stresses of life are simply down to what is going on around you, that you have little control over or that won't really be adding to your life.

"Mindfulness is the practice of being aware of what is happening in the present, at that moment, and focusing on that and everything that is positive about it. It allows you to slow down and realize that happiness is about what you make of your life at that time, and it will let you discover what there is to be happy about. It can promote better health because it can relieve chronic stress and all that goes with that."

Mindfulness is based on ancient Buddhist teachings, and is starting to gain ground among the Western healthcare professions as having a usefulness in the treatment of depression and stress. More information

> **T**
>
> *Tip: Engaging a personal trainer when you start your fitness programme can do wonders for your motivation, and should keep you on course until it's become a habit. This is because not only will a personal trainer gee you up at every opportunity, but if he/she is good, you will not want to fail him/her and you definitely won't want to have wasted the money you've spent on him/her.*

about it can be found at Bangor University's website, bangor.ac.uk/mindfulness, as they play host to the non-profit Centre for Mindfulness Research and Practice.

Be happier at home

As a final point, improve your home life by taking a very simple piece of advice from Sarah Hedley, who maintains there's absolutely no reason why men and women shouldn't get along much better. Providing we put a bit more thought and effort into it.

"Men and women have more in common now than they ever have – social lives used to be a lot more segregated than they are now, women and men do the same jobs and can fit into many areas of society in the same way. But that in itself can give rise to certain problems – men and women don't have set roles, which can lead to confusion.

"It can get difficult for men to work out what they're meant to be. We say that in a relationship, we want a best friend but a lover as well – which is very difficult, because as a best friend you will be non-sexualized. It's difficult to keep a relationship erotically charged and still be able to talk to him about your period problems. And finding both those roles in the one person is difficult.

"It all boils down to keeping that erotic side of the relationship going once you've established that best friendship and that trust. Maintain that erotic side, and to do that you need to spend time creating that erotic space and that erotic time. You have to literally work on your relationship, especially if you've got kids.

"You need to give it the same amount of planning as you do to your career and your hobby. Draw a bar chart of your time on any given week and fill in how much time you have devoted to each aspect of your life, and I'll bet that in every single case the bit dedicated to sex or intimate time with your

T *Changing your life isn't all about beating yourself with health and fitness; take the odd weekend off and revisit some of your old habits. In moderation, of course.*

partner would be tiny. And I'm not talking just about doing it, but planning it, preparing it, thinking about what you will do. Spending time on it. The only effort people do put into this sort of activity is in the early parts of their relationship, so you should think back to then and use that as a model.

"We spend time on our jobs, on our kids, on our hobbies and with our friends, but we underestimate what sex actually means to us. Then every time we have to think about it in these sorts of terms we tend to start thinking about it as a chore, but go back to the benefits. True, you don't get any money for it, you don't get a bigger house, but it'll make life much more enjoyable for you and your other half. I'll bet she won't have it any other way."

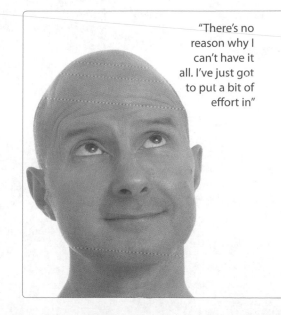

"There's no reason why I can't have it all. I've just got to put a bit of effort in"

Part 3
Reference

How bad could it be?

(17)

The list of ailments that afflict the modern man is a long one, but most of them aren't too serious and can be dealt with at home – usually it's simply a matter of giving up smoking and changing your diet. Here is a handy A–Z of what is most likely to strike you down.

A

Acne
An outbreak of blackheads or whiteheads, creating eruptions under the skin.

Causes
In adolescent males it's the excess of sebum oil produced by the skin, brought on by the surge in male sex hormones, combining with the protein keratin and the clogging up of hair follicles; in adults it is a result of internal toxins not being processed and expelled due to constipation or a malfunctioning liver.

Symptoms
Plentiful facial spots, often merging together into a deep, angry-looking rash.

Treatment
Over-the-counter treatments include chemical skin peels, which dry out the top layer of skin to remove it and release trapped oil. Antibiotics may be prescribed in severe cases.

Self-help
Don't squeeze the spot, as this will disperse some of the oil back under your skin; instead gently stretch the skin around it to create an opening big enough to slowly manipulate all the oil out. Large doses of zinc (3 x 30mg per day) and vitamin B complex have been shown to reduce acne, while beetroot juice, kale or celeriac will cleanse the liver and boost its performance.

Prevention
Regular washing of the face with light, unscented soap will keep oil levels down, but over-washing will irritate and inflame the skin. Avoiding processed foods – particularly sugar and saturated fats – will reduce strain on the liver, allowing it to cope better with internal toxins.

AIDS
The Acquired Immunodeficiency Syndrome is the last, potentially lethal, phase of the Human Immunodeficiency Virus (HIV).

Causes
HIV has invaded the body and multiplied to destroy enough of the body's immune system (CD4 lymphocytes) to render it useless. This may take weeks, months or even years.

Symptoms
Initially there are none, then fatigue, swollen lymph nodes, loss of appetite, weight loss, increasing susceptibility to infections and viruses and purple lesions on the skin.

Treatment
As yet there is no cure for AIDS, although there are drugs that will help maintain the

immune system and slow the onslaught of the virus. Infections that come about because of a compromised immune system can be treated with drugs as they would otherwise.

Self-help

Short of attempting to keep yourself as healthy as possible, there is little you can do.

Prevention

Practise safe sex, do not share needles and never ever get a blood transfusion in an at-risk country.

Alcoholism

Psychological dependence on alcohol, leading to continued use regardless of adverse effects – alcoholism is now classified as a "chronic disease".

Causes

Prolonged heavy drinking.

Symptoms

Drinking to feel "normal" rather than intoxicated; needing rather than merely wanting a drink; drinking regardless of the appropriateness of the time or place;

losing interest in activities that don't involve drinking; ignoring – or simply being unaware of – the problems your drinking is causing in the rest of your life. Physical symptoms of advanced alcoholism include liver damage, which can affect the rest of your system as it will process toxins less effectively; gastric problems as alcohol damages the stomach lining; general nutrition issues as you will not be absorbing vitamins and minerals properly; heart disease, as your blood pressure will be raised; diabetes because alcohol impedes the release of glucose into your system from the liver.

Treatment

After determining the level of your addiction there are residential treatment programmes available for the more seriously addicted. These involve detoxification periods, treatment of the different alcoholism-induced conditions, psychological support and therapy addressing the compulsion to drink and drug treatment which will prompt severe reactions to alcohol such as vomiting or headaches.

Ageing (the effects of)

The symptoms of your getting on in years include a general slowing down, getting weaker, organs not functioning as efficiently and skin looking drier and wrinkly. While there isn't that much you can do to stop this – your body was only designed to last about eighty years and will start to wear out a couple of decades before that – you can minimize the effects by tackling the different manifestations individually.

Cardiovascular exercise will keep your heart from stiffening up and make sure it beats with strong strokes, and it will also maintain the lung capacity that is naturally starting to fall. Strength and flexibility training staves off the decrease in muscle strength, the toughening of muscle fibres and stiffening of the joints. If your regime involves an impact exercise such as running, it can help keep the bones strong to guard against osteoporosis.

Maintaining a healthy diet will be vital, as your body will not be able to cope with processed foods as well as it used to, plus you will need every bit of nutrition you can get. In later life because the amount you are eating will have gone down, but you will need the same amount of nutrients, you may need supplements. Drinking plenty of water is crucial, as is dietary fibre, because the likelihood of constipation increases with age, and the antioxidant vitamins A, C and E will slow down cell damage by free radicals, which contributes enormously to the ageing process.

Keep your brain in shape too, with daily workouts such as crossword puzzles, quizzes or sudokus, and don't stop thinking about things.

T

Tip: Research in the USA discovered that nearly every allergy sensitive subject benefited hugely by switching from drinking tap water to bottled mineral water.

Self-help
Be aware that you might have a problem. If you do accept it, then you can work to do something about it.
Prevention
Don't drink so much so often, and be aware of what you are doing while you are.

Allergies
Physical reaction or sensitivity to an ingested food or a substance breathed in or brought into contact with the skin.
Causes
Pollen, pollution, food additives, pesticides, wheat, dairy, animal fur, nuts, shellfish… the list of substances that bring out an allergic reaction in somebody in the twenty-first century is pretty much endless. Allergies are very likely to be passed on down the generations.
Symptoms
Sneezing, running nose, rashes, coughing, breathing difficulties, watering eyes; severe allergic reactions may trigger anaphylactic shock which is potentially fatal as it can cause a massive drop in blood pressure and difficulty breathing because of bronchial constriction.
Treatment
Allergies are usually determined by skin testing, in which a minute amount of various substances is injected into marked areas of skin with reactions observed and recorded. There is a range of drugs used to inhibit the actions of many allergens – these include cortisone, antihistamine, hydrocortisone and adrenaline – or immunotherapy may be applied. This introduces progressively larger doses of the allergen to the system in order to build up antibodies, much like vaccination.
Self-help
As regards food allergies, there is some evidence to show that maintaining healthy gut flora, through probiotic supplements, will reduce susceptibility.
Prevention
Avoid whatever it is you are allergic to.
(For hay fever see p 333)

Alzheimer's Disease
A progressive, irreversible disease that destroys brain cells.
Causes
Old age, but there is also increasing evidence

Allergies: facts and figures
Over 20 million of the UK's population will suffer from some form of allergy at some point in their lives.
Allergies account for over 10 million visits to the GP per year.
One in three people suffer from some kind of food allergy – this is rising as the number of additives in everyday foods increases.
The UK has the highest prevalence of allergies in Europe – this is rising as air quality falls.
Women are more likely to suffer allergic reactions than men – the ratio is around 60/40.

Figures from the AAIR Charity (Asthma, Allergy and Inflammation Research).

of genetic disposition. In a proportion of people over the age of 65 some brain cells stop working properly, which affects their communication with others, internal circuitry starts to break down and without the stimulation cells die.

Symptoms

Alzheimer's is the biggest single cause of senile dementia, and causes problems with long- and short-term memory and thinking in general.

Treatment

There is currently no cure for Alzheimer's, although there are drugs available to strengthen the connections between brain cells and so offset the effects of the initial stages.

Self-help

You can't really help yourself; you have to trust those around you to look after you.

Prevention

Alzheimer's cannot yet be prevented, but merely slowed down in some cases.

Anaemia

Deficiency in haemoglobin – can either be qualitative or quantitative – the oxygen-bearing molecule inside red blood cells.

Causes

Deficiency in iron or the nutrients needed to absorb it into the system – folic acid, vitamin B12 and vitamin C – or internal bleeding from gastric ulcers or in the colon.

Symptoms

Fatigue, pallor, inability to concentrate, irritability, brittle nails. Gastrointestinal bleeding will cause black or bloody faeces.

Treatment

A blood test will determine if you are anaemic or not – your GP should be able to do this – and that will be addressed with iron or nutrient supplements; if it is the result of internal bleeding those causes will be treated separately.

Self-help

If you think you might be anaemic, step up your intake of iron, folic acid and vitamins B12 and C with a course of supplements. However, be careful not to overdo the iron, as this can cause constipation and in severe cases damage your liver.

Prevention

Make sure your diet includes plenty of leafy green vegetables, wholewheat flour and wheatgerm, red meat and liver. Avoid excess black coffee and tea, as it inhibits the absorption of iron into your system.

Angina

A symptom of coronary artery disease establishing itself.

Causes

Due to a narrowing of the arteries, the heart muscle is not getting enough oxygen-rich blood and attacks will often be brought on by physical exertion when the oxygen requirements increase.

Symptoms

Pain in the centre of the chest, feeling like a weight pushing down on it or a band squeezing it. This pain may spread upward to the neck and it will often be accompanied by breathlessness, dizziness and sweating. If you have such an attack, seek medical attention immediately.

Treatment

Glyceryl trinitrate, as a spray or tablets, is

F

Fact: The average man has around 25 trillion red blood cells in his body, which make up about one-third of his total cell count. They have a surface area larger than other cells to maximize oxygen absorption, yet are flexible enough to squeeze into the tiniest blood vessels.

Anorexia vs bulimia

Both result in a dangerously low body weight. Anorexia sufferers avoid eating and exercise obsessively; bulimics eat either normal or abnormally large amounts of regular food then induce vomiting before it is digested. Bulimics will also take laxatives and diuretics, but generally do not lose weight as radically as anorexics.

used to relieve attacks as it immediately relaxes the blood vessels, increasing blood flow; cholesterol-lowering drugs may be prescribed to help clear your arteries.

Self-help

Taking an aspirin every day reduces the blood's stickiness to allow it to flow more easily; root ginger and freshly ground black pepper improve the circulation; garlic and omega-3 fatty acids thin the blood.

Prevention

Avoid cholesterol-rich foods, don't smoke (it thickens the blood) and eat plenty of fibre, which will help you regulate your cholesterol levels.

Anorexia nervosa

Refusal to eat in order to lose weight. Not as uncommon among men as you might think – an estimated ten percent of cases are male, which means around nine thousand in the UK every year.

Causes

Specific causes have yet to be agreed upon, but the psychological pressure of wanting to be thin, therefore, good looking, is the firm favourite, and inherent low self-esteem will make this worse. There is a theory that a sufferer could be genetically predisposed to the condition, and some evidence that, because the condition is so self-harming, the area of the anorexic's brain that regulates metabolic function must be faulty.

Symptoms

Radical loss of weight, fatigue, hair loss, erratic sleep patterns, irritability, withdrawal,

constipation, low blood pressure, renal failure, depression.

Treatment

Weight gain is most important in the treatment of anorexia, then therapy or counselling to address the causes of the problem. Hospitalization may be necessary for advanced cases.

Self-help

Admit to the fact you might have a problem – doctors say the biggest hurdle to treating anorexics is that they refuse to believe there is anything wrong.

Prevention

Accept yourself and your body shape as being exactly what it should be. The most important thing is that you are healthy – as we've discussed elsewhere, perfection is overrated.

Anxiety attacks

Also known as panic attacks, they are sudden episodes of intense alarm or fear.

Causes

The system is reacting to what it perceives to be a threat, and releases adrenaline to prompt the fight-or-flight mode. But because there is nothing to physically react to – the cause of an anxiety attack is often irrational – the adrenaline is not used up and its internalization causes the physical symptoms.

Symptoms

Breathlessness, difficulty swallowing, accelerated heartbeat and raised blood pressure, dizziness, chest pains, blurred vision. Anxiety attacks will often be followed by spells of melancholy.

Treatment

Therapy or counselling will establish the root cause of the attacks, then work to understand and eliminate the anxiety caused.

Self-help

Relaxation techniques can assist you being less anxious in general, breathing exercises will help if an attack comes on.

Prevention

Addressing the cause of the panic is the only way to stop the attacks; avoiding whatever it is will only put them off.

Apnoea

Obstructive sleep apnoea is the temporary cessation of breathing while sleeping.

Causes

Hypopnoea; fatigue.

Symptoms

The muscles of the throat relax so much during sleep they collapse inwards causing a complete blockage of the airways; hypopnoea is a partial blocking of the airways that reduces airflow by around fifty percent. Breathing stops for around ten seconds at a time, resulting in fractured sleep patterns as this will be enough to bring you out of deep sleep into lighter sleep or briefly wake you up completely.

Treatment

Turning to sleep on your side can help.

Self-help

Avoid alcohol within two hours of going to sleep, as it will overly relax the muscles in the throat. Smoking during the evening will contribute to increased mucus production, which in turn will contribute to the blocking of the throat.

Prevention

Lose some weight: if you are obese you are much more likely to suffer from OSA.

Appendicitis

An infection of the appendix, which is an apparently pointless side-turning of the intestinal system.

Causes

Either a bacterial infection in the appendix, or a piece of digestive waste becomes lodged in it.

Symptoms

An early sign, often missed, is a mild ache in the lower stomach. This then develops

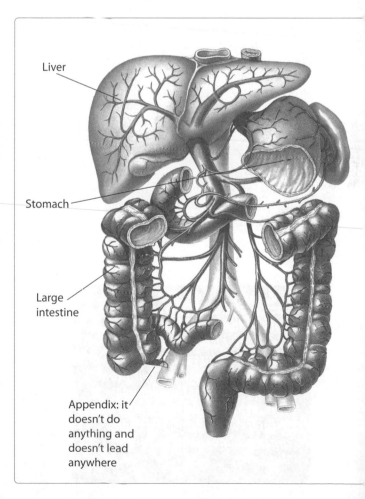

Liver

Stomach

Large intestine

Appendix: it doesn't do anything and doesn't lead anywhere

Arthritis: osteo vs rheumatoid

Osteoarthritis is by far the most common form of arthritis in the West and is a degenerative condition; rheumatoid arthritis is a chronic disease in which the body's own immune system starts eating away at joint tissue.

into a sharp, persistent pain in the lower right abdomen, accompanied by accelerated heartbeat and mild fever. Advanced symptoms include a visible swelling in that area.

Treatment

The appendix has to be removed by surgical procedure. Untreated appendicitis is potentially life-threatening, as it may burst and expel poisonous faecal matter into the abdominal cavity.

Self-help

There is little you can do if you feel you have appendicitis, other than get to casualty as soon as possible.

Prevention

Because appendicitis is entirely random, there is nothing you can do to prevent it.

Arthritis (osteo)

Stiffening and degeneration of the body's joints, particularly the load-bearing ones such as knees, ankles and fingers.

Causes

F

Fact: In the UK 55 percent of the population who are over the age of 65 suffer from arthritis, with a third of adults exhibiting some form of arthritic symptoms in at least one of their joints. This includes those as young as in their twenties, and women are much more likely to suffer than men.

The regeneration of the joints' cushioning cartilage can no longer keep up with its breaking down, so it becomes thinner and less flexible.

Symptoms

Stiffening of the joints and the likelihood of feeling pain when they are flexed.

Treatment

Anti-inflammatory drugs may be prescribed to arthritis sufferers, and the pain will be medicated.

Self-help

Avoid acid-forming foods – processed flour and sugar, alcohol and coffee – while tomatoes and oranges can cause the condition to flare up. Losing weight will reduce the strain on your joints.

Prevention

Light exercise and stretching – yoga is very good – keeps the bones healthy and prevents the joints stiffening.

Asthma

Sudden constriction of the bronchial tubes.

Causes

Air pollution and airborne allergens such as pollen, dust or fur can trigger asthmatic attacks, as can sudden incidences of stress.

Symptoms

Constricted, wheezing breathing and shortness of breath; severe attacks leave the sufferer unable to speak and with a feeling of being suffocated, and this will be accompanied by a quickening pulse and sweating.

Treatment

A bronchial inhaler will reopen the airways during an attack, and a course of inhaled anti-inflammatory treatment can reduce any underlying swelling.

Self-help

Sit upright during an attack as this will ease breathing, while daily deep breathing exercises will keep your bronchial tubes in better condition.

Prevention

Don't smoke and avoid secondary smoke, drink plenty of water to keep mucus production to a minimum and, using a process of elimination, try and identify anything you may be allergic to.

Athlete's foot

Fungal infection of the feet, not restricted to athletes.

Causes

The fungus can be transmitted from other people – the damp floors in changing rooms are notorious – or picked up from micro-organisms in the soil. It then thrives in warm, dark, dank conditions, i.e. your socks and shoes.

Symptoms

Itchy, cracked and flaking skin between the toes and on the soles of the feet.

Treatment

There are numerous anti-fungal creams and paints available over the counter.

Self-help

Eat garlic and onions as they have anti-fungal properties, while live yoghurt will help if it is a problem starting in your gut. Avoid anything fermented or sugary.

Prevention

Dry your feet properly, put talcum powder in between your toes; change your socks regularly; go barefoot as much as possible.

B

Bad breath (halitosis)

Causes

Bad dental hygiene, in which insufficient attention paid to brushing and flossing has resulted in a plaque build-up and infections in the mouth. Or a slow digestive system means food is purifying in the bowel, and toxins are being reabsorbed into the blood to reach the lungs where they create a rotten smell.

Symptoms

People recoil when you talk to them.

Treatment

Clean your teeth after every meal and before you go to bed, and stop smoking, as it dries the mouth out, meaning there is less saliva

Back pain

Eighty percent of all adults will, at some point in their lives, suffer from back pain serious enough to inhibit something they are doing – in the UK over 20 million working days a year are lost to back pain, in the US that figure is nearer 250 million. There are probably as many different causes and specific types of pain; as there are sufferers, and although people in general seem more aware of how to lift correctly and assume the correct posture at their desk, these figures show no sign of going down.

The problem is we were never really designed to walk upright, thus after thirty or forty years of doing so your back will start to complain, and before it does you should get it looked at. Every man over the age of thirty should visit an osteopath at least twice a year for maintenance, repositioning and advice on what you might be doing wrong. It will save so much grief and pain by the time you get to be fifty.

available to combat bacteria. Stay away from processed foods, caffeine and sugar they will all serve to slow down your digestion, and if you can't speed your digestion up by changing your diet and lifestyle, have an enema.

Self-help

Parsley, coriander and mint have an anti-bacterial effect in your mouth so freshen your breath; leafy green vegetables are rich in chlorophyll, therefore, freshen your breath while aiding your digestion.

Prevention

Visit your dentist and oral hygienist at least twice a year and change your toothbrush regularly. Eat smaller meals as this is less likely to overload your bowel.

Bleeding gums

Causes

Overenthusiastic brushing – this will be more likely among older men – or gum disease, prompted by a build-up of plaque.

Symptoms

Blood in the toothpaste you spit out, or blood on your pillowcase in the morning.

Treatment

Try a softer toothbrush and a less vigorous brushing technique; the gum disease may be the result of a vitamin C deficiency, so an increase in your intake may stop it and if that doesn't clear it up visit your dentist.

Self-help

Fresh sage is an effective mouthwash for healing bleeding gums or soothing inflamed tissue inside the mouth – chop a handful of leaves and steep in a cup of boiling water, allow to cool and use as mouthwash, then keep what is left in a closed container in the fridge.

Prevention

Particular attention must be paid to brushing, flossing and rinsing, while you will need regular dental checkups and visits to the oral hygienist.

Body odour

Causes

Poor hygiene leaving a build-up of dead bacteria on your skin, or toxins being expelled through the skin, which could be caused by constipation.

Symptoms

Nobody is keen to stand next to you.

Treatment

Washing away the dead bacteria, paying particular attention to the groin, armpits and feet where the build-up will be greatest, and thoroughly washing clothes. Speeding up the digestion to remove toxins from the system quicker.

Self-help

Drinking a large amount of water to flush out toxins, spraying armpits and groin with an antibacterial spray before applying deodorant.

Prevention

Regular washing, changing your clothes and underwear, thoroughly washing dirty clothes, cutting down on constipation-inducing, low-fibre foods and drinking plenty of water to flush toxins out of the system.

Boils

Causes

A bacterial infection causing a blockage of a hair follicle. Regular outbreaks of boils are a sign that you are generally very run-down and your immune system isn't functioning properly.

Symptoms

Angry-looking, tender spots, probably a fair bit bigger than your everyday blackhead.

Treatment

Goldenseal root applied to the boil will kill the infection; apply tea tree oil once it has been drained.

Self-help

Take zinc to stimulate the immune system and vitamin A to keep the skin in good condition. Drink plenty of water.

Prevention
Eat plenty of fibre to avoid constipation; stay away from processed foods and hydrogenized fats; exercise to keep the metabolism moving.

Brain tumour
A growth of abnormally formed cells on the brain tissue or the membranes surrounding it.

Causes
Metastatic brain tumours are cancer spread from somewhere else in the body; primary brain tumours originate in the brain and their cause is not known.

Symptoms
Headaches, blurred vision, confusion, then, depending on which part of the brain they are in, they can affect coordination, speech, memory or any of the senses.

Treatment
If the tumour is near the surface of the brain it can be removed by conventional surgery; if it is deep within the folds then it will be treated with laser surgery or radiation therapy. There may be chemotherapy involved in either case.

Self-help
Curcumin – found in turmeric – has tumour-inhibiting properties, as it boosts the immune system and prevents the growth of blood vessels within the tumour, thus stopping it expanding.

Prevention
Get checked regularly for all cancers, and eat organic as it reduces the amount of cancer-friendly toxins you may be ingesting.

Bronchitis
Inflammation of the bronchial tubes – the narrow airways leading from the trachea to the lungs – resulting in excess mucus production which further obstructs the pipes.

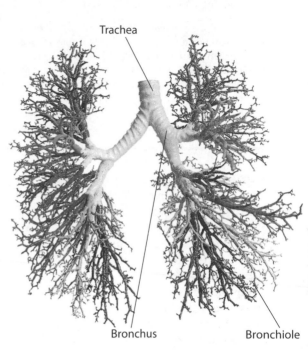

Inside your lungs

Trachea

Bronchus

Bronchiole

Causes
The most common cause of bronchitis is smoking, but it is also caused by bacterial and viral infections and airborne pollutants.

Symptoms
Persistent hacking cough bringing up cloudy mucus – at its worst first thing in the morning – fever, breathlessness.

Treatment
Antibiotics will be prescribed for the infection, while cough medicine will suppress the cough and help you sleep.

Self-help
Try not to get cold; the steam from taking a hot shower will help loosen mucus deposits; drink plenty of water to keep the mucus as thin as possible. Papaya and mango are very good for your lungs.

Prevention
Stop smoking.

Cancers

Cancer occurs when a group of cells within one area of the body start growing uncontrollably due to genetic mutations in their DNA. There are over two hundred different types of cancer. Most are named after the organ or cell type in which they originate and most cause tumours from the mass of unwanted cells they produce. These tumours are either self-contained – benign – which means the cancer cannot spread to other parts of the body, or they are malignant, meaning it will invade other tissues. Benign tumours can usually be surgically removed; malignant cancers require chemo- or radiotherapy. Cancers are the biggest single killers in the world, with lung, breast, bowel and prostate cancer being the most deadly.

Bunions

Bony growth on the outside of the joint at which the big toe joins onto the foot.

Causes

Shoes that are too tight across the toes, as the pad of bone grows to protect the toes from being squashed.

Symptoms

Apart from the growth, the big toe will be pushed inwards, often under the toes next to it, and it will result in pain and tenderness.

Treatment

Bad bunions will have to be surgically removed with the big toe and, maybe, the one next to it realigned. It's a relatively simple, total anaesthetic, outpatients operation.

Self-help

Pads fitted inside the shoe to ease pressure.

Prevention

Wear shoes that fit properly.

Bursitis (tennis elbow)

The inflammation of the bursae – the sacs of fluid that lubricate the insides of your joints.

Causes

Continued jolting of that joint – it is very common in sportsmen, particularly runners

F

Fact: Perhaps unsurprisingly, ten times as many women than men suffer from bunions.

– or the general bashing housework or labouring would give it.

Symptoms

Pain and stiffness in the affected joint; particularly bad if it has remained immobile for some time or first thing in the morning.

Treatment

Your doctor may prescribe anti-inflammatory drugs, or even draw fluid from the bursae with a syringe.

Self-help

R.I.C.E. which stands for Rest, Ice, Compression and Elevation. Wrap a tight bandage around the affected joint, apply an ice pack and sit down with that limb raised.

Prevention

Be careful of your joints, try not to rest on them or leave them bent at a sharp angle for long stretches of time.

C

Carpal tunnel syndrome

Afflicts the median nerve, which runs from the palm of the hand to the wrist.

Causes

As this nerve passes in between the wrist bones (the carpals) it is pressed upon by the surrounding bones and tissue. This can be caused by repeated unnatural or awkward bending of the wrist – RSI – such as when operating a computer mouse.

T

Symptoms

Numbness and pain in the fingers and hand; weakness in the fingers; the fingers will feel as if they are swollen when they do not appear so.

Treatment

Painkillers, repositioning of hands while working to avoid the strain, and, in severe cases, diuretics may be prescribed to reduce swelling around the carpals.

Self-help

Take breaks from repetitive tasks and gently flex the wrists.

Prevention

Ergonomic wrist supports for typing or computer work.

Cold sores

The effects of the herpes simplex virus.

Causes

A viral infection that can lie dormant in your body to activate itself when you feel stressed or are run-down, or can be triggered by excess amounts of the amino acid arginine, found in nuts and chocolate.

Symptoms

Clusters of small, painful sores in and around the mouth, swollen glands, sore throat, headaches, nausea, fever.

Treatment

Antiviral creams will speed the sores' healing, while prescription antiviral tablets will clear up the virus. Regular use of an antiseptic mouthwash will help fight sores inside your mouth.

Self-help

Organic lean meat and poultry, fish and soya products are all rich in the antiviral amino acid lysine.

Prevention

Stay well nourished and with an efficient immune system; if you have cold sores don't fiddle with them as that will spread the infection.

Common cold

Infection of the upper respiratory system, inflaming the mucus membranes inside the nose and throat.

Causes

Infection by one of the many cold viruses – because there are so many of them and they are constantly mutating, it has proved impossible to find a cure that will deal with all of them.

Symptoms

Sore throat, nasal congestion, running nose, coughing, fever, chills, headache, constipation, fatigue, muscle ache.

Treatment

Bed rest, plenty of fluids, keep warm; take paracetamol to bring your temperature down.

Self-help

Echinacea or vitamin C will shorten the duration of a cold; garlic and onion will fight the infection.

Prevention

Keep your immune system in tip-top condition.

F

Constipation

Inability to have bowel movements.

Causes

Lack of fibre in the diet; not drinking enough water; stress.

Symptoms

Lack of bowel movement or the necessity to strain; painful bowel movement; hard, compacted stool.

Treatment

A warm drink first thing in the morning will stimulate the colon; vitamin C powder dissolved in water with magnesium will soften stool; psyllium husks with plenty of water act as a super-fibre.

Self-help

Early morning exercise prompts the colon to work more efficiently during the day.

Prevention

Avoid processed foods and opt for a diet that is high in fibre, and drink plenty of water.

Coronary artery disease (CAD)

An advanced form of angina, whereby the artery becomes completely blocked.

Causes

Extensive narrowing of the arteries that feed oxygenated blood to the heart, caused by smoking, high cholesterol or lack of exercise; a family history of CAD will mean you are more susceptible.

Symptoms

Angina is a symptom caused by your arteries clogging up, but they only complain during exertion. With CAD the chest pains, breathlessness, dizziness and sweating will happen when you are at rest too.

Treatment

Hospitalization will be required, and maybe a bypass operation to flow blood around the blocked bits. Nitroglycerin tablets administered at the start of an attack may expand the blood vessels.

Self-help

Daily doses of vitamin C and lysine (an amino acid) will, over time, reduce the congestion within the arteries.

Prevention

Lead a healthy lifestyle, avoid food that is high in cholesterol or saturated fat, and don't smoke.

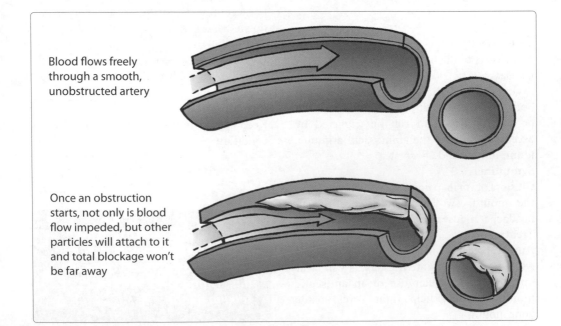

Blood flows freely through a smooth, unobstructed artery

Once an obstruction starts, not only is blood flow impeded, but other particles will attach to it and total blockage won't be far away

Cramp

A contracted muscle that goes into spasm and will not relax.

Causes

Fatigue, dehydration, salt deficiency, restrictive positioning of the muscle to compress nerves or blood supply.

Symptoms

Sharp pain in affected muscle and an inability to straighten it.

Treatment

Massage, gentle stretching and rehydration.

Self-help

Maintain mineral levels, especially during sports or in hot weather.

Prevention

Remain hydrated.

D

Dandruff

The flaking of dead skin from the scalp.

Causes

Excess of skin oil (sebum) secretions, encouraging the growth of the malassezia fungus that feeds on it and causes accelerated cell turnover – hence the large amount of dead skin.

Symptoms

Clearly visible flakes of dead skin falling from the scalp.

Treatment

Anti-dandruff shampoo, but these are not all the same and will carry out different functions – combat the fungal infection, prevent oil build-up or scrub away dead skin. Talk to the pharmacist to find out which is best for you, then only use as directed.

Self-help

Maintain a healthy diet – zinc and the B vitamins work against dandruff – and get some sun on your head: not too much, but a little sunlight will help prevent the fungus getting a hold.

Prevention

Daily washing of hair with a gentle shampoo will prevent excess sebum on the scalp and remove any dead skin. Regular application of tea tree oil will combat infection.

Deep vein thrombosis (DVT)

Causes

A blood clot forms in one of the large veins deep below the surface – usually in the legs – the most common cause is lack of movement slowing down the blood flow in your veins and inviting it to clot. Long haul airline passengers are particularly susceptible.

Don't ignore DVT

The most dangerous aspect of deep vein thrombosis is the risk of a chunk of the clot breaking off to form an embolus, which will then travel through your bloodstream. Because the veins deep in the leg have such a large diameter, even part of a clot formed in them can be enough to totally block a smaller artery.

An embolus will be transported to the heart, and from the heart to the small arteries of the lungs, at which point it becomes a pulmonary embolism, which can do serious damage. A small clot might pass through causing little more than chest pains; a medium-sized embolism could partially block the artery and result in breathlessness or chest pains. If it's sufficiently large it will block the blood flow to the lungs, which will probably be fatal. Around one in ten of the people who don't get DVT treated suffer a pulmonary embolism severe enough to hospitalize them, or worse.

Symptoms

Swelling, redness, sharp pains and the skin in that area feeling warmer than what is surrounding it.

Treatment

Anticoagulant medicine will be administered to prevent clotting or dissolve a clot that has formed.

Self-help

Compression stockings that squeeze the calf to increase blood pressure in the veins in your lower leg reduce the risk of clots forming in the most vulnerable area.

Prevention

Don't stay in your seat for long stretches of time; the obese and smokers are far more vulnerable to this condition as their blood flow will not be all that it should be.

Depression

A pervasive and persistent lowering of the mood.

Causes

The causes are manifold, and can be genetic, or a chemical imbalance in the brain, or outside factors such as situation or environment.

Symptoms

Constant feelings of sadness, worthlessness or hopelessness; an inability to make decisions or concentrate; chaotic sleep patterns; loss of appetite.

Treatment

Psychotherapy or drug treatment (antidepressants) or a combination of the two. Electroconvulsive therapy may be used in the most extreme cases.

Self-help

St John's Wort will reduce anxiety and assist sleeping, and eating foods containing tryptophan (turkey, avocados, bananas, cottage cheese) will raise your serotonin levels, which will help to lift your mood.

Prevention

Alcohol is a depressive and prolonged use can precipitate depression, while regular exercise releases endorphins, which will make you feel better about yourself.

Diabetes

The body either produces too little insulin (type 1 diabetes) or it is producing too much and has become resistant to it (type 2 diabetes).

Causes

Type 1 is a lifelong condition, because the pancreas is not functioning properly; type 2 is the result of too much sugar in the diet.

Symptoms

Thirst, frequent urination, fatigue, increased appetite, tingling in the feet and hands; dangerously low levels of blood sugar could lead to collapse or coma.

Treatment

Type 1 requires daily insulin injections on strict timetables, and dietary regulation that keeps fat and salt to a minimum; type 2 will be treated with medication to reduce insulin

The sugar trap

Taking a world average, adult males eat nearly 30kg (66lb) of sugar per year, and, according to the World Health Organization, this is one of the reasons they expect the number of diabetics in the world to more than double from 140 million to over 300 million during the next 25 years. And the vast number of these cases will be type 2 diabetes, which is self-inflicted and is rising because of the shift in lifestyle towards a sugary, processed diet and a decline in the amount of exercise we take. In the UK, nine out of ten diabetics are type 2, seventy-five percent of them are obese and it is the fourth biggest killer of men.

resistance, strict dietary controls and an exercise regime; it may also require insulin injections.

Self-help
Cinnamon reduces blood glucose levels and foods with a low glycaemic index (GI) – green vegetables, fresh fruit, wholewheat products – will produce the smallest blood glucose fluctuations.

Prevention
There is nothing you can do to prevent type 1 diabetes, but oily fish, raw fruit and vegetables, exercise and dumping the sugary junk food will lessen the likelihood of type 2.

Diarrhoea

Fluid is not being absorbed into the body through the intestinal walls.

Causes
Food poisoning, viral infection, large amounts of alcohol, adverse reaction to certain food additives and tap water that has not been thoroughly treated is a frequent cause.

Symptoms
Liquid stool, frequent and uncontrollable bowel movements, stomach cramping, dehydration.

Treatment
Anti-diarrhoea medicine is available over the counter, but try not to take it immediately, as the diarrhoea may be the result of the system trying to rid itself of bacteria. Drink plenty of water as you will have been dehydrating since the attack began. After it has cleared up take probiotics to make sure your gut flora

T

Tip: You can pick up the bacteria that cause diarrhoea from hands, cutlery or crockery. It doesn't have to be the food itself.

has not been compromised.

Self-help
Camomile tea four or five times a day will settle your stomach.

Prevention
Be as careful as you can with what you eat and your food preparation.

E

Epilepsy

Electrical impulses in the brain operate without control; it affects around one in two hundred men in the UK.

Causes
Epilepsy's causes are identified in only about half of the diagnosed cases, and it is then usually traced to an accident or disease that affected the brain tissue in some way.

Symptoms
Because it is disrupted signals within the brain, epilepsy can affect virtually any aspect of brain activity and symptoms can include blacking out, uncontrollable twitching, jerking limbs, loss of speech or confusion.

Treatment
In most cases seizures are successfully prevented with medication, which, after two or three years of regular dosing, usually leaves the sufferer free from future attacks. Some cases will be treated surgically, but that is only when the abnormal activity is confined to one small part of the brain.

Self-help
Keep a record of your seizures to more accurately inform your doctor of what needs to be addressed.

Prevention
Get plenty of rest – lack of sleep is very likely to trigger seizures.

Not a dry eye in the house

If you suffer from dry eyes as a result of air-conditioned buildings, long-haul flights, smoky atmospheres or long days in front of the computer screen, use natural or organic eye drops for instant relief. To prevent your eyes drying out avoid diuretics like coffee or alcohol, and don't eat foods rich in saturated fats as they prevent your natural oils from lubricating your body and so speed dehydration. Eat foods rich in carotene (carrots and leafy green vegetables), which boost the eyes' overall wellness, drink more water and keep up your vitamin B intake as that prevents eyes drying out.

Erectile dysfunction

Also known as impotence.

Causes

Fatigue, stress, anxiety, advancing years, depression, alcohol, hormonal problems lowering testosterone levels, cold weather.

Symptoms

The inability to raise an erection or to maintain one during sex.

Treatment

Talk to your partner about what might be the problem, and if it persists visit your GP who may recommend therapy.

Self-help

Try not to worry about it, as that will make it worse.

T

Tip: To establish if erectile dysfunction is psychological or physiological, before going to sleep place a thin strip of paper around your flaccid penis and secure the ends with a small piece of adhesive tape – do not put the tape all the way around. This band should be tight enough not to fall off, but not restrictively so. If you have an erection during the night, and most men do, the paper ring will have broken, proving there is nothing mechanically wrong.

Prevention

Don't drink too much and give up smoking.

Eyes – dark circles under them

Causes

Lack of refreshing sleep, allergies, food intolerances (particularly wheat), iron deficiency, kidney problems.

Symptoms

Er, dark circles under the eyes.

Treatment

A good night's sleep is the most obvious step. If that doesn't work cut wheat out of your diet for a week or take a course of iron tablets.

Self-help

Foods rich in vitamin K (seaweed, lentils, leafy green vegetables) will reduce the discolouration; carotene nourishes the eyes.

Prevention

Get enough rest, and eliminate any allergens.

F

Food poisoning

Causes

Contaminated or undercooked food – reheated dishes are a common source.

Symptoms

Diarrhoea, vomiting, stomach cramps, fever, chills, headaches.

F

Fact: Over 25 percent of men currently have gallstones, but fewer than 20 percent of sufferers will ever notice them. Women are twice as likely as men to develop them.

Treatment
Usually nothing, as the vomiting or diarrhoea will be ridding your body of the toxins, but be careful not to dehydrate. If it lasts longer than four or five days, see your GP who may prescribe antibiotics.

Self-help
You may need to top up your gut flora when the symptoms have passed.

Prevention
Pay attention to food hygiene; always wash your hands before and after handling food; don't risk eating anything remotely questionable.

G

Gallstones
A small solidified mass in the gall bladder.

Causes
Hardened excess cholesterol produces over three-quarters of all gallstones; the others are produced within the bile itself by a chemical imbalance.

Symptoms

Although most gallstones produce no symptoms, the bigger ones, and they can be the size of apricots, will block the bile duct from the gall bladder to cause sharp pains in the right-hand side of the abdomen.

Treatment
In more serious cases the gallbladder will be surgically removed, otherwise non-surgical procedures involve medication, sound waves or chemicals introduced via a catheter to dissolve the stones.

Self-help
Take extra vitamin C, as this will turn cholesterol into bile in the gall bladder.

Prevention
Don't put on too much weight and keep your cholesterol levels down.

Gout
It isn't only an aristocrat's complaint.

Causes
Elevated levels of uric acid in the blood, forming crystals that collect in the joints. This is brought on by too much rich, hard-to-digest food. The obese are more susceptible and it is much more common among men than women, although the rates among women are rising rapidly.

Symptoms
Painful swelling and discolouration in isolated joints, usually the big toe.

Treatment
Bed rest, anti-inflammatories and painkillers.

Self-help
Pineapple speeds the body's excretion of uric

Frostbite: what not to do
If you or somebody you are with is suffering from frostbite do not attempt to thaw the affected area out over a naked flame or hot air stream as you may, literally, start to cook it and because the nerves are frozen any overheating will not be noticed. Slapping or rubbing the affected area is wrong too, as it may cause the ice crystals in it to damage surrounding tissue, and rubbing it with snow is on a par with cutting snake bites and sucking out the poison, i.e. just plain daft.

acid, while anything rich in bioflavonoids (blueberries or blackberries) will reduce residual levels.

Prevention
Lose weight and eat sensibly – but be careful to avoid oily fish and other high-protein foods as they can prompt uric acid production.

Glandular fever
More common among men under thirty, but often misdiagnosed merely as fatigue.

Causes
It's a viral infection.

Symptoms
Swollen lymph nodes in the neck, armpits and groin, sore throat, fever, general tiredness.

Treatment
Antibiotics don't work, and there is no cure as such – rest and healthy eating will clear it up, but it might take a month. Because the symptoms are flu-like and sufferers will seem much better after a week or so's rest it's often assumed to have been a bout of flu that has cleared up, but if it is glandular fever it will continue to come back.

Self-help
Completely cut out processed food and go on a whole food diet that is rich in protein to boost your immune system.

Prevention
It can't be prevented, but if your immune system is in good condition you will be able to fight it off more easily.

T

Tip: A spoonful of organic local honey once a day from early spring onwards can stop mild cases of hay fever as the small amounts of pollen in the honey can develop your immunity. This is why it has to be local honey because it will contain the same pollen you will be exposed to.

R.I.C.E. a reminder
This is the sports physio's chicken soup – and application of it is a starting point for practically any sporting injury.
Rest Ice Compression Elevation

Groin strain
Stretching or tearing of the muscle at the top of the inside of the thigh – where the thigh bone connects to the pubic bone.

Causes
Lateral overstretching of the leg.

Symptoms
Pain in that region when the leg is moved upwards or outwards, tenderness on the inside of the thigh.

Treatment
Rest. Ice. Compression. Elevation. And no sport or exercise until it is fully recovered.

Self-help
Don't attempt to run this one off or you will make it much worse. Stop immediately.

Prevention
Warm up and stretch the muscle out properly before exerting it.

H

Haemorrhoids
Inflammation of the blood vessels in the anus (external haemorrhoids) or rectum (internal).

Causes
Straining during a bowel movement – the likelihood of this increases with age.

Symptoms
Very tender swellings either inside or outside the anus, possibly the size of grapes.

Why hay fever is worse in cities

Remarkable as it may seem levels of hay fever are higher in urban environments than they are in the countryside. This is because the large amounts of residual pollution in cities keeps nose membranes slightly inflamed as a default setting. As a result they are on high alert and when something extra like pollen comes along they immediately switch into allergic mode as a defence. This is why hay fever has become more prevalent in recent years as pollution levels, rather than the pollen count, rise.

Treatment

Wash anus with a soft cloth and warm soapy water after bowel movement and pat dry; over-the-counter creams are available to ease the pain and in serious cases your GP may prescribe anti-inflammatory ointment. Usually, though, they clear up by themselves.

Self-help

Ice packs will reduce the swelling, or sitting in a warm – but not hot – bath will soothe the pain and itching.

Prevention

Avoid constipation, and keep stool soft by eating enough fibre and drinking plenty of water.

Hay fever

Causes

Allergic reaction to pollen or house dust, usually during the spring or summer.

Symptoms

Sneezing, blocked or running nose, streaming, itchy or swollen eyes.

Treatment

Antihistamine sprays or tablets, or steroid sprays, minimize the symptoms.

Self-help

Bioflavonoids in dark berries will reduce membrane inflammation; stop smoking and avoid smokers too, as this will aggravate the condition.

Prevention

Long-term, serious sufferers may try immunotherapy, otherwise try to stay indoors on days when the pollen count is high.

Heart attack

Part of the heart muscle packs up because it is deprived of oxygen through the bloodstream.

Cardio-pulmonary resuscitation (CPR) – it may save somebody's life

CPR is a method of "buying" a short amount of time for a heart attack victim by artificially stimulating their breathing and heartbeat with a combination of mouth-to-mouth resuscitation and robust heart massage. Give two good breaths into the victim's lungs, then place one of your palms on their heart, and the other on top of that, and push down thirty times in quick succession. Repeat the cycle of two breaths and thirty chest compressions until the emergency services arrive. This may be enough to keep the sufferer going until the paramedics get there, so it is vital it is applied immediately to anybody who is not responding to people around them or is breathing fitfully or not at all.

F

Fact: Nearly one in five heart attacks go undiagnosed as they are so mild the sufferer doesn't realize they are happening.

Causes

A sudden blockage in one of the coronary arteries supplying oxygenated blood to the heart – usually caused by a blood clot.

Symptoms

Crushing chest pain, difficulty breathing, dizziness, nausea, clammy and pale skin, possibility of collapse and the feeling that you are about to die.

Treatment

Call the emergency services immediately you suspect yourself or somebody else to be having a heart attack. Clot-busting drugs may be administered to clear the blockage, while post-attack treatments include medication to reduce the viscosity of your blood, beta-blockers to reduce strain on the heart and cholesterol-lowering drugs. If the heart has been seriously damaged it may require surgery.

Self-help

If you experience angina (see p.317) or other heart disease symptoms (see p.326) go and see your doctor immediately, as these may be overtures to an impending heart attack.

Prevention

Stop smoking, lose weight, take regular exercise, and make sure your cholesterol levels don't get too high.

Heartburn

An acute form of indigestion that has nothing to do with the heart.

Causes

Stomach acid escaping up through the valve at the top of the stomach and back into the oesophagus where it burns the lining – acid reflux. Excess stomach acid or eating too fast or too much at one go are the most likely culprits.

Symptoms

Burning sensation behind the breastbone; sometimes it feels like food or liquid is coming back up as far as your mouth.

Treatment

Antacid tablets or liquid.

Self-help

Liquorice, fennel or chamomile will soothe restless stomach acid.

Prevention

If it occurs regularly, avoid rich food, black coffee or fried food, and increase your intake of raw fruit and vegetables.

Hepatitis

An inflammation of the liver, and it is divided into five main types – Hep A, B, C, D and E.

Causes

It is a viral infection. A and E are typically caused by contaminated food or water; B, C and D are spread by bodily fluids – usually contaminated blood; B is most frequently transmitted by unprotected sex.

Symptoms

Yellowing of skin and eyes, fatigue, fever, nausea, brown urine, chronic stomach pain.

Treatment

Except for Hep C, the virus usually clears up by itself after a few weeks of rest, good nutrition and no alcohol. About twenty percent of Hep C sufferers will recover naturally, but the vast majority will carry it, and remain infectious, for the rest of their lives.

Self-help

Green tea has powerful antiviral powers, while vitamin B will boost your liver.

Prevention

Take all necessary precautions as regards sex and needles, especially in developing countries; it is possible to get vaccinated against Hep A.

Blood pressure: what do those figures mean?

The two figures given in a blood pressure measurement – 120 over 80, for instance, written as 120/80 – refer to, respectively, the systolic pressure while the heart is contracted and actually pumping blood, and the diastolic pressure when the heart is at rest between beats. The numbers refer to millimetres of mercury (mmHg), which is a unit of pressure measured by the movement of a precise column of mercury.

Hernia

An organ or tissue pushes out behind a weakened area of muscle, usually the groin.

Causes

Heavy coughing, ill-advised lifting technique, straining during a bowel movement or while urinating.

Symptoms

Soft lump under the skin, which may cause pain or not hurt at all.

Treatment

Hernias are usually treated with minor surgery; trusses are rarely used for anything other than comedy sketches.

Self-help

Even if it doesn't hurt it should be dealt with as untreated hernias get bigger and will eventually interfere with your regular life.

Prevention

Don't strain yourself.

Symptoms

Heart palpitations, breathlessness, persistent headache, nausea, dizziness.

Treatment

If you are young enough and healthy enough, your GP will recommend lifestyle changes as the initial treatment. For older people or those with very high blood pressure there are a number of drugs that can lower it. These are usually prescribed as a last resort because once you start on them you will probably have to continue on them for the rest of your life.

Self-help

Potassium-rich foods like bananas or celery lower blood pressure.

Prevention

Stay away from stimulants – legal and otherwise – and reduce the amount of salt in your diet as it increases your blood volume.

High blood pressure

Also known as hypertension, it is when your blood pressure is persistently measured at more than 140/90 – 120/80 is normal. (See box above for explanation of figures.)

Causes

If your high blood pressure is not a reaction to medication or a symptom of an illness (secondary hypertension) then what causes it has yet to be identified – this primary hypertension accounts for around 95 percent of all cases. Lifestyle issues – weight, lack of exercise, smoking, drinking, stress, bad diet – are believed to contribute.

F

Fact: Nobody knows why, but those of South Asian, African or African-Caribbean descent are much more likely to suffer from high blood pressure than any other ethnic groups.

I

Indigestion (dyspepsia)
Disturbance in the upper abdomen.
Causes
Acid from your stomach gets into the oesophagus (acid reflux or heartburn) or the upper part of your small intestine and attacks the lining; a bacterial infection.
Symptoms
Stomach pains that could be a dull ache or a sharp stabbing or anything in between, an uncomfortable feeling of being full, gas attacks, nausea.
Treatment
Antacids provide immediate relief, while for chronic indigestion your GP may prescribe drugs to reduce the residual acid levels in your stomach. If it is a bacterial infection prescription medication will also be required.
Self-help
Tea made from grated root ginger steeped in boiling water aids digestion, as does fresh pineapple.
Prevention
Lose weight if you are obese, as that will remove pressure from your stomach, reducing the likelihood of acid being pushed out. Eat smaller meals and consume them less quickly.

F

Fact: Although no definite figures exist, infertility is not uncommon. In approximately half the cases treated it is female infertility, in around one-third it is male, and in the remaining seventeen percent the causes are unknown.

Infertility
Inability to produce enough or mobile enough sperm to fertilize your partner's egg.
Causes
Men can have a naturally low sperm count or produce sperm with little mobility. Testicular infections can affect sperm production (both quantity and quality), as can the side effects of anabolic steroids, some anti-inflammatory medication and chemotherapy. An unhealthy lifestyle can also contribute, and it is believed the high levels of pesticide residue on food is a factor.
Symptoms
Failure to conceive – 85 percent of couples with no fertility problems will conceive within a year of having regular, unprotected sex.
Treatment
Surgical procedures can help if the problem is a blockage, and there is medication available to increase sperm count.
Self-help
Zinc is a sperm count booster, as are nuts and whole pulses and grains.
Prevention
Stop smoking and cut down on the drinking, as both hugely reduce levels of healthy sperm, as does chronic stress.

Influenza (flu)
A viral infection of the lungs and respiratory tract.
Causes
The flu virus is highly contagious and spread on saliva through coughing and sneezing, which is why epidemics are not uncommon.
Symptoms
Coughing, sneezing, aching muscles, fatigue, high temperature, chills, loss of appetite, nausea.
Treatment
Bed rest, plenty of fluids and over-the-counter medication will usually clear it up in about a week. In severe cases a GP may

prescribe antiviral medicine.
Self-help
Vitamin C and echinacea are both highly effective against the flu virus.
Prevention
Flu vaccination is widely available and very effective.

Insomnia

The inability to sleep restfully.
Causes
Stress, alcohol, eating too late at night, stimulants, depression, exercising late at night, not exercising enough, anxiety.
Symptoms
Regularly having trouble falling asleep, waking after a couple of hours and having difficulty getting back to sleep, general fatigue during the day.
Treatment
If the cause is psychological, counselling may help you get around that, and only take sleeping medication as a temporary measure. Don't lie there willing yourself to go to sleep as this will activate your brain and make dropping off even less likely.
Self-help
Tryptophan-loaded foods like turkey, chicken, wheatgerm, and cottage cheese will help you produce more serotonin, which will help relax you. Valerian root prevents chaotic sleep patterns.
Prevention
Eliminate as many of the possible causes as apply, and make sure your bedroom is as sleep-friendly as possible.

Irritable bowel syndrome (IBS)

The most common gastric complaint among men in the Western world.
Causes
The muscles that line the intestine and ripple to push food in its various broken-down stages through the digestive tract

T

> Tip: An effective remedy against jet lag is to take a serotonin supplement. These are only available on prescription in the UK but widely sold in US airports or larger pharmacies.

go into spasm and move it through to the bowel either too quickly or too slowly. It may be brought on by high-fat foods, excess of dairy products in the diet, undiagnosed food allergies or even stress.
Symptoms
Nausea, stomach pains, excess gas, constipation, diarrhoea, abdominal cramps.
Treatment
Modify your diet, eat smaller meals and don't rush them. If diarrhoea is a symptom you may be depleting your nutrient reserves so you will need to replenish them.
Self-help
Linseeds taken daily will help regulate your bowel functions and return them to normal.
Prevention
Reduce fat and increase fibre intake, address any causes of stress and, if IBS persists, get tested for food allergies.

Jet lag

Causes
Travelling across different time zones faster than your body can adjust.
Symptoms
Disrupted sleep/wake cycle, fatigue.
Treatment
Don't dehydrate; stay up as long as you can in the new time zone; engage in some light exercise as soon as you arrive.
Self-help
Boosting your tryptophan levels with foods such as turkey or cottage cheese, or with

F

Fact: Kidney stones are more common in the summer because you will be more dehydrated, and therefore your urine will be less in volume but of greater concentration.

supplements that will help you relax into a new sleep cycle.

Prevention

Make sure you have had a good night's sleep before travelling, eat with a view to maintaining even blood sugar levels and don't get drunk on the flight.

K

Kidney stones

Hard pieces of waste matter forming in the kidneys and passing into the ureter.

Causes

Minerals being filtered out of the blood to be passed out of the body in urine collect in the kidneys and solidify. Low volumes of urine can cause these deposits – nearly all kidney stones are mostly solidified calcium or uric acid.

Symptoms

Pains in the lower back that are sometimes very sharp; difficulty urinating; dark or cloudy urine; nausea.

Treatment

Small kidney stones pass out of the body through urination, and water intake should be increased to encourage this – this may happen without you noticing, or could cause considerable pain, depending on the size of the stone. Larger deposits may require painkillers and muscle relaxant medication to get them on their way, and stones capable of completely blocking the ureter will be broken up using sound waves then passed out with urine.

Self-help

Hydrangea root has long been used to dissolve kidney stones, while lemon juice taken every day will smooth the painful jagged edges of the stones.

Prevention

Drink plenty of water to flush minerals out of your kidneys before deposits can build up.

L

Laryngitis

An inflammation of the larynx.

Causes

Usually it is a viral infection, and occasionally it is bacterial. It can also come about through straining the vocal cords.

Symptoms

Sore throat, difficulty swallowing, croaky or

Lactose intolerance

The inability to digest milk or dairy products is a common situation that has been diagnosed far more readily during the last couple of decades. It is the result of a body's insufficient production of an enzyme called lactase that is needed to break lactose down into a digestible form. Unmetabolized lactose can cause abdominal discomfort, bloating, gas and diarrhoea. It is far more common among those of African, African-Caribbean, Asian or Native American descent than in Caucasians, and the only remedy or means of prevention is to remove dairy from your diet.

Liver disorders

The hardest working and only self-renewing organ in your body, your liver is far from immune to the punishment it takes as it filters toxins out of your system and regulates the flow of vital substances. Traditionally, the most likely cause of liver complaint has been cirrhosis, from drinking too much, as the effort involved in dealing with the toxins introduced by the alcohol destroys the liver's cells and replaces them with non-functioning scar tissue. Eventually this leads to liver failure as it no longer has the capacity to carry out its duties, but while it slowly shuts down you will experience fatigue, jaundice, loss of appetite, weight loss and nausea. More recently though, as the obesity crisis deepens, nonalcoholic fatty liver disease is gaining ground – it is currently affecting around twenty percent of American adults. It is caused by a build-up of fat in the liver as poor diets lead to such an ingestion of fat and cholesterol the organ cannot process and clear it away quick enough. When this occurs the liver functions far less efficiently, resulting in weakness and fatigue and, in advanced cases, chronic abdominal pain.

Fatty liver disease does not cause permanent damage. Changing to a healthy diet will clear it up and prevent it coming back. Cirrhosis, however, is irreversible. The only way to stop its advancement is to stop drinking completely and switch to a healthy diet, and in severe cases a liver transplant might be necessary.

weak speaking voice.

Treatment

Viral laryngitis will clear up by itself; take it easy and don't talk, write things down to give your vocal cords a complete rest; drink warm, soothing drinks and ease the pain with over-the-counter throat lozenges. Antibiotics will only be prescribed if the infection is bacterial.

Self-help

Steam inhalation, maybe with a menthol infusion.

Prevention

Don't smoke and try not to strain your vocal cords.

Low blood sugar

Also known as hypoglycaemia.

Causes

The liver does not release enough glucose into the system, which can prompt increased adrenaline production.

Symptoms

Fatigue, irritability, lack of concentration, dizziness, hunger, headaches, anxiety, the shakes; severe hypoglycaemia can bring on partial paralysis.

Treatment

Eating a sugary snack or drinking a fast-

T Tip: If you have laryngitis don't make any vocal sounds at all, especially not whispering as rather than saving your vocal chords, it actually puts more strain on them than shouting does.

T Tip: You don't have to be a heavy drinker to adversely affect your liver – regular light drinking or two or three consecutive nights on the lash can start to overload it and make you feel tired and weakened. Make sure you have a couple of non-drinking days every week to give it time to recover.

acting carbohydrate like fruit juice or a sports drink. If it is a lasting condition brought on by diabetes or liver disorders, the sufferer should keep sugary products on hand for emergencies and make sure people know to administer them if they are having a serious attack.

Self-help

Regular dosages of magnesium will keep blood sugar levels stable.

Prevention

Eat regularly and healthily, and don't skip breakfast.

M

Meningitis

Inflammation of membranes covering the brain.

Causes

It is a bacterial or a viral infection, and highly contagious.

Symptoms

Severe headaches, confusion, fatigue, fever, sensitivity to light, stiff neck.

Treatment

Bacterial meningitis will be treated with antibiotics, while viral meningitis usually clears up by itself after a period of bed rest and good nutrition. The symptoms of the latter may be treated individually to ease discomfort.

Self-help

Homeopathic remedy Belladonna (deadly nightshade) will assist your recovery after the antibiotics have done their job or while you are getting over viral meningitis.

Prevention

You can be vaccinated against meningitis and this is recommended if travelling to a high-risk area or if you are an AIDS sufferer.

ME (myalgia encephalomyelitis)

Also known as chronic fatigue syndrome, neurological disorder that affects around 0.3 percent of the UK population and 0.5 percent in the US. It is twice as likely to occur in women than in men.

Causes

Changes in the hormonal and chemical balance of the brain, disrupting the internal sleep/wake rhythms, as well as blood pressure and temperature control, which affect the desire to be active. These changes can be the aftermath of a previous infection, hormonal disturbance or even hereditary.

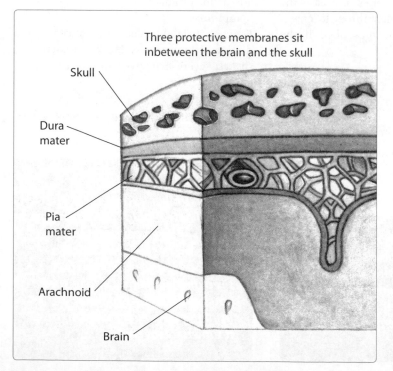

Three protective membranes sit inbetween the brain and the skull

Skull

Dura mater

Pia mater

Arachnoid

Brain

Symptoms

Fatigue after any form of exertion, lack of energy, aching joints and muscles, low blood pressure, headaches, fitful sleep patterns, lack of concentration.

Treatment

There is no cure for ME, although medication will be used to treat the symptoms. There is a commonly applied therapy called pacing, that encourages the sufferer to undertake physical and mental tasks within their limited capabilities, then gradually increases the amount of effort needed.

Self-help

Don't attempt to combat any feelings of tiredness with caffeine – especially energy drinks that may have very high levels – as ultimately they will compromise your immune system, disrupt your blood sugar levels and interfere with your adrenal gland.

Prevention

Apart from maintaining your immune system there is little to be done to prevent ME, although the majority of sufferers also have previously undiagnosed food allergies, so it may be worth exploring that avenue.

Migraines

Intense headaches, a condition that affects one in twelve British men on a regular basis – the figure for women is three times as high, so she may really have a headache.

Causes

Low levels of serotonin can send blood vessels in the brain into rapid contraction and expansion mode, creating the conditions for a migraine, which can then be triggered by a

F

Fact: Because of hormonal changes that take place during the menopause, women are four times as likely as men to suffer from osteoporosis.

number of factors. These can be emotional (stress, shock, depression), environmental (bright or flickering lights, loud noises, airless rooms) or physical (tension, fatigue, dehydration, food additives), and will be unique to everybody.

Symptoms

Severe headache, lack of coordination, problems speaking, heightened sensitivity to light or sound, visual oddities – vivid lights or patterns in your vision – numbness in shoulders or limbs, nausea.

Treatment

There is no cure, as such, for migraines. Painkillers may treat the headache and lying down in a cool dark room may help relieve other symptoms. In some cases, doctors may prescribe triptan, a medicine that stabilizes the blood vessels in the brain.

Self-help

If the blood vessels in your brain have gone into spasm, ginkgo biloba will stop them constricting.

Prevention

Avoid dehydration, maintain stable blood sugar levels (hypoglycaemia can bring migraines on) and learn to recognize the signs and avoid your particular trigger points.

Multiple sclerosis (MS)

A degenerative condition of the nerve cells in the brain and spinal column.

Causes

The causes of MS are unknown.

Symptoms

Loss of mental and physical control – balance and coordination difficulties, slurred speech, bladder control problems, mood swings, confusion, lack of concentration, memory loss, muscle weakness and stiffness, blurred vision, partial paralysis.

Treatment

There are medications to limit the severity and frequency of the attacks, but no actual cure, and the symptoms will be addressed individually.

Self-help

Keep cool – avoid hot environments, and attacks may be relieved with a cool shower or resting in a cool room.

Prevention

There is no way to prevent MS.

0

Obesity

Dangerously excessive fat accumulation.

Causes

Bad diet, lack of exercise, glandular disorders.

Symptoms

A body weight of over twenty percent more than it should be for your height, which can lead to heart disease, diabetes, liver failure, strokes, exhaustion, strain on every part of your body, decreased life expectancy.

Treatment

About two percent of obesity is a glandular problem (usually the thyroid or the adrenal gland) and that will be medically treated, otherwise it's a matter of lifestyle changes or such drastic measures as stomach stapling or gastric banding to limit your food consumption.

Self-help

Do more exercise, eat less.

Prevention

Do more exercise, eat less.

Osteoporosis

Weakening of bone density and strength.

Causes

Old age, calcium deficiency, lack of exercise.

Symptoms

Propensity to bone fractures, progressively stooping posture, chronic lower back pain.

Treatment

Your doctor may prescribe medication that assists the body's processing of calcium (bisphosphonates), or even recommend

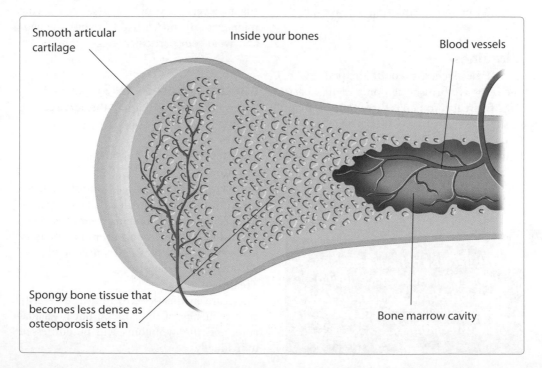

Smooth articular cartilage

Inside your bones

Blood vessels

Spongy bone tissue that becomes less dense as osteoporosis sets in

Bone marrow cavity

calcium supplements.

Self-help

Regular weight-bearing exercise – running is very good – will keep your bones strong.

Prevention

Maintaining levels of calcium and vitamin D in your diet as you get older will keep your bones healthy, and don't smoke or drink to excess, as this will affect the production and utilization of calcium in your body.

P

Peptic ulcer

Ulceration in the stomach or digestive tract.

Causes

Infection, massive excesses of stomach acid, side effect to some medication, especially long-term use of anti-inflammatories.

Symptoms

Stomach pains, often immediately after eating, nausea, weight loss, black or bloody stool and sharp pain are the signs of a perforated ulcer and emergency treatment should be sought.

Treatment

Ulcers usually heal themselves within a couple of months, but it will ease the pain and assist healing if you take an antacid. More serious or persistent cases may require

prescription medication to reduce stomach acid or combat infection.

Self-help

The bark of the slippery elm tree brewed into tea soothes the intestines and speeds internal healing.

Prevention

A healthy, fibre-rich diet will keep your digestive system moving, preventing bits of food hanging about to irritate the walls.

Pneumonia

Inflammation of the lungs.

Causes

A viral or bacterial infection of the lungs, or caused by inhaled foreign bodies or poisonous gases. Pneumonia can also result from other conditions such as bronchitis, asthma, diabetes or leukaemia, and AIDS sufferers are particularly vulnerable.

Symptoms

Breathlessness, chest pain bringing up opaque phlegm, coughing, fever, fatigue.

Treatment

Antibiotics or antiviral drugs will be prescribed to treat infection; bed rest and in severe cases oxygen may need to be administered to assist breathing.

Self-help

A regular dose of magnesium (about 400g) may contribute to keeping your lungs healthy.

Repetitive strain injury (RSI)

Any injury to the joints, tendons, muscles, nerves or ligaments that is caused by the repetition of an action that is causing unusual strain. This can be occupational – operating machinery, equipment vibrations or a computer mouse – or as the result of a leisure-time activity – regular golfers and tennis players frequently suffer RSI. Carpal tunnel syndrome and bursitis, covered earlier in this chapter, are the most common examples of RSI. Others include rotator cuff syndrome (inflammation of the shoulder) and trigger finger (inflammation of the tendons in the index finger or thumb).

The symptoms of pain, swelling and, sometimes, immobility are best treated with R.I.C.E. Then the movement itself should be isolated and ceased, or adapted to avoid the symptoms coming back.

The prostate gland sits just below the bladder and in front of the rectum. Hence it is examined through the anus

What causes it is not known, but it is believed to be sexually transmitted bacteria – it is far more common among young men with patterns of risky behaviour.

Symptoms

Painful urination, blood in urine or semen, lower back pain, bladder still feeling full after urination.

Treatment

Antibiotics, bed rest.

Self-help

Coffee should be avoided, as the diuretic properties will irritate your symptoms.

Prevention

Practise safe sex.

S

Prevention

Don't smoke as it irritates the lungs; don't snort cocaine as you will be putting all sorts of pollutants directly into your lungs; maintain a healthy immune system.

Prostatitis

Inflammation of the prostate gland.

Causes

F

Fact: Although there are around 150,000 diagnosed male SADS sufferers in the UK, there are over five times as many women, while it is estimated around one percent of American adults are afflicted, with the same men/women ratio.

Schizophrenia

A chronic psychotic disorder that tends to appear much earlier in men (teens and twenties) than in women.

Causes

The cause is unknown, but it is thought to have a genetic element to it. Brain damage can contribute, and although excessive drug use may produce schizophrenic-like episodes, it will not cause the condition.

Symptoms

Paranoia, delusions, hallucinations, erratic and inappropriate behaviour, obsessive and compulsive behaviour.

Treatment

Antipsychotic drugs will be prescribed, combined with psychotherapy.

Self-help

Seek help as soon as you realize you may be a sufferer and work to trust those who will be trying to help you.

Prevention

Although schizophrenic episodes may be controlled with antipsychotic medication, there is no way of preventing the condition occurring in the first place.

Seasonal affective disorder

Also known as SADS, this is a lowering of the mood that tends to coincide with the coming of autumn and persists through winter.

Causes

When there is less sunshine and daylight, the pineal gland produces more melatonin to disrupt the internal sleep/wake rhythms. This is believed to be a hangover from a primeval hibernating past, but can make some people feel very under-energized both physically and mentally – suicide rates are considerably higher in countries that have very little daylight in the winter.

Symptoms

Feeling down for no apparent reason, lack of energy, difficulty concentrating, irritability, weight gain.

Treatment

Get out in the daylight as much as possible, exercise to generally boost your system and eat serotonin-boosting foods such as turkey, avocados and bananas.

Self-help

Full spectrum light bulbs in your home will help to replicate sunlight, but tanning beds will not.

Prevention

Take your summer holidays in winter and go somewhere sunny.

Sexually transmitted diseases

Genital herpes, gonorrhoea, non-specific urethritis, syphilis, HIV, pubic lice, thrush and so on.

Causes

Unprotected sex with an infected partner.

Symptoms

Different infections will have different symptoms, but any of the following should prompt you to get checked out at a sexual health clinic: burning sensation during urination; discharge through end of penis; itching around or inside penis opening; blisters or sores in genital area; rashes, redness or swelling around the end of the penis; tiny black deposits in your underwear.

Treatment

Antibiotics or antiviral drugs, and don't have sex again until you are sure it is cleared up.

Self-help

Dark berries will boost your immune system and speed your recovery.

Prevention

Practise safe sex.

Slipped disc

One of the cushioning discs in between the vertebrae slips out of place.

Causes

Incorrect lifting or chronic bad posture, and the obese are much more likely to suffer slipped discs as their excess belly weight puts enormous strain on the lower back.

Symptoms

Progressively building pain if the disc is slipping out gradually, then sharp pain, which will be accompanied by increasing immobility; sudden excruciating pain if it just pops out, and the back will often lock.

Treatment

Painkillers and physiotherapy.

Self-help

Vitamin C aids collagen production to assist with the healing, and has anti-inflammatory properties.

Prevention
Glucosamine supplements keep all joints healthy and protected.

Snoring
Excessively loud breathing through the mouth while asleep.
Causes
Airways obstructed by internal collapse causing tissue in the throat to noisily vibrate against itself.
Symptoms
Resonant, rumbling sounds created by breathing.
Treatment
Try to avoid sleeping with your mouth open, which usually comes about through sleeping on your back, or there are several devices on the market to keep it closed.
Self-help
A couple of drops of eucalyptus oil on your pillow will ease nasal congestion, which may be why you are sleeping with your mouth open.
Prevention
Don't smoke close to bedtime, as this inflames airways, and drinking will relax the throat muscles; check you are not allergic to the feathers in your pillow or duvet.

Stroke
Part of the brain is deprived of oxygen and those cells cease to function and start to die.
Causes
A blood clot in the brain or in one of the arteries that supply blood to the brain or a burst blood vessel in the brain.
Symptoms
Partial paralysis or numbness, coordination and muscle movement problems – this may manifest itself in speech or walking difficulties – blurred or obstructed vision, intense headaches.

Treatment
Blood pressure lowering or anti-clotting drugs will be administered immediately, and stroke victims may require physical therapy to restore muscle activity and control.
Self-help
There is very little you can do, as this is a medical emergency and must be professionally treated as soon as possible to prevent lasting brain damage.
Prevention
Address the three major risk factors, which are high blood pressure, high cholesterol and smoking.

T

Thrombosis
See deep vein thrombosis, above, as it is the same condition, occurring in veins that are not so deep in the body.

Tinnitus
Not only the preserve of rock stars and roadies.
Causes
Usually it is the result of prolonged exposure to loud noise, but it can be a bacterial infection, a side effect of age-related hearing degeneration, or caused by a head injury or partial ear blockage.
Symptoms
Ringing or buzzing in the ears when there is no corresponding external sound, partial hearing loss, disrupted sleep.
Treatment
Antibiotics will treat any infection; there is no cure for noise-induced or degenerative tinnitus – simply address the main symptoms to try to mask or hear around the ringing.

The demon drink

By now it will have seemed that the cure or prevention for nearly everything that could be wrong with you is to pack up drinking. At the risk of sounding like a killjoy, this will be the case. And not because anybody connected with this book has got anything against having a drink either; simply that alcohol is a poison. To take in even the responsible amounts will interfere with your healing process, because your body has to be functioning at the peak of its powers to give it its best chance. To have to deal with even a small amount of self-induced toxin will detract from that. Also, you should never drink while on antibiotics.

Self-help
Vitamin B12 helps reduce the ringing, and ginkgo biloba increases blood flow in the ears.

Prevention
Don't stand so close to the Marshalls.

V

Varicose veins

Patches of veins visible through the surface of the skin, almost uniquely in the legs.

Causes
Defective valves within the veins disrupt blood flow and allow de-oxygenated blood to pool. Standing for prolonged periods of time, lack of exercise and being overweight contribute to the condition.

Symptoms
Swollen and discoloured veins, swollen and aching legs and ankles.

Treatment
They are not a serious health risk, but look unsightly and can be easily surgically removed. Raising your legs above the level of your hips when going to sleep will help the circulation in them.

Self-help
Rosehip tea contains a bioflavonoid called rutin, which maintains strong, healthy veins. It is also present in apple peel.

Prevention
Avoid standing for long periods, maintain a healthy weight and exercise regularly.

What's the problem?

Assess yourself with this handy, easy-to-use guide. Select whatever your main cause for complaint might be from the list of man's most common ailments – in some cases you will need to read down a particular category to further define it – then follow the row from left to right. It will offer a selection of subsidiary symptoms, in different combinations, which will bring you to what is most likely to be wrong with you. The following column provides basic treatment advice. It must be stressed that, useful as this service is, it is not intended to replace your healthcare professionals, and is merely an initial guideline.

Appetite, loss of

Visit your GP if loss of appetite, with no other symptoms, persists for more than a couple of weeks.

Accompanying symptoms	Condition	Treatment
Anxiety, irritability, lack of concentration, fatigue, sleeplessness, loss of appetite	Stress	Address whatever might be causing the stress
Fever, chills, fatigue, aching muscles, headache, nausea, excess mucus production, sore throat	Flu	Bed rest, plenty of fluids, over-the-counter medication
Fever, chills, fatigue, aching muscles, headache, nausea, brown urine, yellowing skin, abdominal pain	Viral hepatitis	Usually clears up by itself
Weight loss, constipation and infrequent urination	Early signs of cancer	Visit your GP
Fatigue, pallor, inability to concentrate, irritability, brittle nails	Anaemia	Iron, folic acid, vitamin B12 and C supplements
Fatigue, swollen lymph nodes, weight loss, increasing susceptibility to infections and viruses, purple lesions on the skin	AIDS	Visit your GP
No other symptoms	Side effect of prescription medication	Consult the professional that prescribed the medication

Back pains

Type	Accompanying symptoms	Condition	Treatment
Sharp pain spreading out from spine, considerably worse when coughing or sneezing	Muscle spasms or paralysis, numbness in legs	Slipped disc	Painkillers, gentle exercise, possible physical therapy. See GP, osteopath or chiropractor if pain continues
Chronic, in the lower back on either or both sides	Fever, nausea, blood in urine, painful urination	Kidney infection	Antibiotics, painkillers. See GP, osteopath or chiropractor if pain continues
Sharp within a clearly defined area, and maybe only during certain movements	Muscle may lock	Strained or sprained muscle; pinched or irritated nerve	Painkillers, anti-inflammatory medication, R.I.C.E., gentle manipulation. See GP, osteopath or chiropractor if pain continues
Chronic, across the centre of lower back	Large stomach	Obesity	Lose some weight

Bleeding gums

Accompanying symptoms	Condition	Treatment
Bad breath, bad taste in mouth, loose teeth, abscesses in mouth	Periodontitis	Antiseptic mouthwash, improve dental hygiene, don't smoke
Fatigue, very bad breath, metallic taste in mouth, excessive saliva production, sore throat	Gingivitis	Antiseptic mouthwash, improve dental hygiene, don't smoke

Chest pains

Type	Accompanying symptoms	Condition	Treatment
Tightness in chest	Inability to breathe or a wheezing shortness of breath, increased heartbeat, perspiration	Asthma	Bronchial inhaler
Weight pushing down in centre or band squeezing around it	Breathlessness, dizziness, sweating, possible collapse	Angina or coronary artery disease	Seek medical attention immediately

Chest pains (continued)

Type	Accompanying symptoms	Condition	Treatment
Sharp pain when coughing	Deep, hacking cough, greenish-yellow sputum, fever, breathlessness	Bronchitis	Antibiotics, drink plenty of water, steam inhalations
Sudden pain, spreading out to neck or shoulders	Inability to breathe, perspiration, vomiting, collapse	Heart attack	CPR and call the emergency services immediately
Burning sensation behind breastbone, usually right after eating	Pain and difficulty swallowing, acid reflux and possible minor regurgitation of food	Heartburn	Antacid liquid or chewable tablets
Wheezing, aching, worse when coughing	Fever, chills, aching muscles, fatigue, loss of appetite, excess mucus production, sore throat	Flu	Bed rest, plenty of fluids, over-the-counter medication
Tightness around chest	Intense fear or anxiety, increased heartbeat, perspiration, difficult or shallow breathing	Panic attack	Sit down, breathe deeply, consult your GP if symptoms recur
Pain deep within chest when coughing	Fatigue, fever, breathlessness, cough, opaque sputum	Pneumonia	Antibiotics, bed rest

Constipation

Accompanying symptoms	Condition	Treatment
Abdominal pain, dehydration, loss of appetite, nausea	Calcium excess	Cut down on calcium – probably dairy products
Excess mucus, headache, fatigue, cough, sore throat, fever	Cold	Bed rest, plenty of fluids, vitamin C, echinacea
Painful stomach cramps, vomiting, gas, bloating, bad breath, tender localized swelling	Gastric obstruction	Consult your GP; surgery may be necessary
Very painful defecation, blood on toilet paper after use, tender swellings inside or outside anus, itching	Haemorrhoids	Ice packs, over-the-counter ointments, wash with warm soapy water and pat dry
Abdominal cramps, gas, bloating, bouts of diarrhoea alternating with the constipation	Irritable bowel syndrome (IBS)	Modify your diet, eat smaller meals, linseeds
Stool is black and hard	Iron excess	Cut out iron supplements, but make sure you continue to get your RDA from fresh vegetables

Recurring, chronic constipation	Poor diet	Increase intake of fibre, drink more water

Coughing

Type	Accompanying symptoms	Condition	Treatment
Dry cough	Sore throat, nasal congestion, running nose, fever, chills, headache, constipation, fatigue, muscle ache	Common cold	Bed rest, plenty of fluids, keep warm
Dry cough bringing up opaque phlegm	Breathlessness, chest pain, fever, fatigue	Pneumonia	Antibiotics or antiviral drugs will be prescribed to treat infection, bed rest
Dry, tickling cough	Hoarseness and possible loss of voice, sore throat, fatigue, fever	Laryngitis	Try not to speak, plenty of fluids, throat-soothing gargles or lozenges
Wet cough	Sneezing, aching muscles, fatigue, high temperature, chills, loss of appetite, nausea	Flu	Bed rest, plenty of fluids, over-the-counter medication
Hacking cough bringing up cloudy mucus	Breathlessness, fever	Bronchitis	Antibiotics, cough medicine

Erectile dysfunction

Type	Accompanying symptoms	Condition	Treatment
General erectile dysfunction	Frequent attacks of chest pains, breathlessness and dizziness	Coronary artery disease	Visit your GP; hospitalization may be required
General erectile dysfunction	Thirst, frequent urination, fatigue, increased appetite, tingling in the feet and hands, blood sugar fluctuations	Diabetes	Visit your GP
General erectile dysfunction	Muscle weakness, decreased sexual appetite, fatigue, shrinking of testicles	Hypopituitarism (disorder of the pituitary gland)	Steroid treatment, hormone replacement therapy

Erectile dysfunction (continued)

Type	Accompanying symptoms	Condition	Treatment
If you still wake up with an erection most mornings, but can't always rise to sexual stimulation	Anxiety, irritability, lack of concentration, fatigue, sleeplessness, loss of appetite	Stress	Address whatever might be causing the stress

Fatigue

Practically every infection will be accompanied by fatigue, as the body will require you to rest to give it the best chance to fight off invaders. Exhaustion will also be a symptom of stress or depression. However, there are some everyday conditions in which tiredness is the principal manifestation, and a few aspects of fatigue that are not merely side effects of something else.

Type	Accompanying symptoms	Condition	Treatment
After any form of exertion	Aching joints and muscles, low blood pressure, headaches, fitful sleep patterns, lack of concentration	ME (chronic fatigue syndrome)	Visit your GP; don't try and combat it with caffeine
Constant tiredness	Pallor, inability to concentrate, irritability, brittle nails	Anaemia	Iron, folic acid, vitamin B12 and C supplements
Constant tiredness	Regularly having trouble falling asleep, waking after a couple of hours and having difficulty getting back to sleep	Insomnia	Counselling if the cause is psychological; sleeping medication should only be used as a temporary measure

Chronic fatigue caused by lifestyle

Cause	How to tell	Remedy
Poor nutrition	Keep a food diary to work out if you are not getting enough nutrition	Change your diet
Lack of physical fitness	Write down how much exercise you actually do over the course of a week	Draw up an exercise programme and stick to it
Obesity	Take your shirt off and look in the mirror	Lose some weight
Breathing badly	Devote about fifteen minutes to relaxing and taking deep breaths, holding them in your lungs for a while before breathing out. If you feel a little light-headed during this, you are unused to breathing properly	Continue these breathing course every day until breathing deeper becomes natural

Genital discomfort

Type	Accompanying symptoms	Condition	Treatment
Itching at penis opening	Painful urination, milky discharge	Chlamydia	Antibiotics
Itching around pubic hair and genitals	Infestation of insects one millimetre in size, possibly tiny blisters, swelling	Crabs (pubic lice)	Medicated shampoo
Itching in genital or anal area	Small circular blisters	Genital herpes	Antiviral medication
Burning pain at opening of penis during urination	Thick yellowish discharge, inflammation of the anus	Gonorrhoea	Antibiotics
Itching at end of penis	Small white bumps on end of penis	Genital warts	Application of medicated cream
Itching in genital area	Itching spreads all over the body, ulcers on penis	Syphilis	Penicillin

Headaches

Type	Accompanying symptoms	Condition	Treatment
Constant dull ache	Inability to concentrate, fatigue, dry mouth, apparent hunger	Dehydration	Drink more water
Escalating dull throb	Dizziness, weakness, thirst, confusion, muscle cramps, nausea, possible passing out	Heatstroke	Bring down body temperature, rehydrate
Constant mild headache	Sore throat, nasal congestion, running nose, fever, chills, dry cough, constipation, fatigue, muscle ache	Common cold	Bed rest, plenty of fluids, keep warm
Fuzzy-feeling headache	Sneezing, aching muscles, fatigue, high temperature, chills, loss of appetite, nausea	Flu	Bed rest, plenty of fluids, over-the-counter medication
Constant dull ache	Constant tiredness, pallor, inability to concentrate, irritability, brittle nails	Anaemia	Iron, folic acid, vitamin B12 and C supplements
Headache over the eyes	Hunger, anxiety, elevated heart rate, confusion, anxiety, shakes	Low blood sugar (hypoglycaemia)	Eat or drink something with a high glucose content

Headaches (continued)

Type	Accompanying symptoms	Condition	Treatment
Throbbing pain at the front, spreading to the sides	Lack of coordination, problems speaking, heightened sensitivity to light or sound, visual oddities – vivid lights or patterns in your vision – numbness in shoulders or limbs, nausea	Migraine	Painkillers, lie down in a cool, dark room
Low-level, constant headache	Aching joints and muscles, low blood pressure, constant fatigue, fitful sleep patterns, lack of concentration	ME	Visit your GP; don't try and combat it with caffeine
Constant mild headache	Breathlessness, fever, hacking cough bringing up cloudy mucus	Bronchitis	Antibiotics, cough medicine
Throbbing, thick-headed feeling	Thirst, fatigue	Hangover	Rehydration, rest
Low-level, constant headache	Fatigue, waking up feeling unrefreshed	Obstructive sleep apnoea	Sleeping on your side can help
Severe, constant headaches	Confusion, fatigue, fever, sensitivity to light, stiff neck	Meningitis	Antibiotics, swiftly! This dangerous condition can worsen very rapidly
Pain behind the eyes and at the side of the nose	Congested sinuses, headache, fever	Sinusitis	Drink plenty of water and hot water beverages like fruit teas, steam inhalation

Muscle aches and pains (acute)

Type	Accompanying symptoms	Condition	Treatment
Acute aches and pains	Muscle may lock	Strained or sprained muscle; pinched or irritated nerve	Painkillers, anti-inflammatory medication, R.I.C.E., gentle manipulation
Pain only during certain movement	Muscle has little strength	Pulled muscle	Rest, gentle massage

Muscle aches and pains (general)

Type	Accompanying symptoms	Condition	Treatment
Muscle weakness	Decreased sexual appetite, fatigue, shrinking of testicles	Hypopituitarism (disorder of the pituitary gland)	Steroid treatment, hormone replacement therapy
Aching joints and muscles	Low blood pressure, headaches, exhaustion after any form of exertion, fitful sleep patterns, lack of concentration	ME	Visit your GP: don't try and combat it with caffeine
Muscle ache	Sore throat, nasal congestion, running nose, fever, chills, dry cough, constipation, fatigue, headaches	Common cold	Bed rest, plenty of fluids, keep warm
Aching joints and muscles	Sneezing, headache, fatigue, high temperature, chills, loss of appetite, nausea	Flu	Bed rest, plenty of fluids, over-the-counter medication

Muscle cramps

Accompanying symptoms	Condition	Treatment
Dizziness, weakness, thirst, confusion, headache, nausea, possible passing out	Heatstroke	Bring down body temperature, rehydrate

Nausea/vomiting

Type	Accompanying symptoms	Condition	Treatment
General nausea or vomiting	Symptoms vary but could include fever, chills, diarrhoea, abdominal pain	Food poisoning	Bed rest, plenty of fluids
General nausea or vomiting	Sneezing, headache, fatigue, high temperature, chills, loss of appetite, aching joints and muscles	Flu	Bed rest, plenty of fluids, over-the-counter medication
General nausea or vomiting	Lack of coordination and balance, fatigue, dizziness, headache	Alcohol poisoning	Bed rest, plenty of fluids
With stomach pains, often immediately after eating	Weight loss, black or bloody stool and sharp pain are the signs of a perforated ulcer	Peptic ulcer	Antacid

Nausea/vomiting (continued)

Type	Accompanying symptoms	Condition	Treatment
With stomach cramps	Excess gas, constipation, diarrhoea	Irritable bowel syndrome (IBS)	Dietary modification
With stomach cramps, just after eating	No other symptoms	Indigestion	Eat more slowly

Nose and sinus congestion

Type	Accompanying symptoms	Condition	Treatment
Yellowish-green mucus brought up by coughing	Breathlessness, fever, hacking cough, headache	Bronchitis	Antibiotics, cough medicine
Mucus flowing through the nose	Sore throat, nasal congestion, muscle ache, fever, chills, dry cough, constipation, fatigue, headaches	Common cold	Bed rest, plenty of fluids, keep warm
Running nose	Sneezing, rashes, coughing, difficulty breathing, streaming eyes	Allergies	Avoid whatever it is you're allergic to
Mucus runs down throat behind nose	Pain at the side of the nose, headache, sore and inflamed throat, fever	Sinusitis	Drink plenty of water and hot water beverages like fruit teas, steam inhalation
Mucus flowing through the nose	Sneezing, headache, fatigue, high temperature, chills, loss of appetite, aching joints and muscles	Flu	Bed rest, plenty of fluids, over-the-counter medication

Skin rash

Type	Accompanying symptoms	Condition	Treatment
Dry, red itchy patches	No other symptoms	Irritant contact dermatitis	Usually caught from soap, detergent or cosmetics. Check what caused it and avoid
Rash with pimples and bumps, sometimes blisters	No other symptoms	Allergic contact dermatitis	Usually caught from perfume, inexpensive jewellery or plants. Check what caused it and avoid

Dry, itchy inflamed skin, most frequently on backs of knees	No other symptoms	Eczema	Visit your GP
Clusters of tiny red bumps	No other symptoms	Heat rash	Avoid restrictive clothing, keep cool
Swathes of tiny, red, fluid-filled spots on arms, legs, body or face	Fever, headaches	Shingles	Calamine lotion, ice, antiviral medication
Raised patches of dry red skin, itching and flaking off	Aching joints, discoloured finger nails	Psoriasis	Visit your GP for prescription skin cream

Sleeplessness

Type	Accompanying symptoms	Condition	Treatment
Waking during the night or feeling unrested in the morning	Fatigue, headache	Obstructive sleep apnoea	Sleeping on your side can help
Unable to drop off or sleeping very lightly	Fatigue	Insomnia	Valerian root is a natural sleep aid
Unable to drop off	Anxiety, irritability, lack of concentration, fatigue, loss of appetite	Stress	Address whatever might be causing the stress
Involuntary jerking of the legs keeps waking you up	No other symptoms	Restless leg syndrome	Do some mild leg exercise – walking or running – before going to bed

Sore throat

Type	Accompanying symptoms	Condition	Treatment
With a dry, cough	Nasal congestion, running nose, fever, chills, headache, constipation fatigue, muscle ache	Common cold	Bed rest, plenty of fluids, keep warm
With a dry tickling cough	Hoarseness and possible loss of voice, fatigue, fever	Laryngitis	Try not to speak, plenty of fluids, throat-soothing gargles or lozenges

Sore throat (continued)

Type	Accompanying symptoms	Condition	Treatment
General sore throat	Fatigue, very bad breath, metallic taste in mouth, excessive saliva production	Gingivitis	Antiseptic mouthwash, increase dental hygiene, don't smoke
General sore throat	Difficulty swallowing, swollen glands in neck, fever, swollen throat	Tonsillitis	Antiviral medication
General sore throat	Pain at the side of the nose, headache, mucus runs down throat behind nose inflamed throat, fever	Sinusitis	Drink plenty of water and hot water beverages like fruit teas, steam inhalation

Stomach pains

Type	Accompanying symptoms	Condition	Treatment
Cramping	Watery stool, frequent, violent bowel movements	Diarrhoea	Over-the-counter medication
Cramps in centre or at one side only of lower abdomen	Excess gas, constipation, diarrhoea	Irritable bowel syndrome (IBS)	Dietary modification
Sharp stabbing pains or cramps	Other symptoms vary but could include fever, chills, diarrhoea, abdominal pain	Food poisoning	Bed rest, plenty of fluids
Specifically located sharp pain	Bloating, gas, nausea	Intestinal obstruction	Seek emergency assistance
With back pain	Burning sensation when urinating, sex is painful, frequent urination	Bladder infection	Antibiotics
Stomach cramps just after eating	No other symptoms	Indigestion	Eat slower
With very sharp pains in the lower back	Difficulty urinating, dark or cloudy urine, nausea	Kidney stones	Painkillers, visit your GP
Sharp pains in right-hand side of the abdomen	No other symptoms	Gallstones	Visit your GP

Wind

Accompanying symptoms	Condition	Treatment
Abdominal cramps, constipation, diarrhoea	Irritable bowel syndrome (IBS)	Dietary modification
Constant feeling of fullness, bad breath	Undigested food in the gut	Colonic irrigation
Bloating immediately after meals	Too much air taken down with food or too many fizzy drinks	Eat more slowly, chew food more thoroughly, drink water instead of pop
Nausea, abdominal cramps, diarrhoea	Lactose intolerance	Cut out dairy products
Bloating, sharp abdominal pain, nausea	Intestinal obstruction	Seek emergency assistance

For your information

(19)

Although this book is pretty good, it can't do everything. Here is a handy rundown of what else is out there and worth your while if you want to find out more about men's health.

Magazines

Men's Health (international)

Monthly

The US edition of this magazine carries the tag line, "Tons of useful stuff", and it won't find itself troubled by any form of Trades Descriptions Act. Published in over two-dozen different countries, in almost as many languages, each different edition mirrors the American original, taking a local approach to a lively mix of men's health, fitness, fashion, sex, cookery and life in general. As well as making sure you look and feel better, it's packed with tips, shared experiences and straightforward advice, so it is a bit like having a sensible older brother, who drops in once a month to help you sort your life out.

menshealth.co.uk
menshealth.com

Men's Fitness (international)

Monthly

Another widely franchised international operation, *Men's Fitness* claims to be "Making your best even better" and carries everything you'll need for it to do so – fitness, health, muscle building, sex, grooming, style, gadgets and clever, life-enhancing tips. But it does so with a certain swagger that comes through in the persistently good-looking design, easy-to-understand practical application and an overall approach that seems not to expect you to behave like a choirboy quite all the time. If *Men's Health* is your sensible older brother, then *Men's Fitness* is your rather rakish cousin. It is worth noting that in terms of breadth of subject matter, presentation and overall tone, the UK edition is by far the best.

mensfitnessmagazine.co.uk
mensfitness.com

Best Life

Ten issues per year

Men's Health's older brother, providing essentially the same mix of health, fitness, sex, style and sound advice, but with the more mature gentleman in mind (See cover to get the idea). And it takes the notion of "mature" to an interesting end – sure, *Best Life*'s guidance and information focuses on what is more likely to affect a man who won't be seeing any more of his thirties – more on heart disease, less on impressing "chicks" and an approach to style that won't confuse your clothes with your son's – but in its very readable grown-upness it is somehow far more relaxed than its stable mate and, therefore, gets its points over with wit and verve. Unfortunately, at the time of writing, there are no plans to publish it in the UK.

bestlifeonline.com

healthy page count to environmental issues. It's a great read for your head as much as your body. There is a German edition, and it is widely available in the UK's bigger magazine outlets on import from the US.

mensjournal.com

Men's Journal

Ten issues per year

Part of the same American publishing house that gives us *Rolling Stone* magazine, *Men's Journal* is less about the quest for health and fitness as what to do with it once you've acquired it. A laid-back compendium of wide-open spaces, adventures across the world's last wildernesses and the sort of gadgets that will put you on a par with nature at its fiercest – and make sure you can still enjoy your record collection while you do. It carries plenty of in-depth articles about the effects of health and fitness regimes and trends, plus the stories behind the stories behind sports and sportsmen and devotes a

Runners World (UK)

Monthly

Although very UK-centric in terms of the events it covers, the British edition of *Runner's World* is probably the greatest running magazine on the planet – it's worth it even for those not living in the UK. With its training features and tips, running gear reviews, sports nutrition, expert race advice, competition calendars, race reports and in-depth pieces on runners and running culture, all written in an accessible, easy-going tone, this magazine totally understands what it is to be a runner on any level from Olympic to round-the-park jogger, and everybody will

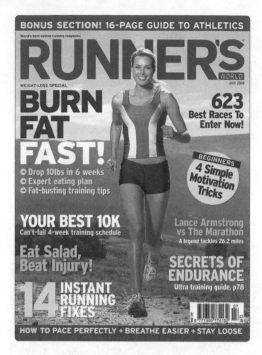

get something out of it. Probably the closest you could get to hanging out with a bunch of really good runners, whenever you liked.

runnersworld.co.uk

Runners World (US)

Ten issues per year

Worth a mention by itself, as while it, largely, offers the same training, running, competition and nutrition advice as the UK edition, because the US is so vast it offers far fewer race details – these can be found on its website. Cleverly, the magazine makes use of the space with a range of general health, fitness and nutrition advice, which makes it worth seeking out by those running as part of a general fitness programme rather than an end in itself.

runnersworld.com

Scarlet

Monthly

Not just the token chick in our otherwise testosterone-fuelled magazine rack, *Scarlet*

is edited by our own sex and relationships expert Sarah Hedley and is a witty, engaging, dead sexy window into the world of women and women of the world. Reading it probably won't get you laid more or give you mysterious powers to know what they're thinking, but the insight it provides might well surprise you and promote a better understanding.

scarletmagazine.co.uk

Muscle & Fitness

Also internationally franchised, this comes from bodybuilding legend Joe Weider's publishing and nutrition supplement empire and is probably the most accessible, least freaky, bodybuilding magazine on the newsstands. It's best for those with a less-than-competitive interest in packing on the muscle, but who still want to take it a little more seriously than, say, *Men's Fitness* or *Men's Health*. Crammed with workout and lifting tips, features on what to eat and how to prevent injury, it also contains a good deal of science, meaning it provides a solid understanding to what you are doing.

UK at muscle-fitness.co.uk
US at muscleandfitness.com

Men's Fitness and Men's Health specials

Throughout the year, both of these titles publish special editions devoted to single aspects of health and fitness – predominantly bodybuilding – put together by their editors. It's worth keeping an eye on the newsstands for them, as they provide ideal slightly-above-entry-level advice for those wanting to go a bit further, but it will be presented in a tone that the magazine's regular readers can instantly relate to.

Books

The Rough Guide to Running

Lloyd Bradley (Rough Guides)
This engrossing work devoted to putting one foot in front of the other, just a bit faster than most people, will take you from your sofa to 10K to marathons in a way that will be fun, not too painful and as effective as possible. It covers what to eat, what to wear, how to set a training schedule, how to avoid and recover from injuries, how to keep safe when you're out by yourself and how to get ready for and run a marathon. All levels of runner should gain something from reading it, as it's probably the best book about running you're ever likely to find. But then I would say that: I wrote it.

The Herbal Drugstore

Linda B. White and Steven Foster (Rodale)
This comprehensive guide to natural remedies stays very true to the dictionary definition of "alternative", as it devotes an entire section to matching commonly prescribed medication to its herbal equivalent. And it does so by condition, thus you can look up what is wrong with you, find what you are likely to have been prescribed, then discover its natural alternative. The bulk of the book proposes and explains herbal remedies for a comprehensive range of symptoms, going into the theory and science of how and why they can work, then looks at the plants themselves to cover how they grow and their history of use. It also offers information on how to use natural remedies safely. Although an American book, which means some of the terms and brand names will not apply elsewhere, there is still a great deal on offer for readers everywhere.

Men's Health: Book of Muscle

Ian King and Lou Schuler (Rodale)
This book announces itself on the cover as "The world's most complete guide to building your body" and it's a claim it seems to live up

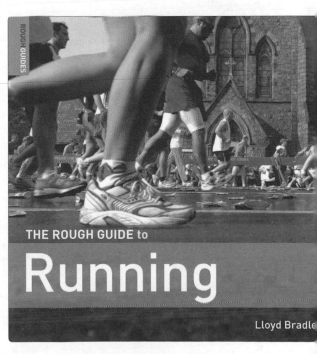

THE ROUGH GUIDE to

Running

Lloyd Bradle

to. Lou Schuler is *Men's Health* magazine (US) Fitness Director and fellow author Ian King is a former power-lifting champion. Together they discuss every muscle group separately and in detail, explain the theories behind muscle growth, run down what you need to eat to make that happen, how to make sure you don't do yourself more harm than good, and, of course, provide a full set of clearly illustrated exercises and routines. If you're just getting into it, or want to take your lifting up a level, this book will have something for you.

The Good Back Guide

Barrie Savory (Random House)
Osteopath Barrie Savory has a client list that includes Sean Connery, Eddy Grant, Roger Moore and HRH Prince Andrew, who wrote the foreword to this book. He takes the approach that we are not functioning efficiently in the modern world as the

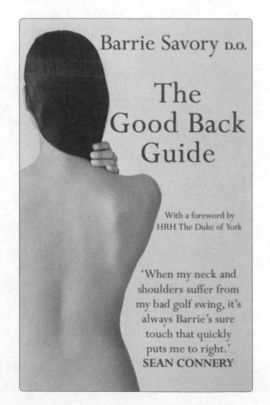

Barrie Savory D.O.

The Good Back Guide

With a foreword by
HRH The Duke of York

'When my neck and shoulders suffer from my bad golf swing, it's always Barrie's sure touch that quickly puts me to right.'
SEAN CONNERY

environment we have created for ourselves is no longer in tune with our muscular-skeletal selves, and offers solutions to back trouble that acknowledge this. The book helps the reader identify particular problems, then provides self-treatment exercises for existing complaints and preventative advice for those not yet suffering – apparently only forty percent of you.

The Johns Hopkins Complete Guide to Symptoms & Remedies

The Editors of *The Johns Hopkins Medical Letter* (Black Dog & Leventhal)
Johns Hopkins Health Information Network is an American medical company's information network that specializes in providing health and fitness information for the over-fifties. Now stop being ageist and appreciate this book for the all-inclusive family health guide that provides a directory of over five hundred common complaints, with symptoms, and, in many cases, causes, treatments and preventions. Further to this, it provides a self-diagnosis service with a lengthy section that starts with symptoms and then lists possible conditions.

Men's Health: TNT Diet

Jeff Volek and Adam Campbell (Rodale)
The TNT of the title stands for Targeted Nutrition Tactics and the eating plans and exercise regimes contained within cover what to eat, when to eat it and how to eat it, in order to maximize fat loss and put on the most muscle. The thing that makes TNT so effective is, once you have grasped the theories, which are explained in some detail, it is an incredibly easy plan to follow as it includes pizza, cream cakes and encourages a glass of wine – it even provides hangover advice. It's all a matter of when you're eating it and how you're balancing it overall.

Sex By Numbers

Sarah Hedley (Piatkus)

Subtitled *Everything You Should Know About Sex and a Few Things You Shouldn't*, this is written by our very own Sarah Hedley and is possibly the most entertainingly informative book you are ever likely to read about the beast with two backs. There isn't a question it leaves unanswered and it will offer advice you didn't even realize you needed, all in an engaging style that leaves you in no doubt whatsoever that sex is supposed to be fun.

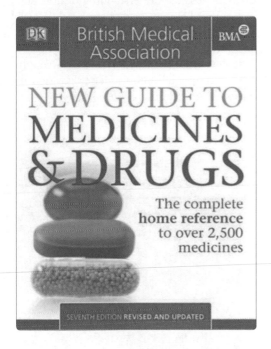

Ancient Way to Keep Fit

Zong Wu & Li Mao (Shelter)

This book explains an ancient Chinese system of keeping the mind and body fit by increasing life forces as you exercise internally and externally by opening the body's energy centres. It's not unlike t'ai chi and can be an incredibly de-stressing experience if performed properly. It explains the history and science behind the 3000-year-old technique, and illustrates some of the exercise sequences with reproductions of ancient scrolls and cave paintings.

The BMA Complete Family Health Encyclopedia

(Dorling Kindersley)

This fourth edition is a subtle update of what is really an old-school medical dictionary, but it is very useful because of that. It has a reassuring, no-nonsense approach, over one thousand pages detailing just about every complaint known to man, complete with hundreds of illustrations and charts, a glossary of medical terms and a list of widely prescribed medication.

BMA New Guide to Medicines & Drugs

John Henry – editor (Dorling Kindersley)

Put together by the British Medical Association, this is the ideal source for anybody in the UK who wants to know what they are taking. It catalogues and explains over 2500 British prescription and over-the-counter medications, going into what's in them, how they work within the body, what possible side effects there might be and how to take them safely.

Eat This Not That

David Zinczenko (Rodale)

A handy sized book with a premise so simple it's beautiful – list around sixty American eating establishments, on the left-hand page display and give nutritional information for the most healthy choices on their menu; on the right-hand page do the same for the most unhealthy choices. Do the same for supermarket food, holiday food, drinks and kids' meals, stir in a section on general

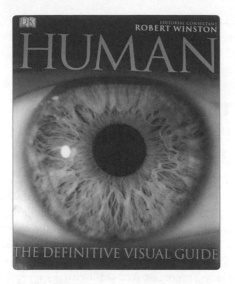

nutrition and calorie intake, and you've got one of the most instantly useful weight watcher's guides. A UK version is scheduled to follow in spring 2009.

Human

Robert Winston – editorial consultant (Dorling Kindersley)
Not strictly a health or fitness book, but a must-read for anybody with any interest in how their body works and what it means to be a human being. Beautifully illustrated and with explanations that limit themselves to bite-sized, layman-friendly chunks, it covers everything from physically being a human to religion, history and different societies around the world. Fascinating.

Pilates for Men: Fit for Sport Fit for Life

Alan Herdman (Gaia)
A male-centric Pilates book that not only deals with the overall fitness advantages such a programme can bring, but targets specific muscle groups in relation to how men play different sports. But while it allows you to improve the strength and flexibility your pursuit might require, it also deals with the

big picture, discussing and remedying the postural problems brought on by modern life, and providing de-stressing help to keep you mentally fit. Highly recommended for anybody who thought pilates was for women.

The Rough Guide to The Brain

Barry J. Gibb (Rough Guides)
Everything you wanted to know about the old grey matter. While it won't directly make you smarter or fitter or healthier, it will give you the best possible understanding of how and why things happen inside your head. Which will help you come to terms with things you and other people do, as by knowing what's inherent, what's learned and what's simply not natural, you'll be in a better position to do something about it.

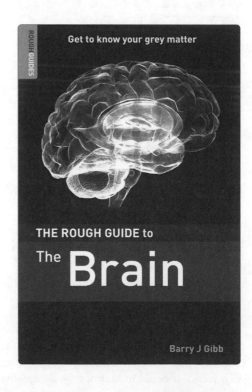

The Testosterone Advantage

Lou Schuler (Rodale)

A somewhat controversial fitness plan when it was first published in 2003, from *Men's Health* magazine's Fitness Director, as it utilizes increased testosterone production to assist in fat burning and prolong exercise sessions. It provides the eating and exercise plans for a pretty intense nine-week schedule, which will reshape your body by turning fat into muscle. It requires dedication and perseverance, but it will give results.

The 100 Simple Secrets of Healthy People

David Niven (Harper)

A light-hearted, useful compendium of health and fitness knowledge that has been culled from the world's medical libraries and is presented here in easily digestible form. Some of it you'll already know, some of it is wisdom of a kind that is also within these pages, but all of it will be entertainingly written and deceptively informative. Did you know that, for instance, dry tea bags placed around a room you are painting will absorb the harmful chemicals the paint has released into the air? Or that playing slow music in the background at meal times will make you eat less?

The Runner's World Complete Book of Running

Amby Burfoot – editor (Rodale)

Very much a compendium of the estimable *Runner's World* magazine, and as such it provides an overview of running that covers everything from starting out to regularly running marathons. A very good-looking book, its section on runners' eating and drinking is worth the price of admission for the recommendation of beer as part of your training diet. You could say this book is like the *Rough Guide to Running*, but, obviously, not quite so good.

500 of the Most Important Health Tips You'll Ever Need

Hazel Courteney (Index)

Probably the most wide-ranging study of alternative medicines on the bookshelves. In straightforward A–Z fashion, it lists commonly encountered conditions and situations from absorption to weight problems via cancer, flatulence, high blood pressure, immune function, memory and panic attacks, then gives a list of herbal remedies that will relieve or prevent. Each entry is introduced by a brief explanation of what the condition is and why it occurs, meaning that even if the supplements don't appear immediately logical, they will make sense once you've read through it. A similarly scientific approach is employed to introduce the book, as Courteney explains the whole alternative approach in a way that leaves you wondering how you ever managed without

367

it. The answer is that you will manage a great deal better if you own a copy of this book.

The Doctors Book of Food Remedies

Selene Yeager (Rodale)

Quite literally eat yourself healthy and fit and out of practically any potentially dangerous condition. This book clearly loves food and while half of it is devoted to conditions and what you should eat to relieve them – cinnamon reduces cholesterol; grapefruit protects against colon cancer; spinach prevents cataracts; and so on – the other half explains exactly how much good certain foods will do you. With a huge range of delicious recipes and kitchen tips, this is a book that will make you feel good about food again.

Alternative therapies

Acupuncture

The cutting edge of this ancient healing art has now dragged itself into the twenty-first century by using high-tech scanners to locate the blockages and bottlenecks in the body's natural flow of energy. Then the practitioner inserts the needles to clear them – makes you wonder what went on before... trial and error?

The British Acupuncture Council: acupuncture.org.uk

Acupuncture and Oriental Medicine National Coalition: acupuncturetoday.com

Aromatherapy

Very good for relieving stress, tension or muscle aches and pains, it uses essential oils as inhalations, for massage and in baths.

International Society of Professional Aromatherapists: ifparoma.org

National Association for Holistic Aromatherapy: naha.org

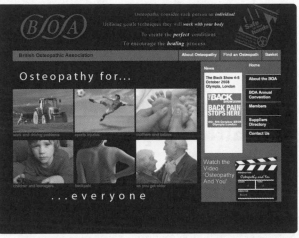

Whys and wherefores: the site 'osteopathy.org' (British Osteopathic Association) explains

Chiropractic/osteopathy

Manipulation of the body to put the bones and joints back where they should be after the stresses and strains of everyday life have moved them out of position. Every man over the age of thirty should visit a chiropractor or osteopath at least twice a year.

The British Chiropractic Association: chiropractic-uk.co.uk

The American Chiropractic Association: americhiro.org

General Osteopathic Council: osteopathy.org

American Osteopathic Organization: osteopathic.org

Colonic irrigation

The pumping of water into, around and out of the colon to clean out any accumulation of digestive crud and potentially toxic fecal matter. Should be compulsory for men once they reach middle age.

Association & Register of Colonic Hydrotherapists: colonic-association.org

The International Association for Colon Hydrotherapy: i-act.org

Homeopathy

Using natural remedies to stimulate the body's immune system and natural defences to heal itself.

The Society of Homeopaths: homeopathy-soh.org

International Academy of Classical Homeopathy: wholehealthnow.com/homeopathy

Hypnotherapy

Can be effective for many things other than giving up smoking, as a good hypnotherapist will relax you so completely it will be much easier to establish and deal with whatever is causing you problems – eating disorders, stress, anxiety, phobias and so on.

National Council for Hypnotherapists: hypnotherapists.org.uk

The Council of Professional Hypnotherapist Organizations: hypnodreams.org

Iridology

A good iridologist will look into your eyes, with a piece of equipment like an optician would use, and be able to tell exactly what is wrong with you and how to fix it. I speak from experience.

The Guild of Naturopathic Iridologists International: gni-international.org

International Iridology Practitioners Association: iridologyassn.org

Reflexology

Working on the theory that everything in the body is connected, this is the stimulation of specific nerve endings in the hands and the feet to have an effect on trouble spots elsewhere.

The British Reflexology Association: britreflex.org

The Reflexology Association of America: reflexology-usa.org

Organizations

The Institute for Complementary Medicine

The smart-looking homepage (see below) is a very good starting point for anybody wanting to find out more about specific alternative practices or to locate an accredited practitioner.

icmedicine.co.uk

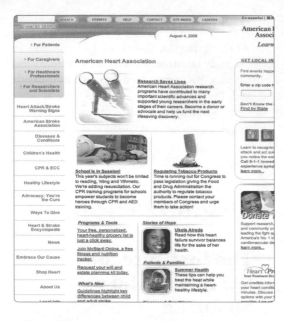

The American Medical Association

A professional body for US doctors, but with plenty to interest those keen on keeping up to date with healthcare developments. Offers a local "doctor finder" service.

ama-assn.org

The American Cancer Society

Devoted to fighting cancer, they offer information for sufferers, help for survivors, advice for families and measures for prevention.

cancer.org

The American Heart Association

Working to reduce death through heart disease in the US, the helpful homepage offers links to local information and a quick course on emergency procedures.

americanheart.org

Cancer Research

The UK's leading cancer charity offers a wealth of information on all aspects of cancer, relevant to anybody who is suffering or experiencing the suffering of a loved one.

cancerresearchuk.org

The British Heart Foundation

A charitable organization dedicated to keeping the nation's hearts beating healthily.

bhf.org.uk

The British Dietetic Association

A professional body for dieticians, set up to advance the science of dietetics, promote training and education in dietetics and to regulate the profession in the UK. They also have a series of highly informative food factsheets that can be downloaded by anybody from this website.

bda.uk.com/foodfacts

Mind (National Association for Mental Health)

The charity dedicated to advancing the views and needs of those suffering from mental health problems and offering advice and information for those caring for them.

mind.org.uk

Mental Health America

They offer information about care, medication and legal issues, and a series of easily understandable, downloadable factsheets about mental healthcare in the US.

nmha.org

The British Counselling and Psychotherapy Association

Will provide information and advice as to what service you might actually need, then help you find an accredited therapist.

bacp.co.uk

Alcoholics Anonymous

An international organization, dedicated to helping those with alcohol problems.

alcoholics-anonymous.org

Narcotics Anonymous

An international organization that functions in the same way as AA, but is dedicated to those wanting to recover from drug addiction.

na.org

Families Anonymous

An internationally focused organization offering support and information to the families of those suffering from drug or alcohol addiction.

familiesanonymous.org

Websites

Healthy Minds

The online resource of the American Psychiatric Association, offering a vast range of mental health information.

healthyminds.org

Menshealth.com

The website for the magazine is lively, informative and useful in every aspect of keeping healthy and manly.

menshealth.com

NHS Direct

The website of the British National Health Service offers such a comprehensive online heath advisory service it is relevant to anybody anywhere in the world.

nhsdirect.nhs.uk

Webmd.com

A highly reliable online medical clinic, this offers a specific men's health department and has a fascinating interactive symptom checker – you never knew there could be so much wrong with you.

webmd.com

Index

A

Accident & Emergency 296
acne 314
acupuncture 368
addiction 196, 197, 229
  addictive personalities 200
  diet pills 93
  natural remedies 204
adenosine triphosphate (ATP) 159
aerobic exercise 166
aftershave 62
ageing
  effects of 263, 264, 315
  immune system 271
  IQ 268
  shrinkage 263
  smoking and obesity 264
AIDS 152, 155, 314
  AIDS/HIV around the world 257
air travel 242–244
  air pressure, in airliners' cabins 242
  air quality, in airliners' cabins 242
  comfort and safety 244
  keeping fit 250
  space restrictions 242
alcohol
  Alcoholics Anonymous 371
  alcoholism 315
  antisocial behaviour 190
  around the world 188

cutting down 191, 192
death rates 185
good points 185
older men 192
overindulgence 188
unit of 182
what to eat before 187
allergies 316
Alzheimer's 270, 271, 316
American Academy of Family Physicians 290
American Cancer Society, the 370
American Heart Association, the 370
American Medical Association, the 370
anabolic steroids 176
anaemia 317
anaerobic exercise 166
Ancient Way to Keep Fit 365
anger management 212
angina 317
anorexia nervosa 318
antibiotics 105
anxiety attacks 318
apnoea 319
appendicitis 319
appendix, the 319
appetite 348
aromatherapy 368
artery blockage 81
arthritis 320
asthma 320
athlete's foot 321

B

C

Index

Index

S

T

Notes